Praise for *The People's Hospital*

"A rare and unforgettable work, *The People's Hospital* takes us deep into the lives of some of America's poorest patients. Following in the tradition of Bryan Stevenson's *Just Mercy* and Atul Gawande's *Being Mortal*, Nuila makes a revelatory passage through a system that is both flawed and primed for reform."

—Andrea Elliott, author of *Invisible Child*

"Like a handful of other storied public hospitals in America, Ben Taub manages to do the impossible: to provide world-class care for the uninsured and indigent; train generations of physicians; pioneer medical breakthroughs; and do it at a fraction of the cost of fancier places. Nuila's lyrical and riveting prose lays bare the dysfunctional, expensive quagmire that passes for our healthcare system. His stories of patients and those who care for them capture the miracle that is Ben Taub. *The People's Hospital* is a tour de force."

—Abraham Verghese, author of *Cutting for Stone*

"Through poignant accounts of his patients, contextualized by medical history and layered with bits of family memoir, Ricardo Nuila has achieved the impossible: writing a comprehensive, personal, and gut-wrenching account of the American healthcare system. Patients, politicians, doctors, insurance companies, and people everywhere will benefit from this insider's description of Ben Taub Hospital in Houston, Texas. In *The People's Hospital* we are given a diagnosis of our current healthcare system but are also offered an imagining of a better future for everyone."

—Javier Zamora, author of *Solito*

"*The People's Hospital* is inspirational and gut-wrenching, thrilling and scrupulous, damning and hope-filled. Ricardo Nuila has seen the potential for our corporatized, profit-driven system to be reoriented around tenets of human dignity and offers readers a glimpse of what is possible when American healthcare recommits itself to the bygone promise of protecting our most vulnerable."

—Francisco Cantú, author of *The Line Becomes a River*

"*The People's Hospital* is that rare book that is as warm and humanely written as it is urgent and necessary. And Ricardo Nuila is that rare writer who doesn't proclaim to be a savior, but rather a caring, knowledgeable doctor with generous ideas and stories to share. These stories are at turns painful, maddening, humorous, and uplifting. They are always powerfully told and colored by the full range of the human heart."

—Jeff Hobbs, author of *Children of the State*

"Ricardo Nuila takes a literary scalpel to the US medical system to reveal the cancer of greed ravaging patients in Houston and throughout the country. Fortunately for us, his skillful, even beautiful dissection of the disease of false hope reveals the healthy, pumping heart of living, breathing, and serving doctors and workers of Ben Taub Hospital. *The People's Hospital* is the antidote to hopelessness in healthcare that prevails."

—Roberto Lovato, author of *Unforgetting*

"In the wake of the COVID-19 pandemic, the impetus for transforming the American health system is more urgent than ever. Dr. Ricardo Nuila offers us a path forward in *The People's Hospital*, grounded in years of caring for patients, bearing witness to their stories, and observing how they link into the mosaic that is modern medicine. With humanity and humility, he guides us from a place of deep understanding, rooted in low-income communities in Houston, to a destination of healthcare as a human right for the entire country."

—Dave A. Chokshi, MD,
43rd health commissioner of New York City

"Ricardo Nuila's *The People's Hospital* is a tour de force. It is a call to action wrapped in powerful storytelling, a book that will prick the consciences of private practitioners while alerting the American public to the care they deserve—and rarely receive."

—Mimi Swartz, author of *Ticker*

The
PEOPLE'S
HOSPITAL

HOPE *and* PERIL *in*
AMERICAN MEDICINE

RICARDO NUILA

SCRIBNER

New York London Toronto Sydney New Delhi

Scribner

An Imprint of Simon & Schuster, Inc.

1230 Avenue of the Americas

New York, NY 10020

First Scribner hardcover edition March 2023

SCRIBNER and design are registered trademarks of The Gale Group, Inc.,
used under license by Simon & Schuster, Inc., the publisher of this work.

For information about special discounts for bulk purchases,
please contact Simon & Schuster Special Sales at 1-866-506-1949
or business@simonandschuster.com.

The Simon & Schuster Speakers Bureau can bring authors to
your live event. For more information or to book an event,
contact the Simon & Schuster Speakers Bureau at 1-866-248-3049
or visit our website at www.simonspeakers.com.

Interior design by Kyle Kabel

Manufactured in the United States of America

1   3   5   7   9   10   8   6   4   2

Library of Congress Cataloging-in-Publication Data has been applied for.

ISBN 978-1-5011-9804-5
ISBN 978-1-5011-9806-9 (ebook)

For the patients and staff of Ben Taub Hospital

Contents

1 Histories   1

PART ONE Life Without Insurance

2 The Dead Parts   21

3 Doctors   41

4 Coverage   59

5 Hospitals   75

6 Wards   93

PART TWO Symptoms and Solutions

7 Assumptions   117

8 Beliefs   143

9 Misperceptions   169

10 Miscalculations   191

11 Algorithmania   211

PART THREE Costs

12 Excess   237

13 Public + Private   251

14 Disaster Syndrome   269

15 Tiers   285

PART FOUR Faith   309

Addendum   329

Acknowledgments   335

Author's Note   339

Notes   341

Index   355

. . . and it occurred to me that there was no difference between men, in intelligence or race, so profound as the difference between the sick and the well.

—F. Scott Fitzgerald, *The Great Gatsby*

For there is no "them," there is only "us."

—Luis Alberto Urrea, "Hearthland"

— 1 —

Histories

The rumor we heard was that patients arrived with hand-drawn maps, our hospital marked like treasure. The stately Nigerian lady who responded, "Yes, Doctor," to everything (metastatic breast cancer). The boy with the black curly hair wearing red Converse All Stars and a Judas Priest T-shirt that screamed Mexico City (acute lymphocytic leukemia). The grandmother with the sari snagged in the guardrails (chest pain, *real* chest pain, might need bypass). We stood at these patients' bedsides; we wrote down their histories; we said we were sorry for examining them with cold hands. We ordered blood tests, interpreted EKGs, scrolled through their CAT scans; we input diagnoses.

We weren't just doctors. Among us were nurses, social workers, X-ray techs, the people who rode up and down the hallways in the middle of the night waxing the floors. Some of us wore white coats with frayed sleeves and busted pockets, others tight-fitting scrubs embroidered with our names. In our bad moments, we became tribal: we weren't "we," we were ortho, medicine, plastics, the 4A nurses; we only covered the unit. More often though, the needs of our patients were so damn immediate, we found a way to work as one.

We ran blood transfusions, heparin drips, a morphine pump when Norco didn't touch the pain. When COVID came, we gave oxygen together, one of us twisting the knob on the valve while the other inserted those tiny prongs into flared nostrils. We consulted one another when things looked dicey: surgery if we found boils, ID for antibiotics, and if anything looked remotely like a seizure—a twitch, a rolling of the eyes—we paged neurology overhead. If Transportation was swamped, we wheeled them ourselves, to MRI, to Special Procedures, to the cath lab, even the ICU (how downtrodden we looked when we did this, like beaten dogs).

We figured out ways to make things work. Not enough money for your meds? We googled the $4 list at Walmart. Muscles too weak? We dug up a refurbished walker from the basement. Dying and homeless and alone? We called in a favor from the hospice that used to be a Tudor-style home. And when our work was done, once we could envision someone not dying within twenty-four hours of our discharge order, once the first chemo had gone in, once we could be sure their chief complaint was addressed, the thought still lingered in our minds: What brought them here? What are their stories?

Ben Taub Hospital. The largest safety-net hospital in one of America's most diverse cities. We are Heathrow if you replaced the Emirates and the Virgin Atlantic planes with Greyhound buses. There are no atriums with pianists here playing "Here Comes the Sun" to welcome you, no soothing sounds of running water from hidden speakers or—*gasp*—from an actual indoor waterfall. There is no Starbucks. Our cafeteria serves some form of barbecue most days for lunch and packaged salads topped with egg or chicken strips. That's unless you prefer the full-menu McDonald's (located inside the hospital) that's open twenty-three hours a day. We do have a gift shop, though it looks more like a convenience store, heavily stocked with greeting cards. Not the pun-filled ones; rather, the kind that get the point across—condolences—available in Spanish, too.

If you type "Ben Taub" into Google Maps, you'll find it crammed between the Houston Zoo and the thirty other institutions that make up the Texas Medical Center, the largest concentration of medical facilities in the world. Some of the field's most important innovations took place in this medical metropolis: the first successful bypass, the first artificial-heart transplant, the first beatless artificial heart (imagine that, no lub-dub, just a constant whirring), the first silicone breast implant, one of the first civilian helicopter ambulances, the Bubble Boy—all here.

Not that the patients at Ben Taub know this. Some may have heard that MD Anderson is rated top in the country in cancer care, or that at Houston Methodist, you might find yourself fortunate enough to have a robot operate on your prostate (the TV ads air in Spanish, too). It's possible that at night, our patients look out their windows and behold the sparkle of so many new glass buildings, some of them named after billionaire sheikhs who sell the oil that becomes their gas. More likely, they're looking out in the direction of the zoo, toward the parking garage and bus stop, wondering how they'll get home.

Ben Taub is Houston's largest hospital for the poor—many working, some not—who cannot afford medical care. That is, after all, the definition of a safety-net hospital: one that serves society's most medically and financially vulnerable. The vast majority of hospitals in the US are either for-profit or nonprofit. Nonprofits receive a tax incentive to provide care to the uninsured, though that care is often limited to stabilizing emergencies due to the high cost of medical care. For-profits behave similarly. Safety-net hospitals have emerged in America's coverage vacuum to give the uninsured a way of receiving healthcare. Ben Taub is a public, locally funded hospital that focuses on the uninsured but that is also open to people with health insurance.

In Texas, the state with the nation's largest uninsured population, and perhaps the worst state in the union to live in if you're poor and chronically ill, scores of people come here. When they do, the community picks up half the tab through property taxes. The rest comes from a variety of sources, including Medicaid, Medicare, and payments made directly by patients. Ben Taub is the flagship hospital for Harris Health, the healthcare system catering to Houston's uninsured patients. Five hundred sixty people stay at Ben Taub or Lyndon B. Johnson Hospital, its sister hospital, *every day*, and thousands more receive primary and specialty care at the county's network of clinics, accounting for more than $1 billion worth of healthcare every year for the indigent.

But there are instances when the insured and even the rich *prefer* Ben Taub. Whenever I mention to locals that I work as a doctor at Ben Taub, I receive a fairly typical response: "That's where I'd go if I got shot." Maybe this sounds uniquely Texan, but I've heard the same about traffic accidents. Whenever there's a pileup on the freeway, it's not uncommon to hear the radio announcer report something like, "Crews on the scene, the victims have been taken to Ben Taub." Ben Taub's reputation in Houston is nothing short of sterling when it comes to trauma care, which is why it's not uncommon to find the crushed, the burned, the dismembered, the stabbed, the shot up, the opened, the clipped, and the repeatedly tased sharing a room with patients beleaguered by mental illness and poverty.

People outside the medical field might wonder why anyone would want to work in a place like this. Why deal with so many social problems and a lack of insurance when you can practice in one of the many hospitals down the road? Aren't you ambitious? You'd have to be some sort of a do-gooder—a bleeding heart—to work here, the thought goes. This sort of characterization, however, while flattering, isn't entirely accurate. Take Dr. Ken Mattox, a trauma surgeon at Ben Taub who served as its chief of staff for over thirty years. Mattox is what you might call a quintessential old-school surgeon—he'll wear scrubs only in the OR and on call nights (*never* at restaurants), he's always cleanly shaven, and he moves methodically down the hallways, even on the way to his patients awaiting exploratory laparotomies for multiple gunshot wounds. Because there's never a need to rush.

Like many Texans, Mattox opposes the federal government's issuing regulations that can encroach upon local practices. The mandate to purchase private health insurance in the Affordable Care Act irked him, for instance, because patients at Harris Health already received coverage without having to buy insurance. He can sound like an ideologue when speaking about welfare—"I don't want to take care of somebody that is indigent who is capable of working and making their own way"— but Mattox has dedicated the bulk of his career to ensuring Houston's indigent patients receive excellent care. This includes undocumented immigrants.

In fact, in 2001, when then–attorney general and current US senator for Texas John Cornyn wrote a legal opinion about how Ben Taub and the county health system might have been breaking federal law by providing nonemergency treatment to the undocumented, Mattox addressed Harris Health's board of managers, who were fearful that federal funding might be cut off. "If I need to be reported for my clinical care, report me," he said, insisting that services to this population ought to continue. "But spell my name right."

A whole array of competing ideologies collide at Ben Taub. But when it comes to caring for uninsured Houstonians, the healthcare workers at Ben Taub—doctors included—put their political philosophies aside, for good reasons.

Ben Taub is an excellent classroom. It's where the diseases and maladies you read about in textbooks come to life, and it's intended as such—Ben Taub is a designated medical education site, and many of the stiff white coats you see scuttling down the hallways are those of students and young doctors in training. You might spend a lifetime with patients at private hospitals without seeing belly tuberculosis, or even cardiac sarcoidosis, where all the cells infiltrating the heart glimmer on the ultrasound. If you spend enough time at Ben Taub, you'll see most everything. It's why many young doctors with meticulously mapped-out careers, who are on their way to Harvard or San Francisco or the

National Institutes of Health, make a pit stop here. The illnesses you see and deal with at Ben Taub make you a better doctor.

But more than this, healthcare workers feel *useful* at Ben Taub. Much of this sense of utility stems from helping those most in need, but another part comes from working in a system that takes healthcare spending seriously. America spends a larger percentage of its gross domestic product on healthcare than any country in the world, more than double, in fact, what Japan, Canada, or any western European nation spends. What that money buys is expansive and comprehensive healthcare for some—including the newest combination pills and robotic surgeries and transplants—and expensive but mostly ineffective emergency care for those who cannot afford high-end care. In 2015, Ben Taub Hospital and Harris Health spent a little less than half the national average, around $3,365 per patient, costs that included emergency, specialty, and primary care. Compare that to national health expenditure data that showed nearly $10,000 spent per patient (Medicare spends nearly $11,000 per patient). To put that in perspective, a healthcare system in Texas dedicated to the poor has found a way to buck the American trend and treat patients as efficiently as French, German, and other healthcare systems regarded as the best in the world. Some doctors, like me, are proud to work in one of the few systems in America that doesn't make healthcare more expensive for those who pay already-inflated prices and premiums—which is to say, all of us.

These savings wouldn't amount to much if Ben Taub provided subpar care. But expensive care doesn't mean better care. In fact, at Ben Taub, you often find the opposite: the best medical care is the most affordable. In 2015, Ben Taub demonstrated itself to be the *best hospital in the country* for treating heart attacks. Heart attacks are essentially like a dying lawn: Imagine a kink forming in the hose you use to water your yard so that only a trickle of water comes out the nozzle. In the hot and dry summer, unless you fix the kink, the grass will start to turn yellow and slowly die. Now imagine that same process happening over not days but minutes.

Imagine the blades of grass are individual heart muscle cells, the hose a coronary artery. Heart cells start to die when the artery is kinked with a clot. A patient feels stabbing chest pain, and so she comes to the emergency room, whereupon a stopwatch starts—how long does it take for the hospital to identify the coronary artery and unkink it? This is how the quality of heart attack care is measured: the sooner the coronary artery is unkinked (through a procedure called a percutaneous coronary intervention), the more heart cells are preserved, the greener the lawn.

On average, it takes hospitals around ninety minutes to figure out if a coronary artery is kinked and to unkink it. Top-rated centers equip themselves with numerous suites to perform this unkinking—called cath labs—and enlist armies of cardiologists. These well-funded sites tout their *US News and World Report* ranking in heart attack care, but the actual outcomes say otherwise. With only four cath labs—two permanent, two convertible labs—and three full-time interventional heart doctors, Ben Taub unkinked arteries in an average of forty-five minutes, the fastest time in the nation. Greener—no, green*est*—lawns.

The question is, how? How is Ben Taub able to provide these scores of patients with this level of lifesaving care? How does it provide primary and specialty care, including chemotherapies and expensive HIV medicines, to patients who can't otherwise afford it or who don't qualify for insurance through the Affordable Care Act? If you consider that only 7 percent of Ben Taub's patients have private health insurance and another 20 percent have government-sponsored coverage through Medicare or Medicaid, leaving a full 63 percent of its patients completely uninsured, how is it possible that a hospital without ample private funding and chandeliers and a pianist in the atrium can give its poor patients great heart attack care?

Is expensive healthcare better or is it just more expensive? Can we trust public hospitals in America? Why can't people access healthcare when America has so many entitlement programs? This book attempts to answer these questions and more. In my twelve years at Ben Taub,

I've found that good care comes from connecting with your patients in whatever way you're able. As a medical student, connecting meant translating for the Spanish speakers. It meant occasionally dropping hints about my own roots ("What part of El Salvador are you from?") and always referring my patients' questions to my bosses, the real doctors. As an internal medicine resident scurrying through Ben Taub's halls, it meant being physically present for my patients when they needed me. It also meant learning more about people's lives, asking questions—"Did you cook with wood inside your home?"—and being honest when I didn't know the answers to *their* questions.

Since I became a teaching attending and hospitalist at Ben Taub, connecting has meant not only performing all my duties as a doctor but also uncovering and understanding the policies that both limit and enhance my patients' care. Why doesn't Mr. Oregón qualify for Medicaid? How often should I tell Rogelio to visit the ER for recurring lifesaving treatment? Is it helpful or harmful to recommend that Christian apply for disability? Will prescribing a more costly medication roil Roxana's already all-too-difficult life? Would a lesser-quality medicine be better, all things considered? By telling the hospital's stories of illness, poverty, loss, convalescence, hope, and more, this book will delve into how Ben Taub and Harris Health provide affordable and excellent care.

This isn't to say that Ben Taub is a panacea. After all, Texas is Texas, quite possibly the most restrictive healthcare environment for the poor in the country. Ben Taub and safety-net hospitals like it are good at providing a basic level of healthcare to the greatest number of people. But some treatments, like transplant surgeries, are still too expensive, and some specialty care, like kidney stone surgery, is too scarce. There are larger issues as well. The safety net's latticework is extremely fragile in its dependence on local politics. Ben Taub serves as a model for how to blend conservative values with compassionate care, which is vital for a blue city in a red state. In many ways, the county has figured out a way to hit the bull's-eye of providing excellent care at cut-rate prices.

Other times, the Texas Legislature's refusal to expand Medicaid, which pushes more responsibility and costs onto the local safety net, leads to broken lives. These patient stories will show the individual realities of political decisions.

This book will not be the first to chronicle how Ben Taub provides care to Houston's indigent. In the early 1960s, Houstonians unable to afford healthcare faced obstacles of epic proportions:

> The smell of poverty cannot be described, although it is the same all over the world. I had smelled it in India, in Paris, in prison camps during the war, but most unforgettably when the first inmates of the Nazi concentration camps came home after their liberation . . . I had seen well-intentioned humanitarian officers start out by trying to treat them as unfortunate human beings. Before the day was past, they were yelling at them, herding them, pushing their milling, mindless mass around as cowboys push a herd of cattle. I suppose they ended up that way because of the impossibility of identification. It was impossible for normal, civilized men to identify with those stinking, unshaven, dirt-caked, lice- and disease-ridden human wrecks . . . I had forgotten their smell; it hit me again, after all of those years, as I entered Jefferson Davis Hospital in Houston, Texas.

The author of this passage volunteered at Ben Taub's predecessor, Jefferson Davis Hospital, for nine months in 1963, changing bedpans when instructed, wheeling pregnant women to safe spaces, sitting like a blue-eyed fly on the wall when doctors and nurses entered the room and took over. He was also a novelist, a playwright, a nominee for the Nobel Prize in Literature, a ship captain who had rescued flood victims, a Quaker, a Nazi resistance fighter, a Dutch war hero, and a visiting creative writing instructor at the University of Houston. His name was Jan de Hartog, and his book *The Hospital* described the transition from Jeff Davis to Ben Taub, from a dilapidated building manned by trainees to a multispecialty center staffed by some of the country's top doctors, from a house of charity to a civic institution, from segregated wards to an edifice whose name rings with hope in households across Houston. De Hartog's words alerted the city to the deplorable state of its safety-net hospital, and the community responded in the mid-1960s with a vote to give healthcare access to everyone living in the county.

Fifty years later, this is the story of what Ben Taub Hospital has become and what it means. This book is an update to de Hartog's as much as it is a foil. Has a locally funded healthcare system served Houston's uninsured well? Do competing ideologies like universal healthcare—even for the undocumented—and cost-cutting actually coalesce at Ben Taub? Can our system help the country figure out how to extend good healthcare affordably to everyone?

Early in my career, during my internship, I was slated to take care of patients on Ben Taub's general wards, meaning those hospitalized for some degree of organ dysfunction—kidney disease, liver cirrhosis, pneumonia, infections of the skin. Every morning, I pulled into work listening to a Wilco song. I wasn't superstitious, but one particular line seemed to encapsulate all the illnesses I was witnessing and my general feeling of ineptitude, and it comforted me to recite it: "Maybe I won't be so afraid." I have no idea when this ritual stopped.

I arrived on the wards and printed out a list of my new patients. Then I visited each hospital unit and started reading through the charts. Everything was paper back then, meaning you could flip and flip and flip—through orders, test results, the notes of other doctors—and still not get to the bottom of what exactly was happening. One patient had a particularly large chart, actually two charts duct-taped together: Alvaro. It was so heavy and had been flipped through so many times that, like on an old book, cracks had started to show in its gray spine.

I read about Alvaro's many surgeries: hip surgery, belly surgery, large portions of his intestines removed. For months, he couldn't eat, his only nutrition delivered through an IV and then a tube in his stomach. It started as colon cancer. It had spread throughout Alvaro's body to multiple organs and joints. Over the prior nine months, he'd spent only a couple of weeks out of the hospital. Otherwise he was in the ICU, then the wards, then the ICU again with septic shock from an infection of the blood, then a rehab center, then again the ICU. And now Alvaro was here on the wards, in Ben Taub, my new patient. After flipping through the chart, I draped a stethoscope around my neck and went to meet him.

"English or Spanish?" This was the first important question I asked.

"Español," he said.

When I was a medical student, professors used to praise me for the translations I provided. They had no clue. I'm the son of Salvadoran immigrants and, as such, grew up with Spanish everywhere—at the dinner table, at my parents' parties, every summer visiting my grandparents in the hills outside the capital. But apparently reading and studying English influenced me more, and I speak Spanish like a gringo. It is something I'm constantly aware of, a part of who I am and how I'm seen, like a tic. Except at Ben Taub. The patients here rarely mention it. Even *my* Spanish is music to their ears.

"Any bleeding?" I asked.

Mr. Alvaro shifted his head a little. "I don't think so."

"Can you lean forward?" I said, giving him a little push.

He took two short breaths like a weightlifter in the clench and stayed right in place. "Not really," he grunted.

When I was on my way into his room, the nurse had stopped me. There was a decision I had to make, the quicker the better. "MAP is sixty," she said. "Want to give fluids?"

It took me more than a second to realize what she was saying. The mean arterial pressure tells us if our vital organs are receiving an adequate amount of blood and nourishment. If this number is too low, then organs aren't receiving the blood supply needed to survive. My new patient's MAP was right at the cutoff. Patients with low MAPs usually have to go to the ICU. Mr. Alvaro had just come from the ICU, and the nurse wanted to know if we could give IV fluids to bring up the MAP or if we needed to send him back.

I told the nurse to give me a minute. In thinking about what to do about the MAP, I had almost blinded myself to what was in front of me: a scared man, struggling to live as much as to die. I went back into the room, sat down beside Alvaro, and listened to his story.

Alvaro told me about the past nine months of his life—not about the pain or the vomiting or the bloody stools constantly filling the bag attached to what remained of his intestines, but how he had become a burden to his family. His daughter stayed with him in the hospital most nights and worked during the day cleaning offices. She had to. If you're poor and people depend on you, you can't not make money. She had kids at home too, school-aged kids. Alvaro told me she should have been taking care of them, not him.

Somehow, in this moment, my Spanish didn't stumble. "You know that it's okay if you die," I said. As ever, I could hear a note of gringo, but the accent sounded muted, unimportant.

He was the same age as my grandfather; maybe that's why I said what I did. Or maybe seeing the fear in his eyes when we discussed what might happen next, that this could *go on*, gave me the courage to be frank.

When I came out of the room, I saw the nurse talking with a woman I quickly recognized as Alvaro's daughter. I buttoned my white coat and wove my way into the conversation.

"How is he?" the daughter asked.

I told her what Alvaro had told me, that he didn't want doctors to resuscitate him if his heart stopped, that he didn't want a breathing tube inserted under any circumstances. What this meant was that he wouldn't be returning to the ICU again, ever.

"He's been through so much," I said in Spanish. "I think he's tired."

She nodded. It was still summer, the ridiculous Houston heat continued to broil outside, and yet everyone in Ben Taub wore layers and long sleeves. The AC did that to us. The daughter shivered, held her elbows tight. "I know he is," she said.

As I started to walk away, the nurse reminded me about the MAP. "Are we giving fluids?"

"He's DNR/DNI now," I said. "I'll put in the order."

I flipped to the "Orders" section of his chart, wrote "Do Not Resuscitate" with my signature timed and dated, and slid the wobbly chart into its slot. I called my attending and told him about the change. Immediately I turned my attention to the next name on my list, a patient staying on the other side of the hospital. I didn't walk there with my usual quick pace, but I didn't saunter either. Ten minutes later, I was absorbed in a different patient's chart. That's when my pager went off. I cursed having to be so connected and called the number back.

"This is the intern," I said.

"Just wanted to let you know that Mr. A just passed," said the nurse.

"He's dead?"

"The daughter's at the bedside."

I rushed back to the unit and met the daughter in the hallway. She was on the phone, pacing, crying, holding a tissue beneath her nose, getting words out. I didn't want to interrupt her, and so I waited until I had her attention, and then I mouthed to her in Spanish, "Lo siento."

She smiled at me courteously and held her hand over the receiver. "It's okay, it's really okay," she said.

It didn't hit me until after I performed what had to be done next—the death exam, the death note, signing off for Transportation to wheel the body away—that Mr. Alvaro might have still been alive if we hadn't talked. Was that even possible? That words could mean the difference between life and death?

I knew the words I had written—"Do Not Resuscitate"—had that power, but what about our shared words? What about what I had said to Mr. Alvaro? What about what he had said to me? What about Mr. Alvaro's story?

It's been over a decade since Mr. Alvaro died. I've cared for hundreds of patients at Ben Taub in that time, patients from Nigeria, Bhutan, Eritrea, Vietnam, the Fifth Ward here in Houston, even from my grandparents' village in El Salvador. I'm no longer an intern. In fact, now I am the one teaching residents and medical students. Still, I try to find my patients' stories. It's my favorite part of being a doctor. I don't mean their medical histories. I mean the circumstances of their lives. All of this information helps me to better empathize with them, but the stories also make medical care more efficient, more personal, and they reduce the number of tests needed to diagnose and give treatment.

Hearing a patient's story helps me visualize their illness. If, for instance, they tell me they drenched their bedsheets the past few nights and that they nearly passed out this morning while standing to use the bathroom, a vision of a dry creek appears in my mind. This is what the veins inside their body look like, I tell myself: a kidney infection, like a violent summer, has dehydrated them. The image of this illness helps me prioritize what medicines I prescribe: I know I need to write for IV fluids and antibiotics to replenish the creek immediately. Using metaphors like this has helped me understand how the body works.

This book uses stories to think through a problem that goes beyond any one body. It comes from a question formed, in part, by experiences like the one I had with Mr. Alvaro: Why do some people benefit from healthcare in America while others are excluded? The stories appear intertwined, each building on the others. Some take place before the COVID-19 pandemic and others during. I've pieced them together alongside some of my own personal stories in order to think about the basic foundations of our healthcare system in America and uncover for myself how Ben Taub illuminates what is missing in American medicine.

"There ought to be a man with a hammer behind the door of every happy man," Anton Chekhov wrote, "to remind him by his constant knocks that there are unhappy people." Many people know Chekhov worked as a doctor, even as he wrote his short stories and plays in late nineteenth-century Russia, but his devotion to the poor is not so well recognized. Chekhov traveled via horse-drawn carriage from Moscow, which sits on Israel's longitude, three months through the Russian tundra, nearly four thousand miles, to Sakhalin Island, just north of Japan. He did this to write about the deplorable conditions of a penal colony on Sakhalin, as well as the public health failures.

More than anything, however, Chekhov wrote about the *people* living in these desperate conditions. As famous as he was, Chekhov could have worked as a concierge doctor and catered to Moscow's elite. Instead, he wrote stories about the poor so that the fortunate might understand that their plight is everyone's responsibility: "Apparently a happy man only feels so because the unhappy bear their burden in silence."

Chekhov eventually died of tuberculosis, an illness he contracted from the patients he served. He had been born poor. His patients were poor. He had traveled to the poorest part of Russia. He saw in his practice how tuberculosis devastated his fellow Russians with a mortality rate of four hundred deaths per one hundred thousand people, one and a half times that of COVID-19 in the United States more than a century later. Chekhov also recognized how little the government of his beloved Russia cared about tuberculosis and poverty. The authorities had enacted a campaign they called the "Fight Against Tuberculosis," which consisted of nothing more than epidemiological surveys. For all its pomp, the program received no funding from the state. Rather, it relied on charity.

This touched a nerve with Chekhov, and three months after returning from Sakhalin, he wrote a letter to the vice director of the Ministry of Justice, a man who taught law, served as a judge, and, it so happened, had a soft spot for writers. "I believe it is very harmful to have to depend mainly on charity," he wrote. "I think it would be far better if this problem were to be addressed by funding from the state."

Chekhov explained that the problems in Sakhalin went deeper than whatever numbers might appear on a survey: "I encountered no infectious diseases on Sakhalin, and found very little congenital syphilis. But I did see children who were blind, dirty, and covered in sores, all diseases that bear witness to neglect."

Years later, at the height of his popularity, Chekhov sat down in the dining room of the Hermitage restaurant, one of the most exclusive locations in all of Russia. As the meal began, blood began to stream from his mouth. The tuberculosis—which up to that point had for him been more of an annoyance than a debilitating illness—had caused his lungs to hemorrhage.

He lay in bed for days recovering, first at a clinic and then at a hotel. The clinician and master of the written word received what treatments were available, including ventilated air spiked with turpentine and eucalyptus, wine from Hungary, a cognac after dinner. He wrote more letters in his convalescence, including to young authors, giving them advice. "Your task is to be a sincere artist writing only about what exists or what you think ought to exist," he wrote, "painting pictures of life as it is."

This book takes inspiration from the many letters Chekhov wrote as much as from his fiction. Chekhov never got to see his beloved Russia reform the way it treated its sick and poor. The scourge of tuberculosis continued until governments around the world recognized the illness as a public health threat and invested in institutions. Improved social conditions, measures to ensure the poor weren't malnourished, and public education on the illness, as well as the end of World War I, helped cut the death rate from tuberculosis in half in Europe and Russia by the mid-1920s. Had he lived, Chekhov would've been in his sixties by this time. Instead, he died at age forty-four in a sanatorium in the Black Forest.

But his devotion to the poor and to his writing had meaning. The man at the Ministry of Justice to whom Chekhov had written took his words to heart. Russia's criminal code was revised one year before Chekhov died, meaning that fewer people were sent to suffer on Sakhalin

Island. As a patient and a doctor and a person who cared deeply about the suffering of others, he never would've chosen to have tuberculosis, but he also didn't regret contracting it—or, at least, he never said he did in the letters he wrote. Even at the peak of his illness, in the throes of maximum symptomatology, he blamed and reviled no one, not even the patients who transmitted the disease to him. Connecting with people, serving them, making them think and enjoy life for the length of a play or short story, or even an appointment in his clinic, meant that much to him.

So did pushing to change the system that ignored this suffering. Histories were Chekhov's hammer. The tapping on the door we hear in stories of injustice—his and all stories that depict the unhappy living in silence—should awaken us to find more humane ways, in this case, of providing healthcare.

The stories in this book are inspired by Chekhov's portrayal of people hidden from us. But this book also shows what Chekhov didn't live to see: more people working to alleviate this suffering, and government, not charity, helping in this work. It is a love letter to the hospital, my hospital, where people find healthcare and revere it like treasure. It is also a letter to those sitting in positions of authority, to alert them to the consequences of failing to act with immediacy. As Chekhov himself noted, when we hear the hammer tapping upon our door, we should spring up:

"In the name of what must we wait?"

PART ONE

Life Without Insurance

The Dead Parts

If Stephen Hart was good at one thing, it was managing restaurants. For twelve years, he'd resurrected different branches of a burger chain in Houston and made them profitable. Stephen didn't have an MBA or any kind of special training. He had people skills, which, after some twists and turns in life, had bloomed for him in the service industry. The truth was that Stephen enjoyed going out of his way to help customers. He loved becoming the highlight of someone's day. That corporate talk about turning an "Ow" into a "Wow" sounded lame, yes, but, in fact, it made him tick. He wasn't one of those general managers who buried himself in an office tracking avocado prices during the dinner rush. Rather, he preferred striking up conversations with customers the moment they stepped through the door.

One night, while Stephen was taking orders at the counter, a guest mused to him about having eaten the tastiest burger there the last time he came, one with slabs of bacon and Swiss cheese topped with a thick slice of grilled pineapple. Did Stephen know the burger?

"That would be the Hawaiian burger," Stephen said, smoothing out the ends of his 'stache. His silvery voice and appearance—kempt, like a man rising from a barber's chair—helped to soften the bad news that the chain hadn't carried the burger for years.

"Man," the guest lamented. Most general managers would've chalked up the disappointment to part of the job: specialty burgers came, and they went. Stephen, however, was not most managers.

"Would you like one?" he asked.

"That would be awesome."

Stephen warned him it might take a minute, since he knew the kitchen didn't stock pineapple. He picked up the keys to his truck, exited the restaurant, and drove three miles to the nearest grocery store where, for eighty-nine cents, he purchased a can of the prized fruit. Not ten minutes later, the first dribbles of nectar sizzled on the grill. Stephen made sure the char was just right before flipping the pineapple over and then crowning his concoction. As the guest bit into his Hawaiian burger, Stephen knew he'd earned a customer for life.

Pleasing guests was one thing, but to manage a restaurant successfully, Stephen knew you had to be prepared to deal with people every which way. Satisfy a customer on Tuesday and you better have a plan to keep that same customer happy over the weekend. People were complicated. Resurrecting a Hawaiian burger might go a long way one night, but what if that guest found himself in a different part of town? The guest might spot an entirely new branch of his favorite burger joint and feel his mouth water. He might order a Hawaiian burger at the counter, only to be told by this branch's GM that no such burger existed. Oh no no, the guest might insist, he'd just enjoyed one at their restaurant up in Spring, the one managed by that well-put-together and personable GM. Word of mouth like that ought to be a positive—it was business!—but often it provoked frustration and jealousy and maybe even a little GM-on-GM backstabbing.

An email to corporate stated that Stephen had broken protocol. No recipe existed in their handbook for a Hawaiian burger, it noted, and since cooking items outside the handbook was forbidden, Stephen had failed to adhere to company standards.

There were other complaints. The flip side of caring so much about customer satisfaction was that it left you vulnerable to nagging. One diner—the CEO of a local company who ordered his wife a salad—couldn't be sated. The kitchen had run out of romaine lettuce and the CEO wouldn't accept any substitution. Iceberg wouldn't do. If the menu specified romaine, he reasoned, well then, that was what his wife would receive.

Stephen apologized and attempted to placate the CEO, offering to replace the salad, comp it, have one prepared and ready for him at a future date, whatever. Nothing stuck.

"I would be eating dinner with my wife by now," the CEO noted, "if you, Mr. General Manager, had done your job."

That was when Stephen broke. "I get it!" he said, slapping the table.

A hush fell over the restaurant. Guests perked up. Staff stopped in their tracks. Even the sizzle off the grill sounded muzzled. The words from Stephen's mouth came out whiny. "You don't have to be a dick about it," he said.

The CEO sat aghast.

"Did you just call me a dick?" he said.

"No, sir," Stephen replied, "you must have misunderstood." So ended the exchange. He walked away, and after a bit of fuming, the CEO and his wife exited the building, but Stephen knew this wasn't over. At the end of the shift, he called the staff together for a team meeting to make it clear his actions were unacceptable.

"I'm probably going to be fired tomorrow," he announced, his voice whinnying a bit, "because if any of you would've done what I just did, I would've fired you."

As much as his staff supported him—"He really was a dick," many admitted—Stephen understood the final word lay with corporate. He informed his boss, the district manager, who reached out the very next day to the slighted customer. But his mea culpas fell on deaf ears. The irate CEO saw no point in speaking with a district manager about such affairs. Any discussion, he insisted, would have to be CEO to CEO, himself and their head honcho up in Austin. "We speak the same language," he said.

Indeed, feeling most versed in the language of sales, the burger joint's CEO in Austin focused on the numbers. It turned out that, year after year, Stephen boasted sales increases of 10 percent. While other GMs reported 20 percent losses, Stephen's focus on customer satisfaction made his location a proven winner. The CEO of the burger joint knew losing an asset like this made no sense. He heard the angry customer out, hung up the phone, and that was that. Within a year, Stephen earned a raise as well as management of one of their larger restaurants. He commanded a $75,000 yearly salary, which helped him afford the payments on a house in one of Houston's middle-class suburbs. Stephen did more than get by. He did well.

The burger chain offered different grades of health insurance, from Cadillac plans to the bare bones. Ever a bargain hunter, Stephen opted for the cheapest health insurance available, which deducted only $88 from his check every other week. Like buying cheese at the right price point, this was a value-based decision. In his fifty-five years of living on God's green earth he had never needed to see a doctor. Why waste the money?

Then in late March 2020, as the world awakened to the fact that a pandemic was spreading to all its far corners, Stephen phoned corporate with some bad news. After shaking all night with chills, he checked his temperature. Stephen was running a fever. As the only one with keys to a restaurant trying to make do during a COVID lockdown, Stephen knew this presented a problem. He agreed to open the restaurant and return home immediately for a two-week quarantine. This would be the last time he set foot in the restaurant as its general manager.

His insurance plan only provided coverage for a tele-doc visit. Via his webcam, Stephen tried to show this new doctor a lymph node below his left jaw, one that had grown in size over the past year. But Zoom made it hard. The doctor prescribed him an antibiotic, and within a couple days, what had felt like a pea beneath his skin now felt like a baseball. Stephen was sure he didn't have COVID, and he began to worry the mass was causing the fever. Aware it would cost him, Stephen decided to bite the bullet and visit the emergency room of a reputable nearby hospital.

Before even sitting down in the waiting area, he paid the $639 requested—*insisted* upon—by the hospital's clerk. This got him in the door. Next, a doctor examined him, ordered a CAT scan of his neck, and, not long afterward, relayed the results, first that Stephen had cancer in his tonsils, and second that an ear nose throat doctor, or ENT, awaited him at a different branch across town.

Stephen feared what the ambulance ride might cost. "I feel okay," he said. "I can walk. Can't I just drive myself or go tomorrow?"

The hospital followed a specific protocol in these situations, the ER doctor explained.

Stephen walked into the ambulance and sat quietly the entire ride to the branch. Once they arrived, nobody there seemed to know anything about his situation, so Stephen waited patiently for the ENT who was supposedly there waiting for him. Finally, after many hours, the doctor saw him. He'd seen the scans and, yes, there appeared to be cancer in his tonsils. Stephen expected more after this, for the ENT to say, "And so," or "Based on this," or to dive into some plan of action—this was cancer, after all—but the operative word was "however."

"However, you don't have insurance," he said.

He meant *sufficient* insurance. It is a fiction in America that the thin plastic card bearing our name and plan is our panacea. Politicians and journalists pretend it's a tidy little equation: if you're insured, you're okay.

The truth is much more complicated. Even though Stephen had insurance, it covered so little that he had to prepay the ER for a cancer diagnosis. He could live with being on the wrong end of a bad deal—for now, anyway. What he couldn't quite digest was how the people in the ER had treated him. He felt shitty. It seemed wrong that they'd sent him here and there and then kicked him to the curb. He could understand that nothing would take the cancer away today and that his life wasn't immediately in danger, but how could anyone be so callous? Who says "however" in a situation like this?

After the ENT departed, a social worker entered his ER room and gave Stephen some quick and simple advice. Go to the public hospital, she said. "Go to Ben Taub."

Stephen patted the tiny handlebar ends of his mustache. His fingers drifted to the left side of his neck, which felt hard and unshaven. In his mind, these two words—"public" and "hospital"—never belonged together. Wasn't this America? He'd never spent a night in a hospital, and now he would have to step foot in a place he recognized from the ten o'clock news, where gunshot victims recuperated and Houston's homeless took shelter. He imagined drug addicts lining the halls, the dregs of society.

This is gonna be hell, he thought. I have hit bottom.

*   *   *

It was April in Houston, just a few days after Easter, and a full month since Roxana had left the hospital. From morning through the early afternoon, she lay in bed with her trusted companion, her smartphone. Texts from her family back home in El Salvador kept coming in. Cómo estás? *How are you?* Has visto un doctor? *Have you seen a doctor yet?* Inevitably, some of her family started to call on video chat. Roxana struggled up in bed and patted the loose strands of her hair into place. She warmed up the muscles she used to smile. Roxana was sick, but looking elegant had always been important to her.

In 1998, Roxana had been in the prime of her life. She worked as a salesperson at the Saks Fifth Avenue in the Houston Galleria. It was a good job. Every time she walked into work, bright lights hit her from every angle of the showroom. She felt like a star. More important, the Saks job had provided her with health insurance. She hadn't used it much—she'd once received routine gallbladder surgery after a pain in her belly doubled her over—but whenever she needed it, it was there. What she wouldn't have given for health insurance now.

Twenty years had passed since she had worked at Saks. Roxana was forty-eight now and in need of help. Gangrene had overtaken her arms and legs, leaving her bedbound. A tumor arising from one of her major blood vessels—diagnosed within the last year and operated upon in a lifesaving surgery—continued to grow inside of her, like a large tapeworm. Roxana was still trying to piece together exactly how this had all happened. She remembered meeting an old friend in December whom she hadn't seen in a while. She remembered that friend taking her immediately to the nearest emergency room after seeing how much weight she had lost. She remembered signing the consent for a major surgery, the only hope to save her life. After that, the next weeks were a blur to her. Doctors told her after the fact that she had fallen into a monthlong coma following the surgery. When she awoke, she found gangrene covering the areas where she wore boots and a pair of long gloves. Her limbs looked withered, like charred wood. Roxana had suffered a devastating complication from the surgery named vasoplegic syndrome. The surgery to remove the tumor growing in her heart had sent her body into shock.* While medicines kept her vital organs alive, the circulation to her limbs wasn't sufficient. Without oxygen, the cells in her legs and arms perished. The result was that Roxana now carried the dead parts on her body.

Roxana felt the heavy weight of dead limbs even in the smallest of movements, for instance, when holding up the phone for video chats. She tried to keep the camera on her face and not on the limbs. The sight of them on-screen made her sob.

---

* Technically, her body had reacted to the cardiopulmonary bypass machine used in the surgery as it would have a deadly infection. "Shock" here means her circulation failed and her blood pressure plummeted.

When doctors discharged Roxana from the hospital, there was no medical plan for what to do about her dead limbs. This is what happens when people don't have health insurance. The only medical advice she received was that she return home and let all the dead parts "auto-amputate," a process that could take years.

Roxana held her once graceful arms up to the medical staff in disbelief. "Like a dead branch falling off a tree?" she said.

These were wrists that had once modeled diamond bracelets and wafted perfumes beneath the noses of a high-profile clientele. On these feet, she had escaped her war-torn homeland of El Salvador and crossed Mexico to arrive here in the early eighties. These legs had carried her throughout Houston from job to job, allowing her to send *remesas* back home to her ailing mother. Immediately before falling into this whirlwind of illness, Roxana had worked as a personal caretaker. With these fingers, Roxana had changed the diapers of some of the city's wealthy elderly. Service was a part of who Roxana was, and her hands were her tools. She bathed the sick with them. She used them to pour her friends coffee in her humble but tidy apartment. She prayed with these hands. And now they only weighed her down.

Now all of her activities—like eating and washing her hair and virtually everything to care for herself—involved an extra set of hands and feet. Marí had put her job in El Salvador on hold and flown into Houston to help her mother. Going outside every morning was a ritual for them. Roxana planted her two feet atop Marí's and draped her arms around her neck, like she was learning to dance. Then mother and daughter took one stiff step at a time, from the bed to the front door. It took so much effort for Roxana to feel like a person again, but whenever the sunlight hit living skin, they both knew it was worth it.

If only she could have all four limbs amputated. That was what Roxana wanted. She had come to grips with the new reality that she would never use her arms or legs again, and she wanted to move on. Maybe without the weight, she'd be less ungainly, and she could start to take care of herself. Maybe she could receive prostheses. Maybe she could start to work and send her mother more money. How to get started on this new life, however, remained a mystery, since the hospitals nearby required health insurance. Getting a hospital and doctors to focus on her quality of life, rather than how they might be paid, would be a challenge.

Nearly half of all people in the United States receive their health insurance through their job. The way this works is that an employer will negotiate a contract with an insurance company to offer its workers a plan. This is known as "group coverage." Under this system, the worker and the employer split the cost of this insurance. How much the employee pays and what tests and treatments are covered (as well as how much they're covered) depends on what the employer has negotiated with the insurance company. Some employers are more generous than others, and some employees are more risk averse than others. While Saks gave Roxana a good enough plan to cover her gallbladder surgery in the nineties, Stephen, dissuaded in part by the cost of a high-coverage plan, had opted for the burger chain's lowest coverage and found himself with few options when he needed them the most. As healthcare has grown increasingly expensive, employers have shifted more expenses to employees. In the nineties, it was quite common for employers to foot their employees' full healthcare bill. Today, that same arrangement is rare.

Another 7 percent of people in the US purchase their own health insurance. Negotiating one-to-one with insurance companies gives people the ability to decide exactly how much they want to spend on healthcare for what specific services, but this freedom comes with risks and costs. Some policies have deductibles, requiring a person to spend $1,400, $2,800, or even as much as $10,000 before benefits kick in. The Affordable Care Act extended private insurance to those who couldn't find insurance through an employer. Depending on the plan, the government took the employer's role and subsidized a portion of it. Neither of these options, employer-based health insurance or private insurance through the ACA, was possible for Roxana. With the dry gangrene on her body, Roxana was unable to work. She was also expressly forbidden from purchasing health insurance through the Affordable Care Act exchanges because she lacked a green card. According to federal law, those who are not citizens or "aliens lawfully present in the United States may not be covered under a qualified health plan."

As an undocumented immigrant, Roxana also couldn't receive either of the government-paid health insurances, Medicare and Medicaid. Citizens and residents aged sixty-five and older who have paid into the system through paycheck deductions qualify for Medicare. Some people with a recognized disability might qualify at an earlier age if they live with the disability for two years. But since the Social Security Administration denies two-thirds of disability claims, even a green card wouldn't have guaranteed Roxana the basic recognition that her charcoal-colored limbs qualified as disabling.

It's possible that if Roxana had been a US resident, she would have qualified for Medicaid, the coverage intended for the poorest and most disabled Americans. But even this would have been a long shot. Each state runs its own Medicaid program that it funds in cooperation with the federal government. Some states, like New Hampshire and New York, are more generous than others. Texas is the least generous state, not only in who can qualify for Medicaid—earning more than $8,796 *per year*, which is $4,000 below the national poverty line, disqualifies Texans—but also in how much it pays to doctors and hospitals for services provided to the patients it covers. Correspondingly, some hospitals refuse to treat Medicaid patients, preferring patients covered by private insurance or Medicare, which pays better.

Roxana started to feel that she had no options, that she would live with the weight of the dry gangrene for the rest of her life. She was one of the thirty million people in the US lacking health insurance. And another forty million are underinsured, meaning that their deductibles and out-of-pocket costs are so high that they make treatments unaffordable. This amounts to 20 percent of the population without access to care in the US healthcare system. What happens when people like Roxana need healthcare but don't have coverage?

The sick and uninsured basically have three options. Their first is to find a clinic or doctor themselves and pay cash. This is simple enough, and to the healthy, this may seem like an ideal way to afford healthcare—to pay for what you get. If all you have to afford is an urgent-care visit here, a flu shot there, and you have enough money in the bank—and what you're paying isn't exorbitant—then being uninsured like this isn't a problem. And, in fact, Roxana lived like this for many years after she lost her employer coverage: a little here, a little there. What she discovered, however, is that we can't predict when we'll fall ill, and that when severe illness arrives, healthcare is way too expensive. The medical costs snowball into an avalanche. A 2019 article in the *American Journal of Public Health* showed that 66 percent of all bankruptcies in America—affecting more than 530,000 families—were due to medical bills, by far the most of any cause. Roxana had already received an $80,000 bill from the hospital that just released her, an amount well beyond the few hundred dollars she had kept in savings before falling ill and one she'd never be able to repay, especially with a disability that so severely limited her professional options.

People without health insurance can visit an emergency room. Under federal law, *anyone* can visit an ER that accepts Medicare dollars (and virtually all do). Of course, just because you have the right to visit an ER and find out if your life is in danger doesn't mean that this service comes free. ER visits generate bills—big ones. ER doctors charge more for their services than primary care doctors, but since ERs can't refuse anyone seeking an evaluation, the uninsured visit them frequently. Many receive prescriptions for high blood pressure or diabetes through the ER. Specialty care, like the type that Roxana needed and the type that saved her life during her previous hospitalization, happens only in the ER. It's a place designed to give a quick assessment of pressing issues. In return, the uninsured receive bills—mind-boggling ones, the type that bankrupts a family, the type that can't be paid—but what else can they do? You enter whatever doors are open to you.

More often than not, the uninsured take the third option: they endure their sickness. This is especially true for those with a chronic illness like Roxana. "Enduring" can mean a lot of things. Sometimes it means accepting the wheezing and gasping of asthma as normal. Sometimes it means living perpetually dehydrated by blood sugar that's at five times healthy levels, that causes you to faint at work and desiccates your kidneys. Sometimes it means having loved ones in Nigeria or India mail you water pills for congestive heart failure. It can mean taking a day trip into Mexico to visit an affordable doctor or signing up for each and every health fair in town to take advantage of the free samples. Or it can mean accepting charity that isn't necessarily specific to your situation. That was what the hospital that discharged Roxana arranged: for a visit from a home hospice nurse from a local charity. But Roxana *wasn't* dying. The best the hospital could do for Roxana, however, was release her and send her home to die.

Enduring sickness leads to one of two paths: to the emergency room when the muscles and the organs simply wear out, or to the grave, which is much more common for those without health insurance. Either way, these choices make the struggles of life without insurance not only Roxana's problem but also everyone's problem. The $80,000 bill sitting in one of Roxana's old shoeboxes will become part of the $140 billion of medical care doled out annually and left unpaid. Except that this staggering amount *must be* paid for in some way. Uncompensated care increases the amount hospitals charge insured patients in order to recoup costs. More than that, it leads to financial struggles at particularly vulnerable hospitals like those in small towns or in underserved areas. Some hospitals apply for rescue money from the government (i.e., us, the taxpayers); some simply cut staffing and specialty care, thereby reducing the quality and extent of service. Some close their doors, leaving wide swaths of people without any local option at all.

We all pay, somehow.

*   *   *

On the other side of town, Ebonie was busy settling down her family in a new city. It was May, and for a month now, she and her two youngest children had been living with her sister Sharonna on the southwest side. Switching cities like this—and states, for that matter—had sapped Ebonie of all her energy. The last three days had been hectic. She'd spent them running around trying to enroll her daughter Blessn in school, only to confront bureaucracy. These were the times that made her wonder if she should have stayed home.

Ebonie had been born and raised in Southern California and lived her whole life in the LA area, moving from Hollywood to the coast, but when the rent on her Long Beach apartment grew too expensive, she took Blessn and her two-year-old son, Lyse, to Texas. To make the move, she had to leave her two older children back in California with her mother. Sharing the rent with Sharonna gave her a roof overhead and an extra set of eyes and hands for the young children, not to mention more money in her pocket, something Ebonie needed to get by. Ebonie spent the daytime hours picking up after Blessn and Lyse, making them waffles, keeping them entertained with different takes on the alphabet song. Now that it was almost Blessn's bedtime, the two lay in Ebonie's bed, listening to R & B on Pandora.

Ebonie was exhausted and a little nauseated, because on top of everything she was dealing with, she was also nineteen weeks pregnant. Two of her previous six pregnancies had ended in a miscarriage, and Ebonie was worried she'd lose another child. Just before moving to Houston, she'd started to experience bleeding, especially when sitting down. In recent days, the blood had started to soak through the pads she wore and through the seam of her jeans. Sharonna had taken her to the closest emergency room three times in the past month. At the most recent visit, one week ago, doctors had kept her in the hospital overnight to give her a blood transfusion. Beyond recommending that she find an obstetrician, which Ebonie hadn't been able to do since she was uninsured, they dealt with the immediate problem but did little to ensure that Ebonie would receive good care going forward. They released her on Mother's Day. "She had previously received PNC [prenatal care] in California and recently moved to Houston," wrote the doctor. "Has not established care yet."

As she lay in bed, listening to music after another tiring day, Ebonie suddenly felt something wet beneath her. She made her way to the bathroom and Blessn followed. When she reached to turn on the light, a cramp hit her right side. Immediately, a bright red pool collected beneath her, much of it mixed with clots. Blessn looked at the blood and then at her mother.

"Tell your auntie," Ebonie instructed her.

Sharonna called 911. An ambulance arrived quickly, and when the driver loaded Ebonie into the back, he asked her if she had health insurance. Maybe he did this because Ebonie was African American. Maybe he asked because of her neighborhood, Gulfton, with all its working-class apartments. Maybe he saw Ebonie's nose ring and her Afro parted down the middle dyed half red, half green, and made an assumption. Or maybe he simply knew how things worked and he wanted to help her. If he took her to the nearest hospital, as the other ambulance drivers had before him, Ebonie might not receive a thorough assessment because she lacked insurance. The hospital would make sure she was stable, but would it address the root of the problem and prevent the bleeding from happening again?

Ebonie didn't know what to say. She'd already gone through this during her recent hospital visits—in California, she was covered by Medi-Cal, the state's version of Medicaid. But did that cover her in Texas? No one could give her good information, and the healthcare she had received thus far during this critical moment in her life had been impersonal and imprecise.

The ambulance driver gathered from her silence that Ebonie was not insured. He loaded her into the back and started to drive, knowing exactly where to take her. He was used to this, after all. The uninsured rate in Texas was climbing again. It had reached nearly 25 percent, as high as it had been before the ACA started, when health coverage became mandated. An ambulance driver notices such shifts.

The rate of mothers' dying shortly after childbirth was also rising. In Texas, it had nearly doubled from 2011 to 2012, for reasons public health experts and statisticians couldn't explain. The spike in maternal deaths loomed so large that Texas lawmakers added it to an emergency legislative agenda. The numbers looked bad. Only during war or catastrophes had there ever been such a spike. Was there a connection between the uninsured rate and the rate of maternal death? Nobody knew. What experts did know was that African American mothers bore the highest risk.

So much of our healthcare system is mired in discrepancies. While the rate of new mothers dying in Texas was increasing, Ebonie's home state of California was bucking that trend. When the Affordable Care Act was signed into law, California expanded Medicaid to cover more than twelve million Californians, making it the largest public insurer of the poor and near-poor in the country. Right in the middle of a pregnancy, Ebonie had left the country's safest state for expectant mothers—where the mortality rate looked more like that of France or Germany—for one of its most dangerous. Her new home state, Texas, had the same maternal mortality rate as Mongolia.

The disparity was visible in the palms of Ebonie's hands, which were white and wan, not pink and healthy. Ebonie was anemic. She was bleeding. At this moment, when she was most vulnerable, her insurance didn't cross state lines, and her only option, over and over, was to go to the emergency room.

The contradictions of the American healthcare system were evident on Roxana's body as well. Her face was olive colored, her lips pouty and pink, her eyes amber, the vibrant colors of cells receiving oxygen through the blood. Roxana was alive. In any other country, she probably wouldn't have been. What had caused Roxana's sickness in the first place was a tumor winding through her back muscles and invading her heart. It so happened that one of the world's leading heart tumor surgeons practiced in Houston. In all of his years, he had only seen one other patient with such a complex tumor, but he'd decided to try to help Roxana.

The American healthcare system put him in a position to do so. Our system enabled the surgeon to develop his technical expertise. It provided him with a license to practice medicine safely. American medicine also stoked the surgeon's ambition enough for him to give a moonshot like Roxana's tumor extraction a try. It even earmarked funds through Medicaid to care for an uninsured patient under emergency conditions. This is the great paradox of our time: we can decode the genome, but we can't seem to treat the sick. What an awesome feat, saving a life like this. But our healthcare system hasn't found a way to complete the job. After the surgery, Roxana no longer needed a topflight expert. What she needed was good but not necessarily elite surgeons to amputate her arms and legs. She needed physical therapists and primary care doctors to help her regain a level of humanity and self-sufficiency. She needed healthcare access. Likewise, Ebonie needed more than just routine prenatal care through community organizations like Planned Parenthood: she needed access to high-risk obstetricians. And the need extends to all of us, if we believe that healthcare costs should be controlled. In this capacity, our country fails. Roxana's charcoal-colored arms and Ebonie's pale palms testified to this fact.

In 1980, Arnold Relman, then editor of the *New England Journal of Medicine*, repurposed the Cold War term "military-industrial complex" to describe the new world of healthcare. The "medical-industrial complex," according to Relman, was composed of doctors, hospital administrators, insurance companies, medical equipment makers, medical schools, and Big Pharma—essentially, *any* vendor of *anything* remotely medical—who supply healthcare to Americans like clockwork. Forty years later, business and medicine no longer act as partners in supplying healthcare: business has subsumed and digested medicine. Medicine *is* business. The reason Stephen and Roxana and Ebonie could not find proper healthcare in their times of need is simply because they lacked a payer.

We might think we have a healthcare system, but in reality, we have something more sprawling and disjointed and impersonal. There's no one term to describe it. "Corporate medicine" comes close, though it doesn't quite capture our feeling of helplessness when a cancer diagnosis is followed by an onslaught of bills. "Medical-industrial complex" paints the picture of a firing squad, except the squad is disorganized, each of the gunmen—the insurance companies, doctors, hospitals, and Big Pharma—aiming not only for us but also for the other gunmen.

The promise of profit means each of these players is clawing and charging the others: insurance denies claims, hospitals inflate bills for insurance, Big Pharma ups drug prices to scrounge from insurance's profits. Let's call it "Medicine Inc.," then, this amalgam of healthcare suppliers in America, for its level of sheer conscience-less competition. It's not a perfect term, and it's not meant to disparage business or capitalism. Perhaps Medicine Inc. wouldn't be so bad if we were the customers, but we aren't. We might pay for our care, as a customer would, through insurance premiums and co-pays, but our bodies are the merchandise.

It's tempting to imagine that Medicine Inc. was hatched by a small group of moguls gathered together in a secret location—maybe in the cone of a volcano—in a plot to fleece the American public. The truth is far more complicated. Those whom Medicine Inc. benefits most—doctors, hospitals, pharmaceutical companies, and middlemen like insurance companies—didn't create this behemoth on purpose. Medicine Inc. is the product of patchwork and the struggle of these groups (along with policy makers) to accommodate the foundational building block that is private health insurance. Private health insurance is the root of our own healthcare problems.

If we look at Medicine Inc.'s history and how it operates today, five basic assumptions stand out that make it distinctly American:

1. The government should not produce or provide healthcare. It's okay to use public funds to purchase private healthcare for certain people, but only companies or private practitioners should provide healthcare.

2. Those who receive healthcare have earned it, whether through work or through wealth. Fairness means ensuring that the deserving people receive better healthcare.

3. There is no significant conflict between the income a doctor generates and their duty to the public. Doctors can practice simultaneously as businesspeople and as professionals sworn to a code of ethics without major repercussions.

4. Science is impersonal and best aligns with commercial needs, not public ones. Science's primary beneficiaries should be people who can afford to pay for it.

5. The primary goal of healthcare is to generate income for providers. Other goals, like preventing sickness and empowering people, can happen, but only if the first goal is met.

These tenets are so much a part of American healthcare that we don't even realize our political debates reinforce them. Take, for instance, the first principle, the idea that healthcare should be private and available through the market alone. This tenet transcends politics. Those who want the Affordable Care Act repealed and those who champion Medicare for All might beleaguer each other over Twitter, but they actually agree on this most basic tenet. For the last sixty years, every piece of legislation, every regulation, every political debate, has attempted to solve our healthcare problems by preserving private health insurance. Any problems that have arisen we've solved by doubling down on this idea, even at the cost of other institutions. To help seniors access this private healthcare, for instance, we created a separate government-sponsored health insurance named Medicare. To help the poor, we asked states and the federal government to work together as insurers. This is called Medicaid. For the near-poor, we made our tax code even more complicated and founded a whole new insurance market (the ACA). To this day, when we debate whether to repeal the ACA versus passing new legislation to give Medicare to all, we are still trying to fit the square peg into a round hole. What if we removed the middleman of insurance? In other words, we need to rethink the belief that it's distinctly un-American for government—whether local, state, or federal—to provide or sell health services.

Are we the type of society that connects the needy with those trained to help them? If someone has dead arms and legs, and there are hundreds of surgeons within a twenty-mile radius with the technical expertise to remove these limbs safely, do we facilitate this, or do we adhere to the value that business decides? Should we prioritize the healthcare of all soon-to-be mothers, to ensure the next generation has the best chance of thriving without medical problems? Are we able to keep our ambitions and moonshots as well as take care of our most vulnerable outside of Medicine Inc.?

What happens when the government provides healthcare?

What if we defined fairness by how all people received healthcare, rather than by who received it?

If doctors acted less like businesspeople and more like public servants, would it help their patients?

Can science be personal and precise and geared toward the public good?

What if the goal of healthcare wasn't to earn money but to help solve people's medical problems?

Three Houstonians, Stephen, Roxana, and Ebonie, were about to find the answers to these questions and more.

— 3 —

Doctors

When I started working at Ben Taub, I didn't know what it meant that most of our patients had no health insurance. Growing up, I experienced healthcare the way most people in this country do, which is through private insurance. My pediatricians encountered no snags as they kept me on the vaccine schedule and ensured I didn't fall too far off the growth curve. The doctor-patient relationship looked idyllic from my vantage point. My dad delivered babies for a living, and every Saturday morning, he brought me to the hospital for his rounds. I was my most docile self during our short car rides, which ended in the parking garage. From there, it was a couple of quick turns into back entrances and service elevators before we were on the labor and delivery floor.

"This is my son," he'd tell the L & D nurses.

"Yes, we've met," they would respond graciously.

After the intros, my dad would punch a couple of numbers into an electronic keypad to open a door down the hall, and for the rest of the morning, I parked myself in front of the television in the doctors' lounge, where I watched TV while he visited his patients inside the hospital.

It was glorious. Being at the hospital made me feel fortunate, like my dad's assistant. Aesthetically, the lounge could have used a little love. Every table or countertop had granules of sugar speckled over it, and of course, the heavy aroma of burned coffee hung in the air. I spent hours in there. Sometimes his doctor friends would come in, sit down, and make me chat to them about my family and school. Other times, they'd see me presiding over the TV and leave as quickly as they came in.

These Saturdays with my father started in America's heartland, Wichita, Kansas, where my dad worked for a private clinic owned by a group of doctors. The clinic used the hospital we visited for all its deliveries, which was how my dad had his special standing. Having joined the group fresh out of his residency, and less than five years after immigrating from El Salvador, he worked overtime the way a young lawyer working their way up in a firm might. The established partners gave him a base salary plus incentives for productivity. His schedule included plenty of overnight calls and undesirable shifts, though my dad never complained much. It must have helped that he was young, but my dad also saw his work as a doctor as more than just a job. Medicine was his calling. Those scrubs in the OR and that suit in his clinic were his identity. To my dad, the privilege of talking with people about their problems and thinking about and sometimes operating on them was priceless. The partners set all the rules for the patients he saw and the payments he received; my dad didn't have to do anything but work. "Estoy de turno," *I'm on call,* became a common refrain around the house.

Virtually all of the patients the clinic scheduled for him had private health insurance, which may have been one of the reasons the hospital seemed so impressive to me. The women in Wichita who didn't have insurance used a charity clinic—a site I never visited—where my dad volunteered three hours every week.

In 1986, sensing he might never make partner, he opened a private obstetrics and gynecology practice in Houston. His brother, my godfather, was also an ob-gyn, and so the two worked in tandem, sharing office costs while keeping their patients separate. They used a hospital on the northwest side, in what was a predominantly Hispanic neighborhood, for the vast majority of their surgeries and deliveries. As a demonstration of confidence in their future business relationship—and as a sign of the times of the 1980s—the hospital gave my father a $100,000 line of credit at 0 percent interest to start his practice, the only requirement being that he bring in patients.

My dad had moved from a group practice to a private specialty practice. He was no longer an employee of the doctor group in Wichita. Now he could decide what shifts to work and which patients to see. He opened his practice with an entrepreneurial sentiment: every cent generated from every surgery would funnel back into his practice and improve the level of care he could provide his patients. The money would also help his family grow.

This was how buoyant the world looked to a young doctor from El Salvador. In the Texas of 1986, anything was possible. The hospital had given him a discounted rate on an office on the sixth floor of the adjoining professional building, provided he walk next door for surgeries and deliveries.

"It's beautiful," he said. The view was of nothing more than six lanes of freeway going in either direction, but to him, it could have been Mount Kilimanjaro.

What my dad couldn't have realized was that over the next thirty years, healthcare costs would double, and health disparities would widen. Without a system to accommodate the growing number of patients disconnected from healthcare, he'd have to pause every time a patient without insurance asked him to be her doctor. As more money flowed into healthcare and into his own practice, he would have to reconcile his love of medicine and surgery with the headaches of running a business.

Career Days at my elementary school presented special opportunities to my dad. The questions my classmates posed to him about their bodies and where babies came from ("The butt?") required the right mix of humor and grace and fatherly distance to keep things enlightening for everybody. My dad was always game. The teachers fed off his energy. "Ask him to come next year," they insisted after each go-round, and each time, he put it on his calendar.

One year, a scheduling conflict made it impossible for him to attend. As luck would have it, the ob-gyn father of another classmate took his spot.

I broke the news to him that evening at the dinner table.

"Really?" he said, a little flabbergasted. "Did your friends like it?"

"He gave us this."

To accompany his talk, the replacement ob-gyn had distributed a menu of services and procedures he offered to his patients. Some of the procedures listed, like "C-section," I recognized, but there were others that sounded painful, like "hysterectomy."

"Interesting," my dad said, a bit amused.

"Do you do these?" I said, pointing to the entry "VBAC," which my dad explained stood for "vaginal birth after cesarean."

I was in fifth grade.

"Tu que crees?" he said. *What do you think?*

"Is this how much you make?" I asked.

I pointed to the dollar amounts listed beside the procedures, which my dad hadn't initially noticed.

"Interesting," he repeated, his attention now fixed on the page. The way he nodded, it looked like he was absorbing an insult.

When I reached out my hand to retrieve the paper, he pulled it away and said he was going to keep it.

"This is good," he said, nodding more assuredly now. "We're going to update our charges."

At the time, in the late eighties, most doctors in private practice were able to offer one menu like this with one set of prices, what's called a fee schedule. The amount he billed a patient's private insurance for performing a VBAC was no different than the cash price he charged those without insurance. The growth and domination of private health insurance over the next forty years rendered the universal fee schedule obsolete. Instead of offering one menu, doctors would have to develop hundreds, each unique to a patient's particular insurance and plan. They would also have to describe the menu items, or procedures, with increasingly complex terminology and codes. What was once a one-page menu would become a binder filled with numbers.

The handout from Career Day might not have appeared as anything more than a photocopied piece of paper, but, in reality, it represented one of the central struggles in American medicine: Who decides what a doctor charges?

Historically, doctors in America have insisted on keeping their own fees separate from the costs incurred by a hospital or other healthcare workers. Doctors are uniquely privileged workers in this manner. We don't buy tickets for a basketball game and then Venmo money to the players, for instance, or cut one check to the mechanic and another to the garage. That my dad was able to print up his own fee schedule for his patients, and that his patients would receive a whole different set of charges from the place of his work, the hospital, is a testament not only to American doctors' authority but also to their collective business sense.

Up until the early eighteenth century, local governments restricted doctors' fees, which made house calls and clinic visits more affordable to those who weren't well-off. But with the Revolutionary War came the free market. In the 1800s, doctors charged whatever fees they wanted so that by the Civil War, fewer and fewer Americans could afford healthcare. Over time, railroads, the invention of the car, and telephones made doctors more accessible. Medicine also became safer: improvements in anesthesia made more complex surgeries possible, doctors spread contagion less as hand washing became the norm, and vaccines prevented illnesses from tetanus to typhoid. Recognizing the benefits medicine provided, and in the midst of a rapid urbanization, more Americans *wanted* to see doctors by the 1920s, but only those with sufficient cash could do so, in large part because doctors maintained independence from healthcare organizations. Hospitals could have employed doctors, but some doctors resisted: they wanted the power to determine their own fees.

Europe played it differently. In the nineteenth and twentieth centuries, many European countries restricted doctors' fees to keep healthcare affordable for the public. Healthcare access became a public good, with the government providing access to doctors and clinics for those who could not afford it. But American doctors lobbied against any such plan.

They had their reasons. When I was in medical school, while professors taught the importance of taking a good patient history or how to give bad news, there was a phrase they repeated nearly as often as they did parts of the Hippocratic oath: "One patient, one doctor." At the time, I understood the phrase to mean that the doctor-patient relationship was a personal and sacred one. That while I was with someone who was sick, I should turn off my phone. It meant my job was to listen and to think and to focus on the person in front of me. It meant medicine wasn't just a job; it was a vocation.

But like so many maxims, "One patient, one doctor" was utilized for not-so-rosy ends. Doctors used it to justify how and what they billed. In 1934, in the midst of the Depression, the American Medical Association published a list of ten principles. Politicians were discussing how to make healthcare more affordable and whether universal coverage should be included with Social Security. Three of the ten rules listed by the AMA would serve as seeds for the cost crisis. Rule two was a reiteration of "One patient, one doctor" made explicit: "No third party must be permitted to come between the patient and his physician in any medical relation." Rule six pushed into financial territory: "The immediate cost [of medical service] should be borne by the patient if able to pay at the time of the service." Rule ten established authority: "There should be no restrictions of treatment formulated and enforced by the organized medical profession."

Practically, what this meant was that doctors could charge patients directly for the costs they incurred, not necessarily for the final product.

If a surgeon accidentally left a rag inside his patient during gallbladder surgery, for instance, he could remove the rag during a second surgery and bill the patient for two separate operations.

This payment method became known as fee-for-service, and it would become the blueprint for how Americans paid for their healthcare.

Throughout the twentieth century, doctors fought hard to preserve this billing method: they organized and lobbied and defeated any potential legislation meant to curtail fee-for-service. Even though healthcare was completely unaffordable for many, the doctors' lobby launched ad campaigns that painted change as tantamount to socialism; they looked more like the NRA than the AMA. Doctors started caring more about business than the actual practice of medicine. As Paul Starr notes in *The Social Transformation of American Medicine** when discussing this unique market power, "The doctors escaped becoming victims of capitalism and became small capitalists instead."

Doctors feared that private health insurance would sap them of the authority to determine their own fees, but in practice, insurance relieved doctors of the pressure of holding prices down. Insurance companies worked with doctors to continue fee-for-service. Whatever extra costs doctors incurred were passed along to patients, allowing insurance companies to reap higher profits. When, in 1964, the US government began paying for health insurance for the elderly and the poor through Medicare and Medicaid, it adopted fee-for-service and allowed doctors to bill for whatever costs they incurred. Instead of handing bills directly to their own patients, doctors found themselves billing faceless insurance companies or the US government. At this point, business really started to boom.

The result was that healthcare costs—including doctors' charges—skyrocketed through the 1970s: now prices were growing at three times

---

* It's hard to overestimate how vital this book has been to the ideas and history detailed in this section.

the national inflation rate. Eventually, politicians on both sides of the aisle began to wonder if fee-for-service was making healthcare way too expensive. President Nixon, when addressing this brewing crisis, noted the "illogical incentive" that stimulated doctors to perform more services rather than fewer. Sickness paid doctors and insurance companies more than keeping patients healthy. The profession turned on its own ideals and bowed toward business.

Medicare only started to cap doctors' and hospitals' fees during President Reagan's tenure in the 1980s, just as my dad's practice in Houston opened. Instead of allowing billers to run up exorbitant amounts, the government began setting reimbursement rates. By this time, however, the damage had already been done. Fee-for-service had served as the principal driver of healthcare inflation. If a doctor's job was to balance serving his patients with business, then fee-for-service tilted it toward the latter.

With age, I began to notice the daily balance my dad struck between serving his patients' needs and running a business. He had grown up hallowing medicine as if it were a calling, and like me, he took his early lessons from his own father. It's very possible that Buenaventura Nuila, my grandfather, was the first Salvadoran doctor to earn a public health degree at Harvard. He didn't stay in 1940s America long after receiving his diploma, though; he returned home to El Salvador to start a private pediatrics practice. Rather than serving the elite with his Ivy League degree, he focused on middle-class children, which in El Salvador meant the working class. Whenever my dad got out of school, he walked to my grandfather's office and waited for him to see his last patients before the two headed home. If a child's cough persisted beyond the salves and the humidified air and the tinctures of tonic water, my grandfather made house calls. Sometimes, my dad would awaken in the dead of the night to find petrified parents staring blankly at the walls of his living room. My grandfather opened his own home to his patients out of a simple belief: the profession of medicine demanded that a doctor take responsibility for the well-being of others. Money came second.

My dad exhibited a similar ethic within his own practice. He wore a suit to the office every day and insisted on meeting all new patients face-to-face from behind his escritoire. This was in contrast to those profit-minded colleagues he reviled, who introduced themselves while inserting the speculum to procure a pap smear, because they "had no time." Courtesy and attention were as fundamental to my dad's practice of medicine as knowing anatomy.

This old-school commitment to patients bore fruit business-wise. Soon after he opened his office, corkboards filled with photos of him hoisting up the babies he delivered lined the walls between exam rooms. The collages grew so plentiful that my dad routinely had me change them out for new ones.

"It's kinda sad," I said, tossing an old corkboard into the trunk of his Mercedes.

"Ricky," he said, "there are too many."

His practice grew. My dad began taking care of the next generations of women; some of the babies he delivered entered his office nearly two decades later. Mothers and daughters visited him together. He earned sufficient income to send all three of his children to a private grade school, then private high schools, then private colleges. Yet the wealth he earned in his practice came at a cost.

In the eighties and nineties, two trends gained momentum in American medicine. Both were responses to the exorbitant costs imposed by fee-for-service, and both jeopardized "One patient, one doctor." My dad, as a small-business owner and a doctor determining his own fees and how his practice ran, despised both.

Saying the letters "HMO" to my father was tantamount to ignoring him when he talked to you in public: little irked him more. These organizations, instead of guaranteeing their patients individual services, focused on overall wellness and keeping costs down, hence the name "health maintenance organization." Patients who joined HMOs paid a subscription fee that allowed them to visit doctors within a network, one that, in turn, provided the doctor with more patients. More expensive care, like visiting an orthopedic surgeon for a hip replacement, occurred at the discretion of a primary care doctor. To combat the "illogical incentive" of prioritizing sickness over health, President Nixon had advocated for HMOs, since they cut the cost of healthcare. Savings were supposed to go back into patients' pockets, but that's not how my dad saw it. HMOs negotiated tough with doctors. To be a part of their network, my dad would have to lower his fees. The sheet of prices my dad offered would grow from one page to dozens as insurance companies started to negotiate doctors' fees the way HMOs did, each requiring my dad to charge different amounts for the same service.

By 1987, 12 percent of the US population received care through an HMO. A new era of "managed care" threatened to strip doctors like my dad of the ability to provide a service and bill for it independently.

My dad ran his practice like a small business. If the office needed printer cartridges, he bought them. He put in extra time on the weekends making sure the supplies were in order, that his little lab had sufficient reagents, that his employees had enough coffee, and that the back-room refrigerator was clean. The second trend transforming American medicine didn't impact his practice directly, but it made this kind of approach more difficult, and it gobbled up practices like his. It was a trend happening not just in medicine but in nearly all American industries.

America was becoming corporatized. Ever since the mid-1900s, corporations aimed to enter a burgeoning and increasingly lucrative healthcare market but found themselves stymied by doctors' monopoly over the industry. The launch of Medicaid and Medicare in the 1960s incentivized corporations to enter the market. The public funds brought stability and a flood of money to the healthcare marketplace. They also decreased financial risk, and the money became a carrot for companies looking to earn profit. Reaganomics, which relaxed government control over the healthcare market, emboldened corporations further to purchase doctors' private practices. The old Wall Street parlance started to leak into medicine: hospital systems "merged"; larger conglomerates "acquired" smaller local hospitals; decisions on what medications would go on formulary were made in a hospital's "boardroom," which was located hundreds of miles away in the corporate headquarters. With fee-for-service as the operative billing system, doctors served up increasing volumes of healthcare with more services and shared in the spoils. In the 1980s, when my father finished his training, nearly two out of ten doctors boasted incomes in the nation's top 1 percent. They earned 80 percent more than their counterparts in Europe. Now doctors were strongly incentivized to behave like businesspeople.

The former CEO of Humana—a hospital firm turned private health insurance corporation and currently ranked number 40 on the Fortune 500—once stated that he aimed for healthcare to be as "reliable a product" as a McDonald's Big Mac. Doctors' responsibilities drifted away from their patients and more toward the company line. Doctors stopped charging set fees. Instead, they charged whatever they could extract from private health insurance to increase their profits. In Medicine Inc., they became charge masters.

Optimizing a bill and gaming the system determined a doctor's success more than their surgical or diagnostic prowess. I once met an ear nose throat doctor at a friend's engagement party who described a patient's first visit with him—which included introductions and a review of past medical problems and questions about personal issues and replacing one's clothes with a gown for the initial examination—as a "loss leader." He just wanted to get patients in the door.

Despite the original intention of HMOs to bring costs down, healthcare continued to become more and more expensive. The trifecta of expensive doctor fees, expensive healthcare workers, and the drive to profit mechanized by corporations—and emulated by nonprofits—made sure of it. As a result, the number of uninsured people grew. When pregnant women started approaching my father and telling him that they needed a doctor but that they had no health insurance, he had to make a choice. Should he offer these women services for free even though he charged others? Should he look away and stretch out that nagging cramp in his flank, the way he always did whenever he said something that troubled him?

He already knew what it meant to volunteer his services. To receive his medical school diploma in El Salvador, he'd had to work a full year in villages where there were no doctors. Doctors in America resisted this kind of mandatory public service. What a difference the year had made. In serving as the village's lone doctor, he'd grown into a true medical man. Dad saw as much of life as he did of pathophysiology during this year. He learned how to solve problems and how to negotiate with patients. Maybe a new young mother couldn't pay him, but she wanted to pay what she could, and so she made him a batch of fresh tortillas.

Initially, he carried that same flexibility with him into his private practice in Houston and negotiated with needy patients. In the late eighties, 85 percent of his patients had private insurance. Ten percent had Medicaid, and 5 percent paid him cash on a payment schedule according to a negotiated fee. Like his father, he tried to find ways to see patients who didn't have insurance. My grandfather found his niche in large part because the Salvadoran government capped fees to make doctors' services affordable to all, but there was no such inclination in America to make healthcare affordable.

But that made it increasingly difficult to help patients without health insurance. My dad had started his practice with a nurse and a receptionist as his only employees. Thirty years later, it took two full-time workers to handle insurance claims, while six others helped him take care of patients. He even sicced his mother, my grandma—a Chicago-born, Depression-era-raised former public schoolteacher who once drove by herself from El Salvador to California—on the insurance companies full-time. During summers, he paid me and my sisters to organize files and insurance claims. Our meetings focused on his office, not the hospital. We weren't medical helpers; we were business office helpers.

By the time I started medical school at Baylor College of Medicine in 2002, more than half of his patients carried insurance through Medicaid. A decreasing number carried private health insurance through their work, as employers avoided offering health insurance as a benefit and hired fewer full-time employees and more contractors. With the cost of supplies increasing, he couldn't afford to treat uninsured patients, and so he turned more and more away. Something had to give, and so my dad decided to return to his roots: he volunteered at Ben Taub. He didn't have the time, but operating with the ob-gyn residents gave him a reprieve: he didn't have to worry about coverage denials or whether his patients' policies covered hospital bills as well. All he had to worry about was the patient in front of him. He could work purely as a doctor again.

As I progressed through medical school, my dad and I discussed whether I might follow in his footsteps and take over his ob-gyn practice. He envisioned the two of us passing each other in the hallway between exam rooms or discussing difficult cases in his office with a view of the freeways.

"Have you thought about it?" he asked me. "It'd be nice."

It certainly would have been from a business perspective. For more than two decades, my dad had done the heavy lifting of building a tried-and-true moneymaker. But my memories of my dad's experience as a doctor didn't entirely line up with his own. His struggles with insurance companies stood out to me as much as the corkboards lining his hallway. I had nearly decided to leave medicine altogether for a career in public health or, possibly, as a writer, but my experiences at Ben Taub had shown me a different side of healthcare. The attending doctors never bogged themselves down with insurance companies. Instead, they spent hours discussing different types of problems encountered by their patients, not just medical or genetic, but also social and personal. I started to see what people meant when they said medicine was more of a vocation than a business.

My dad continued to volunteer at Ben Taub once a month for the next fifteen years. One morning, after I'd finished medical school and residency and started to work in the hospital full-time as faculty, I received a page from a number I didn't recognize. When I called the number back, I heard Spanish on the opposite line.

"Hombre, que tal?"

It was one of the senior anesthesiologists at Ben Taub, who'd been on staff for more than twenty-five years. He specialized in giving laboring women epidurals. There was nothing he liked more than having coffee in between cases.

"If you're not busy, come down now," he said, "have a *cafecito*." His Guatemalan Castilian made his coffees sound delectable, and he was one of those people you always wanted to spend time around, but I knew what this was all about.

"Really busy seeing patients," I said. "I'll see what I can do."

I'd intended to take the stairs down only one floor, but instead, I kept going, until I ended up at the third floor, right outside labor and delivery. My anesthesiologist friend was waiting for me in one of the administrative corridors.

"Hombre!" he said. We shook hands and hugged each other. He put his hand on my back warmly and guided me into his small office.

The smell of the *cafecito* was pungent, like espresso straight from the bag. I would've asked him about his coffeemaking methods, but my attention went directly to the matter at hand and the anesthesiologist's other guest.

"Hola, hijo," said my dad.

"Hola, papi," I replied.

We were two doctors divided by medicine, not by the practice of it, but by its identity. My dad had evolved into the successful business-doctor with a booming practice. I was the academic doctor working with uninsured patients. Needless to say, our political ideas about healthcare didn't align. In fact, we hadn't spoken to each other in months. Each of us raised his Styrofoam coffee cup toward the other and took a short sip.

*   *   *

We disagreed on where the right balance lay between the business of doctoring and the profession's duty to the public. We agreed, however, that how or what a doctor is paid shouldn't affect a patient's experience of medicine. But as healthcare grew more expensive and inaccessible, doctors tailored their diagnostics and treatments to what a patient could afford rather than the best course of treatment. Sick people looking for a diagnosis often encountered confusion with each new doctor they met.

Christian Garza looked like an all-American kid. He was tall and thin and he wore pastel-colored T-shirts with khaki shorts and Vans. His jet-black hair was cut shorter on the sides than on top, where it curled into a tuft that fell naturally to one side of his brow, as if windblown. The stubble on his chin and the pencil-thin mustache atop his lip appeared professionally sketched onto an otherwise perfectly shaven face, much like Cantinflas in *Around the World in 80 Days*. His jaw wasn't exactly square, but it was prominent, like the black-rimmed eyeglasses that sat high on his face and gave him his appearance of bookishness.

He was born in Cypress, Texas, a suburb on Houston's northwest side. When Christian was ten, his parents divorced, leaving him and his younger brother to adjust to the reality of a fatherless home. His mother, Norma, worked with special-needs kids. Whatever she couldn't provide financially to the family, she made up for with tenderness and determination.

Christian was an A student through high school, and he wanted to study architecture, but he knew that he would have to contribute to the family, and so he decided to attend community college. The plan was simple: work hard, rack up the university credits, earn money on the side for tuition and for home, and then transfer to a reputable school for the degree. He took a job at Best Buy. Out went the khaki shorts and Vans, in came the electric-blue polo with the embroidered emblem and name tag. He made it through the probation period required before employees can earn benefits but decided against paying for health insurance. It seemed like a luxury a twenty-one-year-old couldn't afford. After all, he was young and healthy.

That was before the knee pains began. Calling them "knee pains" doesn't capture the debilitation Christian started to feel from these recurrent, crippling ordeals. The process was always the same. First, Christian would feel hot all around his body, then achy, as if the flu was coming on. Then his patella and upper femur started to feel as if they would snap. Soon, he was curled up in a ball, wailing in pain. There was nothing Norma could do but curl up beside her son and cry with him. The episodes could last for hours and they disappeared as mysteriously as they arrived, never leaving a mark, like a Category 5 hurricane that breaks nothing but leaves a city rigid with fear.

After enough of these episodes occurred, his grandfather took matters into his own hands. "Lay down," he told his grandson, rubbing a homemade concoction into his hands. The mixture of rubbing alcohol and green herbs did nothing for Christian's pain. The art of *sobar*, or Mexican massage, had the power to cure many ailments, but not this one.

He visited an ER at a nearby hospital. After a few hours, an X-ray, and some blood work, doctors gave him the diagnosis of "a virus," which made no sense to Christian. They couldn't perform more tests to figure it out, they said, and prescribed him ibuprofen for his troubles. The advice sounded formulaic and impersonal to Christian, like something he could've looked up on the web. For this, he received a bill of almost $3,000.

The bill was enough to dissuade him from visiting the ER after most of the lighter episodes that started happening monthly. But sometimes he just had to go, and when he did, he always received the same diagnosis.

"I started living around the pain," said Christian. "I made contingency plans." He structured his days so that he'd be close to home in the later afternoons when the pains tended to hit. Christian's grades at community college started to go down. He went from being a stellar employee to being an unreliable one. The ER doctors recommended that he see specialists in clinic, starting with a rheumatologist.

"We didn't know where to start," he said.

He called rheumatology offices around town and managed to convince one doctor's staff to accept $60 cash per visit. It was a lot for Christian, and that didn't even include the $20 in parking fees. But at the time, the thought that this expert might figure out what was causing his episodes seemed priceless.

Arriving at their first visit, Norma felt so hopeful she nearly cried. Mother and son were guided to the examination room, one orderly, air-conditioned room among thousands in the Texas Medical Center. It didn't take long before they heard a knock.

The person introduced herself as part of the doctor's staff. Norma didn't understand. What about the doctor?

She listened to the administrator's explanation of the clinic's policy: the doctor doesn't see the patient until at least the second visit.

It took Norma a minute to recover from this news. Wasn't it a doctor's job, or at least, hadn't they sworn an oath, to help someone in need? She felt no one was taking her son's pains seriously. The staff pleaded with her to stay, but Norma wouldn't have it. They left the appointment upset. Was it too much to ask to see the doctor after paying so much out of pocket? What did it take to be treated like a person?

But in the end, they could find no better option. Norma swallowed her pride, and Christian returned to the Texas Medical Center every two to three weeks. He saw the board-certified rheumatologist only a few times. Each visit took ten minutes. They were moved through the office swiftly, like a piece of meat in a processing plant. Pain still there? Any swelling? Can you please extend your arm for vitals? That'll be $60. See you next time!

It continued like that for more than a year. At one of the visits, Christian's frustration boiled over. While pointing out for the hundredth time where the pain started and where it moved, he noticed the doctor using a familiar tone. It was slow. ("I see . . . so . . . you had a-nother pain a-ttack . . .") The staff attempted to express a level of pity. ("That's so terrible, and you were crying for how long?") Christian was no fool, and he was tired of being treated like a child. His suspicions were confirmed when, at the end of the exam, the doctor noted that, yet again, she saw no marks or physical signs of inflammation on any of his joints, "which is kinda weird." She doesn't believe me, thought Christian.

"Would it help if I came in excruciating pain?" he said.

It wasn't like he was asking them for opiates. The strongest medicine he received were T3s, a combination of codeine and Tylenol, a baby in the narcotic world. During intense pain episodes, he took, at most, two of these, nothing more. Christian was well aware opiates caused addiction. The last thing he wanted was another reason to come to the doctor.

He'd had enough. Nothing had changed. The pains had taken over his life. After an interminable series of appointments and ER visits over the course of five years, the knee pain only seemed to occur more frequently.

Then, just as easily as this darkness had enshrouded him, hope appeared on the horizon. Christian applied for an administrative job that offered him health insurance. His employer would pay a portion, and he, another. Maybe I can get specific answers, he thought. Maybe this doctor will take me more seriously.

It was a hope that many others, including one hundred years' worth of US presidents and members of Congress, held too: that health insurance would solve the problem of how doctors and hospitals were paid. Christian felt the area on his knee that had once been covered with a Band-Aid during an ER visit, a ridiculous gesture to suggest something had been done for the pain. As a throb started to rise from deep within his joint, this time Christian felt some relief. He had more options. Maybe with insurance, his problems would be solved.

— 4 —

Coverage

Like most Americans, I've lived most of my adult life with health insurance paid for partially by my work and partially through deductions from my paycheck. Like a fourth of all Americans, I've also experienced gaps in coverage. For a whole year after graduating medical school, I lived without insurance. Thankfully, I made it through that year without requiring healthcare.

I've also experienced the opposite. The day my daughter was born—a "qualifying life event" in the insurance parlance—I added her and my wife to my health insurance. Since my wife already received health insurance through her work, this meant that two health insurances should have covered the birth of our child. You know where this is headed: for reasons I still haven't seen spelled out, both insurances declined to cover the birth. The hospital sent us a bill just north of $15,000. "Why do I even have insurance?" were likely among the first words to escape my mouth.

I know, too, what it means to be underinsured. Halfway through my internal medicine residency, after a grueling night shift in the ICU, I drove to Austin for a friend's bachelor party. The festivities started with a game of eight-on-eight; the sport, Wiffle ball. I felt wary of showing the guys my poor fielding skills, which I hadn't used competitively since the seventh grade, and so I volunteered to play first base. Not long after the first pitch, I was called into action. One of the more eager bachelor party attendees fielded a dribbler down the third-base line. He rifled the ball toward me, except, in midair, the ball changed course, whirling left (I suppose this is what makes Wiffle ball fun). I had seen enough first basemen make the cardinal error of sliding their foot off the base while reaching for a throw. As the ball spun toward me, I decided I wouldn't make the same mistake. I held my foot firm and stretched. Somehow, the ball spun right into my hands. That was the last I remembered of the game.

Some hours later, my friend, the one getting married, said my collision with the base runner hadn't initially looked so jarring. If anything, it made the guys laugh. And why not? We were two men, neither in the best of shape, both nearing middle age and playing a sport we hadn't played since childhood, running into each other. Except the back of my head bore the impact. It had been the third out of the inning. As my team hustled toward the sidelines, I remained on the field, staring off into space.

My friend guided me off the diamond. "You all right?" he said.

"The brain is in a box," I replied. The head trauma may have caused an artery inside my skull to burst, I explained. Blood might have been pooling, slowly pushing against the neurons that kept me breathing, constricting them, strangling them.

I was delirious, unaware of where I was, and somehow, I had started to recite medical facts stored in my concussed brain. I began guiding him through a quick and dirty neurological exam. We needed to see if my brain cells were compromised, I said.

"Are my eyes following?" I asked as he dragged an outstretched finger from one of my visual fields through the next. "Do my pupils look the same size?"

I remember this now like the vaguest of dreams, but my friend felt terrified. He was a schoolteacher pursuing a master's in creative writing. It didn't take him long to realize he wasn't remotely qualified to perform this exam. He decided to rush me to the nearest emergency room.

I don't recall giving the receptionist my insurance card. But as the brain fog lifted and I slowly came to, I remember feeling comforted by the thought that this emergency room visit was covered. The emergency room doctor asked me a few questions, performed a quick exam, and sent me to get a CAT scan. He even let me see the images of my own brain: no blood, no worries. By the time I left the ER, I didn't even have a headache. We headed back to the bachelor party, which, by that time, had turned into a few guys watching college football. The story of my concussion made the rounds. That's all it ended up becoming in the end, and how lucky for me: a story.

A few weeks afterward, the bills started coming in—lots of them. My insurance sent me a statement showing it had paid the hospital and doctor more than two thousand dollars for my visit. It took me a few reads, but I understood that I was responsible for any outstanding balance. My insurance had washed its hands clean.

This isn't a unique story. Look on any news site and you're sure to find more remarkable and poignant ones. They don't always end so innocuously, either. Some people go bankrupt from all the bills. Some are left to wonder if seeing a doctor is worth the trouble.

The first health insurance in America sold access to doctors and timely care, but more than anything, it sold peace of mind. If the pain of appendicitis or gallstones struck in the middle of the night, a patient could visit the hospital, receive surgery, recover, and leave, no bills, no hassles. Credit for the idea goes to Justin Ford Kimball, a name that sounds corporate enough, but, in fact, Kimball was an ex-schoolteacher and superintendent. In 1929, he left a job as a college lecturer to oversee the medical and nursing schools at Baylor University. The most pressing issue to come across his desk had nothing to do with education, however. The university's hospital was going broke.

For decades preceding this problem healthcare had become increasingly expensive, in large part because it was moving into hospitals. Families in the 1800s feared illness because it meant lost wages. That changed in the 1900s. Advances in anesthesia and surgery gave people more faith in medicine and more real healthcare options within the hospital, but these came with a price. In the 1920s, a worker admitted into the hospital might pay half of his yearly income to cover hospital bills.

Many of these bills went unpaid. The result was that more and more hospitals found themselves in the red.

"I did not know a thing about a hospital," Kimball later mused. "My thoughts went back to my days as a school superintendent. I had found that teachers tended to worry too much—and none more so than over illness."

An idea started to take shape. What if he sold the teachers peace of mind? Would that help him save the hospital?

Kimball offered the teachers a deal: if each paid fifty cents a month, or $6 per year, they would be guaranteed twenty-one days of hospitalization paid in full if they fell ill and required treatment.

By the end of the year, more than 75 percent of schoolteachers had enrolled, for a total of 1,500 enrollees. He called it a sick benefit program. It was more than that. Kimball's plan was the beginning of group coverage, one that revolved around a basic financial rule. Covering one person is expensive. The larger the group, the more affordable healthcare coverage is for everyone.

Soon enough, Kimball offered the same deal to a different group, this time, the employees at the *Dallas Morning News*. The plan not only brought steady income to the hospital; it also pleased the patients. "On release from the hospital after surgery, I found that the insurance took care of almost all of the expense," said one of the women in the *Dallas News* circulation department who had joined the plan. She had received exactly the care she needed and had been treated like a person. Purchasing peace of mind had paid off. It seemed like a dream.

Other hospitals followed suit, offering their own prepayment deals to different groups of people. Beyond staying afloat, hospitals repurposed any profit toward improving the services they provided to patients. For a short while, the people of Dallas found themselves in the driver's seat as hospitals competed for their business. That same year, however, the Great Depression hit. People could no longer afford to put money into an insurance plan. It was more important to stay fed. And with so little middle-class income available, hospitals languished. Some feared they'd all go bankrupt. The quest to make healthcare accessible returned to square one, but, as has always been the case in America, the void created financial opportunities for the right investors.

To understand how the peace of mind offered by the first health insurance transformed into the confusion and out-of-pocket expense that we experience today, it's important to remember the teams involved. Justin Ford Kimball wasn't a doctor, and he wasn't an insurance agent. He worked for the hospital. The insurance Kimball offered covered the patient's stay, which was by far the most expensive part of being sick. Patients paid surgeons and other doctors separately. And so, the first health insurance kept two players on the field of healthcare, doctors and hospitals. That would soon change.

Insurance companies had wanted to enter healthcare since long before Kimball's deal with the schoolteachers. A fundamental problem gave them pause. While basic human behavior controlled how much people used traditional insurance products—nobody wants to get into a car accident or cash in a life insurance policy—healthcare was different. Estimating costs had proven difficult. Getting over pneumonia might require a two-day stay in the hospital for one person and four days for another. Different doctors might order different quantities of medicines and tests. Plus, what about that type of person who *wants* to see doctors, who only feels reassured by receiving a consultation with a specialist and a subspecialist and a sub-subspecialist, all wielding the latest technology?

In insurance theory, this is known as "moral hazard." If insurance is paying, and I am paying little or nothing out of pocket, why not get the next test, whether it's truly necessary or not? We encounter this idea in other parts of life. Whenever we ladle an extra helping of butter chicken onto our plates at our favorite all-you-can-eat non-veg Indian restaurant, we're engaging in moral hazard. It doesn't matter if I end up eating it or not; each visit to the buffet communicates: someone else is paying, so you can take what you want.

Some economists argue that moral hazard doesn't really exist, that people consume healthcare only when they absolutely need to, and certainly not like butter chicken. But evidence suggests that the more insurance people have, the more healthcare they utilize. This includes visits to the emergency room.* Consider: if it cost you the same to receive a cast on your hand in an urgent-care center and at your primary care doctor's office, but the cast could be placed immediately at the urgent-care center, whereas you'd have to wait a week for an appointment at your PCP, which would you select? Most would select the fastest service, in the urgent-care center.

In the case of the Indian restaurant, the owner absorbs the cost of my oversize hunger—he accepts the risk of more and more consumption—which might be fine because they've already built this excess into their pricing. But what if someone else picked when and how much I served myself? And what if that person received a dollar for every plate I filled? Fee-for-service not only complicates moral hazard, it amplifies it. It makes insuring healthcare risky. Insurance companies had been wary that healthcare might wipe them out.

Kimball's success with the schoolteachers showed there was a real need and a market for coverage. And so, a third player entered healthcare.

---

* One argument in favor of universal health insurance coverage had been that it would decrease ER visits by giving patients access to primary care doctors who would solve health problems before they rose to the level of requiring an emergency room. This idea has been proven false. People consume what's given to them.

Insurance companies began to act as brokers. To reduce the risk of moral hazard, they made deals with hospitals, promising to supply patients for a negotiated cost of care. They cut their own costs by constructing larger and larger groups of patients. Ten years after Kimball's plan, ten million Americans had purchased health insurance. This would be the pattern for decades, two diametrically opposed forces dominating how Americans were covered. On one side, fee-for-service pushed for more healthcare; doctors were paid based on the amount of service they provided. On the other side, group coverage attempted to pool risk so that the insurance companies could turn a profit. A collision was inevitable.

Except that more players stepped onto the field. In 1942, with the country steeped in World War II, Congress passed the Stabilization Act. The legislation froze all wages, salaries, and benefits earned by workers. Hefty taxes were levied against companies reporting profits above their prewar intake, all to avoid inflation. The law made it much harder for employers to keep workers, except it left a loophole. Employee benefits could be deducted from profits. And with more and more Americans wanting and buying their own health insurance, companies decided to dangle this as a benefit in front of workers. The age of employer-sponsored health insurance was born.

It's understandable why legislators at the time may have been elated to see business take on the expense of healthcare. Doctors were fighting tooth and nail against insurance and group coverage. There was the financial incentive, sure, but doctors also feared the day when insurance companies wielded so much authority that they dictated how medical care unfolded. Government could have stepped in, as it had in England and continental Europe, and organized healthcare into a system. Politicians going back to Theodore Roosevelt had proposed a social insurance similar to workers' compensation that covered healthcare. The politics were hard, though, not just in the United States, but everywhere. Employers' volunteering to take on healthcare costs for most of the public must have felt like a godsend.

But the great forces driving healthcare—fee-for-service and group coverage—would wear out this new player too. Employers had been lured into the game. They remained for their own incentives. A rewritten tax code in 1954 made health benefits tax deductible, not just for employers, but also for workers. A year later, 70 percent of all Americans had health insurance, mostly through their work. Now employers were forced to walk a fine line. On one side, they had to offer workers health insurance—the tax code incentivized them to do this—but on the other side, they didn't want to pay health insurance companies too much. Some larger companies began insuring workers themselves, meaning that any paid claim came off the employer's profit sheet. It's no wonder that the more expensive healthcare became, the more eager companies would be to pass on the costs to employees by stripping down their plans.

Take Christian's situation. As you'll recall, Christian believed that his rheumatologist's ability to treat him had been hindered by his lack of insurance. Now, with a new health insurance policy obtained through his work, he felt hopeful.

The rheumatologist took Christian's health insurance card and immediately ordered an MRI and an arthrocentesis, or drainage of fluid inside the knee. Lab technicians would examine the fluid beneath the microscope to see if tiny crystals made of uric acid—gout—were causing Christian's pains. Now, this seemed like a more personalized medical plan to Christian. Both tests were prohibitively expensive for someone paying cash. But the new health insurance had reignited the rheumatologist's inquisitiveness.

When his mother, Norma, called to schedule the MRI, an attendant placed her on hold. No big deal, Norma thought, I've waited for years. If necessary, I will wait my whole life; this is, after all, my son. Occasionally, someone would click on the line and ask for more information—the policy number, the group number, when the health insurance went into effect—and Norma relayed the data. Finally, someone at the MRI center explained the holdup. If she wanted the MRI or the arthrocentesis, she would have to pay out of pocket. Christian's new health insurance had denied coverage for either test.

It's reasonable to suspect that his employer hadn't paid for top-of-the-line insurance, or even good-enough insurance to cover the tests. The cost of insurance plans rises every year, and perhaps his employer had recently opted to raise wages and compensated with cuts to employee coverage. Or maybe denying coverage had simply become the default practice for this particular health insurance. This is what's certain: it was not in the insurance company's interest to pay for the test, nor was it in the employer's interest to pay for rock-solid health insurance.

Christian and Norma returned to the rheumatologist's office exasperated. "Don't we have health insurance?" Norma said. "Didn't you, the doctor, order these tests?"

The rheumatologist nodded with embarrassment. Of what use were her orders if they weren't carried out? She attempted to defuse the situation with a couple of white lies, telling the insurance company that Christian had, indeed, despite what the documentation showed, received steroid injections in the knee as well as physical therapy. But the insurance company recognized the old yarn: there would be no MRI and no analysis of knee fluid, not on their bill.

His grandmother couldn't understand how her American grandson could be going through this. "Fuiste nacido aquí, y eres ciudadano," she said: *You were born here, and you're a citizen.* So why the struggle?

Christian thought about this. All these reasons the doctors and insurance companies gave him sounded so arbitrary and vague, like what you might tell a toddler. Why wasn't anyone talking with him like he was a person? "Why do I even have insurance?" he asked himself aloud.

In July 2017, he decided enough was enough. An opportunity arose to see a new doctor in a new healthcare system. He could receive medical care straight from the doctor, no insurance companies, no impediments, no vague advice. Both he and Norma felt confident they could afford it too. And so, after putting on his shorts and Vans and brushing the ends

of his Cantinflas whiskers, he headed out to George Bush Interconti-
nental Airport. From there, it was a short flight to Tampico, Mexico.

I didn't want to pay any more. Financial groups representing the hospital and the doctors' group kept sending me bills. Each time a new one
arrived in the mail, I'd place it on my bed and try to understand the
charges. My eyes kept returning to my insurance company's statement
that showed it had already paid two thousand dollars for my emergency
room care. How was it possible that this amount hadn't sufficed for my
short visit?

The night before the concussion, while covering the ICU, I had
spent hours with extremely sick patients. I had ordered CAT scans and
antibiotics and even inserted a pressure gauge into a patient's artery. If
someone had asked me what I would've charged for that work, I wouldn't
have known where to begin. Something seemed off. The amount I had
been billed didn't seem in line with the work necessary to deliver my care.

I fought. I refused to pay. Instead of giving me peace of mind, the
insurance had made me belligerent and argumentative, especially in the
responses I mailed back to the hospital. "I reviewed the record, and it
shows that the ER doctor did NOT test for dysdiadochokinesis before
ordering the CAT scan," I wrote. "This is concerning."

Included in my correspondence were guidelines written by the American Academy of Neurology for what constituted a thorough neurological
exam. The components of the exam that the doctor hadn't performed—
for instance, making me clap my hands in the motion of making a tortilla
to check the function of my cerebellum—I starred and highlighted. I
argued that I should not be held responsible for any extra payments since
I had received less than the standard care. The doctor and hospital had
jumped to perform the CAT scan, I insisted.

I didn't really believe that. I believed that the doctor had done a good-
enough job of ruling out a brain bleed. He'd ordered the right test. I told

people close to me about the fight and my strategy. One friend wasn't at all surprised by my responses. "Seems a bit self-righteous," she said.

When I told my dad, he was uncharacteristically silent. For a moment I thought he wasn't even paying attention, but then a look of disgust swept over his face and he began reaching for that elusive cramp in his flank.

"Que se vayan a la miércoles," he said, *Tell them to go to Wednesday*, except he didn't say "miércoles." The thought of my paying the hospital and doctor anything more angered him. He didn't want me to give either a single dime.

On the surface, this seemed like a contradiction. Over the years, my dad raised the co-pays he required from his patients. He—or, rather, my grandma—regularly sent outstanding-bill reminders to women. Insurance companies had negotiated harder and harder with doctors over the years, and he had followed suit.

This wasn't private practice. It wasn't medicine. It was Medicine Inc. at work.

Back in the middle of the twentieth century, insurance companies were interested but hesitant to enter the healthcare business in a bigger way. Corporations waited for a signal from the market. It came when President Lyndon Johnson signed Medicare and Medicaid into law.

In the early 1960s, the fundamental problem of linking health insurance with work began to manifest. People who didn't work or who worked part-time or for employers that didn't offer insurance found healthcare too expensive to access. Retirees posed the first problem. The moment they left their jobs, they were expected to pay whatever the market demanded. The price of hospital care had doubled during the 1950s. One in six Americans over the age of sixty-five had been admitted to the hospital. Their stays lasted twice the length of someone sixty-five or younger. Something had to give.

Medicare paid for healthcare for the elderly, and Medicaid for the indigent. Except the government didn't offer these services itself. Rather, the government paid for these groups' health insurance to access care on the expensive healthcare market. The result was predictable: doctors charged these government programs for every individual service they provided. Hospitals followed suit. Both started to look at empty hospital beds as money slipping through their fingers. Healthcare not only grew even more expensive; it was now lucrative. Between 1960 and 1965, national health expenditures had increased from $142 to $198 per capita. By 1970, that number had grown to $336. Government spending on healthcare increased 250 percent in those five years. Corporations took notice. Not only was the government invested in healthcare, there were government dollars out there to be taken. Medicine Inc. was born.

That's not to say Medicare and Medicaid didn't help people. Without question, the sick were better off with Medicaid and Medicare than without health insurance. Those with Medicaid, previously unable to afford healthcare, started to see doctors more often. African Americans in particular gained access. Prior to Medicaid, white people saw doctors 42 percent more often than Black Americans. The government-sponsored insurance narrowed this disparity to 13 percent by 1973. But Medicaid only covered one-third of the poor, and Medicare covered less than half of the expenditures on the elderly. Qualifying for either was difficult, especially for Medicaid. Many earned too much to qualify and too little to afford the out-of-pocket expense for doctors or hospitalization. Many people still couldn't afford healthcare.

The vulnerable had been plugged into a system that rewarded treating sickness over maintaining health. Corporations saw that the government now held a stake in keeping these programs running. The extra money in healthcare not only stabilized their investments; it was also there for the taking.

Over the next fifty years, these corporations, some of which sprang from insurance companies, would corner the healthcare market and make life difficult for independent practitioners like my dad. A few started by buying hospitals, at first in rural areas and then in the cities. An early insurance plan grew into a nonprofit insurance conglomerate named Blue Cross, which, in 1994, voted to allow its franchises to become for-profit companies. Today, a direct descendant of Kimball's plan, Anthem, ranks number 20 on the Fortune 500 list. The corporation not only offers thousands of different types of insurance plans, it also owns dozens of hospitals nationwide and multiple doctor practices.

This has been the major effect of corporations' entering healthcare: integrating the major healthcare players under one roof. Theoretically, organizing the players on the healthcare field into a unit like this could have cut the cost of healthcare. But with fee-for-service as the basic means of financing healthcare, the corporate drive for profit thrived. It made healthcare increasingly exorbitant through a very discernible pattern: hospitals were incentivized to procure more expensive devices and medicines; doctors were incentivized to order these; and insurance companies were incentivized to absorb costs temporarily and raise premiums, which companies and workers paid.

In other words, doctors, insurance companies, hospitals, and pharmaceutical companies—the major players in American healthcare—might occasionally seem at odds, one billing the other, each *blaming* the others for prohibitive costs, but they share a unified purpose: to solve sickness through the mechanism of business. The healthcare we experience today is the most extreme version of business driving care.

As a result, independent doctors like my dad have had to compete with very large companies. But doctors aren't the only ones who have felt overwhelmed by corporate medicine. Have you ever wondered why cholesterol medicines are cheaper in Canada or Mexico than they are in the United States? Or why a colonoscopy costs more in the United States than anywhere else?

We are charged—whether for an expensive medication, a visit to the ER, or a doctor's opinion—whatever the market permits. We're not charged the actual cost of the goods we receive; rather, we're charged high amounts because we pay high amounts through co-pays and higher premiums. Medicine Inc. demands that patients act as consumers. It expects us to know precisely what we're buying for what cost while obscuring those costs. When we don't know the product or the cost, we can be convinced to pay more. Health insurance companies, pharmaceutical companies, hospitals, and many doctors count on this.

I didn't know any of this history when the first bills for my ER visit came in, but as someone who depended on hospitals for my paycheck, I had a clear sense of the work that was performed and how this work did or did not align with the charges on my bills. After two years of my fighting the charges, both the hospital and the doctors' group adjusted my balance to $0. I also fought the $15,000 hospital bill that arrived years later when my daughter was born, and this balance, too, was adjusted to $0. I happened to be a very good healthcare consumer. What this required of me was a medical degree, ten years of clinical experience, and a working knowledge of health policy, not to mention the inclination to go toe-to-toe with corporate medicine. Who but very, very few patients are equipped to do this? Most, like Christian, are forced to find another way around.

Within a day of his arrival in Tampico, Christian had scheduled appointments with six different specialists, including four bone specialists and two general practitioners. He paid around $15 for each appointment.

One of the doctors, who offered him a knee surgery for $30,000 without so much as a scan, struck Christian as a charlatan. But another doctor seemed honest. This doctor had ordered a simple blood test, called a basic metabolic panel. When he received the results, he called Christian and told him to go to the nearest hospital immediately because of the severe and potentially life-threatening abnormalities he'd seen in the labs.

Christian called his mother. Norma took the news hard. Six hundred fifty miles and a border separated her from her son. She wanted to take the next flight to Tampico to be with Christian through whatever came next, but Christian tried to appease her. "I don't feel that sick," he said. It had been weeks since his last pain episode. Norma wanted him to follow the doctor's advice. We'll figure out the payments later, she implored. Christian couldn't say no.

He went to the nearest private hospital. There, emergency room doctors informed him of two items: first, that his kidneys were failing and required urgent testing, and second, that Christian would have to pay at least half of the estimated cost for admission into the hospital up front in cash. The total would be around 50,000 pesos, or $2,700, an amount lower than Norma expected, even adjusting for buying power.

Kidneys? What, Christian wondered, could this have to do with his knee pains? Christian's rheumatologist had mentioned something to him in passing many months ago, he remembered. "Your creatinine is high," she'd said. "You should see a nephrologist." But that was it. No alarm in her voice, not even a referral. There wasn't even an explanation of what the word "creatinine" meant. Just a lone fact, blurted out of context, followed by the acceptance of sixty dollars in cash.

Now Christian was being told his kidneys looked terrible. But he didn't feel ill. Was it possible that the hospital stay wasn't worth the money?

"Do you have bubbles in your pee?" one of the doctors in the ER asked him.

Christian nodded. Whenever he urinated, there was so much frothing that it looked like someone was pouring out detergent. He called his mother, and Norma wired him the money.

Over the next days, as doctors ran a slew of tests on his urine and blood, Christian tried to get his health insurance to cover some of the costs. US health insurance companies, however, rarely pay for healthcare in Mexico, and when they do, the tests and treatments must be preapproved. The diagnosis was elusive and so was Christian's insurance company. It started to employ typical resistance methods. It wasn't enough that the Mexican doctors wrote letters in English explaining the problem. Documents had to be translated officially and then faxed to the appropriate office at the appropriate time. The paperwork grew so cumbersome that, for Christian, having insurance became a full-time job.

Christian's new doctors couldn't help but shake their heads. Of what use was insurance if you couldn't use it when you were sick? That isn't to say that they expected anything different. One of the doctors confided to Christian that 30 to 40 percent of his patients came from the United States, so seeing this escape to Mexico and the paper chase was nothing new. Here was someone who at the age of twenty-six had lived the last five years—a fifth of his life—with excruciating pain. His health insurance and his doctors—their actions guided at each turn by Christian's level of coverage—had provided him with no answers and no relief. In order to break the cycle of pain and confusion, the young man had fled his home country, and here he was, in a foreign hospital, FaceTiming his mother, visited occasionally by cousins and aunts, but otherwise, alone.

If only you were Mexican, one of the doctors told him. If Christian were a Mexican resident, he could access the public hospitals and clinics. The doctor feared that all the diagnostic care Christian received there would be for naught back in the United States, where his insurance company might not approve the necessary tests and treatments. He had seen as much in his other American patients.

"I'm really sorry you're from the United States," he said.

— 5 —

Hospitals

There were plenty of hospitals nearby Roxana's apartment in West Houston. In fact, one of the largest hospitals in the city loomed over her neighborhood. That hospital was a gleaming metroplex boasting more than four hundred inpatient beds, an Amputation Prevention Center, and a thirty-three-story executive tower, the top six floors of which were decked out with ice-blue glass and aluminum fins to look like an enormous crown. It was less than a mile from Roxana's doorstep. Whenever she and Marí shuffled outside for fresh air, they could see it in the near distance.

I knew that hospital well—its old parts, at least. As a kid I received my vaccines and checkups in one of the squat, brown-bricked buildings around which the fancy new towers had been erected. I'd also spent a summer in college working in the hospital's old MRI department. Every day that summer, I verified patients had no metal on or inside them and wheeled them from the machine table to the waiting area.

The job suited my needs that summer. The previous semester, I had wrecked my knee during a friendly game of touch football, which required surgery once school was out. Taking the summer to recover didn't seem like a good idea at the time, since I didn't want my med school application to show any holes. But I also needed a job flexible enough to allow me to visit my physical therapist. When I told my dad about my predicament, he pursed his lips and nodded confidently.

"Let me talk with Wayne," he said.

Wayne was the CEO of the glittering hospital. My father delivered babies at one of the network's outlets. He had met Wayne in meetings, and they had golfed together on more than one occasion.

My dad's not the type to feel embarrassed about asking for favors—and he fully expected he'd receive a response from Wayne. Sure enough, within a week, I was offered the perfect summer job for someone seeking to look busy while limping.

"Go to MRI and they'll take care of you," said my dad.

"Do I have to fill out any forms or talk with a manager or anything?" I asked.

"Just show up."

For Roxana, there was no similarly easy route inside. No doubt, if she had shown up with good health insurance, Roxana would've been welcomed. Vascular surgeons, plastic surgeons, cardiologists, oncologists, and hospitalists would've puzzled through her many problems. She would have been made to feel worthy of the medical care she would have received. And then, as natural as the breeze, they would've billed her insurance for their services.

But at a hospital like that, having the surgery Roxana needed without insurance or sufficient cash wasn't possible. As it stood, Roxana didn't have coverage, and so she waited for whatever little bit of care she could find. The hospice nurse she'd been assigned would visit occasionally; other than that, she'd been left to sort out her situation on her own.

One afternoon, shortly after her release, Roxana heard a knock that was loud enough to turn her attention from her smartphone toward the door. Marí looked through the peephole.

"Es la enfermera," she said to her mother.

A nurse stood outside. "Would you like water?" Roxana said from bed after the nurse entered her home, an old habit.

"No, thank you," the nurse replied graciously, turning to her work. She removed a piece of paper from a manila folder with Roxana's name on it, sat down beside her, and began asking about the pain medicines—were they doing the job? How often was she taking them? What are you taking, again?

Roxana motioned toward a prescription bottle labeled as tramadol. "That's all I take," she said.

The nurse gave a short nod. Fifty milligrams of tramadol. The nurse had been expecting to prescribe Roxana much stronger painkillers, two-hundred-microgram patches of fentanyl, Dilaudid injections, morphine elixirs, whatever it took. The sort of end-of-life pain management typically administered to hospice patients. But pain, unfortunately, wasn't the problem.

"I'm worried about my wounds," Roxana told the nurse. She lifted her left arm with a crane-like motion. "It's starting to look infected," she said.

"Let me take a look," said the nurse.

The nurse snapped on a pair of disposable gloves. She happily did what she could in these cases, but inspecting the skin and determining whether a wound was infected wasn't a typical part of her job. She asked Roxana to hold up her arm. The nurse picked loose the tape holding the dressing together. One revolution at a time, she began to remove the white gauze.

The gauze didn't stay white for long. After a few turns, a yellow spot appeared on the bandage. It grew thicker and greener and more oblong at each subsequent layer until the nurse reached the final layer, which felt stuck. She peeled away this final swath of gauze and uncovered the living portion of Roxana's arm where it connected to the dead part. As before, the hand was charcoal black, the muscle fibers carbonized. Farther down the arm near the elbow, the flesh was healthy and olive colored. But at the line between living and necrotic flesh, there was cause for concern.

"Is it infected?" said Roxana.

The nurse brought her face close to Roxana's forearm and inspected it as best she could. Then she removed her gloves, rubbed her hands with sanitizer, jotted down some notes, and said something she wasn't supposed to say.

"I think you should go to the emergency room," she said.

The nurse didn't give this advice lightly. In fact, she was bound by duty not to send clients like Roxana to the hospital. She was a home hospice nurse. The whole philosophy behind her work was to help people die with dignity. Whether or not Roxana was actually dying hadn't been established, however. Surgeons had extracted as much cancer from her body as possible, and though she had suffered an awful complication, multiple tests still had to be performed to establish her prognosis. Since Roxana didn't have health insurance, her doctors had had to resort to arranging hospice services at home through a charity. This wasn't ideal, but it seemed better than nothing to them. Sending her home like this carried the added incentive of limiting her hospital bill. It was already unlikely she could afford the care she was receiving, let alone whatever care followed.

There were practical implications to the nurse's advice that she explained to Roxana. "If you go to the emergency room, I can't come see you again." Hospice gives charity services to people without insurance only if patients agree not to seek treatment for their terminal conditions. "This would be our last visit together," she told Roxana.

Roxana's face slackened and her eyebrows drifted low on her forehead. She began to sob. It wasn't easy to hear that she might lose the little help she had. Life was hard enough. In a demonstration of pity, the hospice nurse tried to explain how this had all happened, but the explanation fell flat for the simple reason that none of this made any sense. "You're not dying," she told Roxana. "You're sick."

Referring undocumented patients to hospice just to get them help—any help—wasn't such an uncommon predicament in a city where the uninsured numbered just below one million. The hospital that saved

Roxana's life had recouped a portion of its costs through emergency Medicaid funds, the only funding it could receive from the state or federal government for the care of undocumented immigrants. But to receive these funds, hospitals and doctors have to watch carefully for the moment when a patient's condition no longer constitutes an emergency. As detailed by the *Texas Medicaid Provider Procedures Manual*, giving care to undocumented patients, even for urgent conditions, places costs squarely on doctors and hospitals: "Any service provided after the emergency medical condition is stabilized is not a benefit."

But Roxana couldn't endure her sickness any longer. It was time to get help. The hospice nurse dialed 911 on her phone. One place the ambulance wouldn't be taking her was the very place that US lawmakers hoped would help those lacking insurance. If Americans couldn't afford coverage, the government hoped that tax incentives would motivate nonprofit hospitals to provide charity care to poor patients in need of care, like Roxana. It so happened that one of these hospitals loomed over Roxana's neighborhood, its gleaming crown signaling to West Houston that it was open for business. Roxana, however, knew she was not welcome there.

One morning not too long ago, the following headline appeared on my news feed: "Woman taken to Ben Taub after crashing stolen ambulance from Ben Taub." I couldn't help but shake my head and mutter something aloud: "Yep."

Years ago when I was a student in the ER, something similar happened with one of the patients assigned to me. My shift had ended Thursday at seven p.m., and after two days of rest, I returned Sunday at seven a.m. to find the same patient still in the ER's holding area.

"They still haven't found him a bed upstairs?" I asked one of the residents.

"You didn't hear?"

When I last saw him, the man had been recovering from a PCP intoxication that had caused him to go berserk, running around naked, threatening and terrorizing his neighbors. He was large and muscular, and it had taken multiple cops to contain him and bring him to the ER. Even with handcuffs on his arms and legs, lying on a stretcher, he continued to thrash so much that a police officer threatened, "I'm gonna put a dart in you!"

The injections of Ativan in his deltoid finally settled him. In fact, they snowed him. He was somnolent bordering on lethargic, snoring heavily, when the ER attendings saw fit to assign him to a student. My job was to make sure he didn't descend deeper into sedation and lose the ability to guard his windpipe. People have suffocated to death in such a manner. My note was as short as can be: "Patient unable to respond to questioning," I wrote for "Past Medical History," and "+ PCP" for "Social History."

Every ten minutes or so I walked by his stretcher to confirm he was still snoring. Until seven p.m., when my shift ended. That was when I handed off my duties to another student and went home.

When I returned Sunday morning and saw him again, snoring, I figured he was yet another patient waiting thirty-plus hours to be admitted into the hospital. I didn't notice his stretcher was in a different slot.

As it turned out, the man had awakened not long after my Friday shift ended. The cops had removed his cuffs as a precaution after the Ativan had taken effect, and so he was free to sit and stand up. Very unobtrusively, he slipped out of the ER and found himself at the dock, where a recently unloaded ambulance, still running, awaited him. He climbed in and drove away with nobody the wiser until he crashed the ambulance into a tree. Ben Taub happened to be too full, or "on diversion," at that moment—someone else had quickly taken his slot in the holding area—and so he was taken to another hospital ER that immediately requested to transfer him back to Ben Taub since he lacked health insurance. That process had just finished when I arrived for my

Sunday morning shift. "He's only been here a few hours," the resident told me. While I had been enjoying my weekend, this man had been on an odyssey.

I went to interview him. He was still snoring, though not as heavily as last time.

"You may not remember, sir," I said, "but I was helping out with you the last time you were here."

His eyes fluttered open, a good sign that he was at least conscious. The Ativan and the PCP had left his system. Right now was as good a time as any to interview him, to get a real "History & Physical" down.

"So what brought you into the hospital today?" I said.

With that, his eyes closed again. And that was that. He didn't want to talk with me anymore. To him, I was nothing more than another body in a white coat and scrubs. Some hours later, he was somebody else's patient upstairs in the hospital.

Since that day, I've reflected quite a bit on the chain of events leading to our encounter. Why did law enforcement bring him to Ben Taub when his other issues, like his trouble with the law and his social problems, seemed more pressing? Is it the hospital's job to handle the consequences of drug use and poverty and whatever other factors might have led to this man's taking PCP and behaving erratically? Does the hospital serve a purpose beyond the medical?

These are questions that have been around since the dawn of hospitals, because the idea of dedicating space to the sick and ailing is timeless. "Hospital" in the old French means "shelter for the needy." The Bible notes that the needy will always be with us, so the difficulties of how to provide shelter and deciding who is needy enough for this shelter are facts of life.

For centuries, hospitals served the purely social role of keeping the disabled and abandoned under a roof. It's only been within the last one hundred and fifty or so years that we've linked their mission to medicine, and only within the last century that we've required payment for these efforts. The first American hospitals grew out of almshouses. Large port cities like New York and New Orleans opened these in the 1700s to clear the streets of "infirm immigrants" and workers without homes or family to care for them. Over time, the infirmaries of these almshouses grew into public hospitals.

But before that happened, newer hospitals that accommodated a more technical and sanitary medicine started to spring up across the United States. Most of these hospitals were founded in the early 1800s by religious institutions, which is how buildings bore the names "Presbyterian" and "Methodist" and "Jews' Hospital" (later Mount Sinai). As opposed to almshouses, many of which received public funding, these hospitals relied on their churches or the community for funds. Correspondingly, all hospital care, including nursing, was volunteered: a patient left the hospital with no charges, including from their doctor. Doctors volunteered their time inside the hospital in exchange for the ability to charge for follow-up visits at patients' homes, which is how these hospitals came to be called "voluntary hospitals."

Voluntary hospitals may not have charged patients, but that didn't mean they gave care for free. Patients were often expected to read the Bible and to perform chores, especially if it seemed that the person's physical illness was the product of a vice. Alcoholics, opium addicts, syphilitics—if they were of the hospital's faith and followed the rules—found a roof over their heads and volunteers to tend to their wounds.

At least they did on their first visit. If they returned smelling more strongly of alcohol, with pupils shrunken by opium like slugs in salt, with venereal disease in full bloom, maybe the hospital wouldn't take them in. In any line of work, when the structures you've built and toiled over tumble down, patience wears thin, and workers lose heart; healthcare is no exception. Add to this a more pressing demand for cleaner and more private hospital rooms from working members of the congregation, who might make it a point to tell their pastor or rabbi or bishop how unpleasant it had been staying at the hospital among such riffraff, and it's not hard to see how these hospitals began selecting which patients to let in and which to keep out.

These decisions were made according to a patient's "worthiness," as in, this patient is worthy of care and this one isn't. Today, we shirk such terms, but all eras have attempted to distinguish responsibility from misfortune. It's not uncommon, for instance, to hear a doctor in the present day refer to a patient as "poor protoplasm." Depending on the context, this can mean they're suffering from terrible luck or terrible judgment, from a preponderance of susceptible genes or a bevy of bad choices. Most of the time, the phrase connotes problems with the law, such as drug use—especially crack, meth, PCP, and heroin—or a predilection for STDs. It might sound cruel for healthcare workers to discuss the sick in this way, but it's hard seeing the same patients return to the hospital repeatedly. To continue their labors, healthcare workers need to make sense of their own seemingly ever-failing efforts. Imagining that the person who returns to the hospital again and again is unworthy, or poor protoplasm—a fixed entity destined to wilt—might be a way of coping.

Roxana was on the receiving end of this type of thinking, and she sensed that the medical world had made up its mind about her. This is in part why she didn't think of going back to the hospital that had saved her life. During her time there, she had begun to feel like a burden on the hospital's nurses and doctors. As her medical problems were starting to transition into social ones, it became increasingly unclear to her whether her hardships fell within the healthcare workers' purview. Now, at home and hobbled by dry gangrene, she was at a much higher risk of starving or stumbling to the floor than she was of dying from a slow-growing tumor. Any police officer or firefighter, seeing her in a vulnerable position such as this, would have been compelled to take her to the hospital to ensure her life wasn't in danger. But still, she wasn't certain she belonged there.

One hundred years ago, a voluntary hospital might have taken Roxana in on the basis of her vulnerability alone, pending an interrogation about her faith. It's also true that one hundred years ago, a hospital wouldn't have been able to provide the technical theater necessary for the heroic surgery that saved her life. With time, increasing costs meant that advances in science were—and always will be—at odds with the ideals of fairness and equality: that is the price of technology. The result, as Jeanne Kisacky notes in her book *Rise of the Modern Hospital: An Architectural History of Health and Healing*, was that voluntary hospitals homed in on the problems that science could address rather than people's social problems:

> The American high-rise hospital was no depository for the sick poor, no dispenser of basic unspecialized care, no symbol of pure philanthropy . . . its concentration of medical facilities and practitioners accommodated research and interactive medicine, but made basic healing and recovery quite costly and secondary to treatment. This posed an ominous precedent for future development of an affordable hospital system.

In the late nineteenth century, as science advanced, voluntary hospitals began offering their patients increasing levels of technology. To do so, they had to become even more selective about whom they cared for. The number of people considered unworthy, therefore, grew. Those deemed unworthy were made to depend on public hospitals. These hospitals became dumping grounds.

Neglected by both the community and the government, public hospitals declined even further from their almshouse days. Many were financed, poorly, by either the city or the county, or a combination, and so they became known as "municipal" or "county" hospitals. To draw upon the cheap labor of student doctors, they aligned themselves with medical schools. Students and residents practiced their craft on the poor, often without appropriate supervision.

Local and state governments only worsened the disparity of care found between public and voluntary hospitals. In the early 1900s, in a push to help the middle class afford the increasing cost of hospital care, a quarter of all taxpayer funds spent on healthcare went toward subsidizing voluntary hospitals, not public ones. One system grew wealthy while the other floundered.

The healthcare practices within each type of hospital reflected this. Chekhov, who saw and worked in many public hospitals in Russia, noted how backward these places could feel for a doctor inspired by the new therapies available elsewhere but inaccessible to his patients: "To put the seriously ill in the hospital and care for them according to the rules of science was also impossible, because while there were rules, there was no science." Public hospitals in the United States weren't much better.

This story seems straightforward enough: that public hospitals have remained today what they always were, little more than society's dumping grounds. In some parts of the United States, that might still be true. But as the missions of voluntary hospitals shifted more toward wealth and growth, the rift between them and public hospitals would continue to increase in size, and public hospitals would eventually find their niche. Ironically, the federal government's first piece of legislation to make healthcare more accessible would catalyze the voluntary hospital's transformation.

The dawn of the era of the beautiful, gleaming hospital began with an infrastructure bill. In 1946, Congress passed the Hill-Burton Act, which provided $4.5 billion in grants and another $1.5 billion in loans to help modernize American hospitals. With Hill-Burton money, the institutions of the Texas Medical Center grew into Houston's second downtown, one healthcare skyscraper after another just a few minutes down Main Street from the oil and gas headquarters that make up the city's principal skyline.

Hospitals that accepted funds were supposed to provide "free care" to people who couldn't afford the fees, and free care was provided, but only to a point. Congress gave little guidance on what constituted sufficient charity and didn't police the spending of Hill-Burton funds. There were other rules, too; for instance, bankrolled hospitals couldn't discriminate against minorities. Segregation, however, remained the law of the land and manifested in nefarious ways: hospitals like Jefferson Davis and the Houston Negro Hospital only received limited funds compared to those given to wealthier voluntary hospitals. In the end, the Hill-Burton money, worth nearly $85 billion today, served more as a subsidy for voluntary hospitals looking to grow. The hospitals serving paying customers modernized, while those serving the poor continued to crumble.

A decade after voluntary hospitals began to receive more funds from the Hill-Burton Act and their clients, an opportunity to change their tax status also arrived. In 1956, the IRS allowed hospitals to report themselves as charities if they offered reduced costs and operated "for those not able to pay for the services rendered." The IRS did not police hospitals to ensure they followed these criteria, however. Immediately, voluntary hospitals began reaping the rewards of the charitable tax designation, which allowed them not only to avoid federal, state, and local taxes but also to receive charitable donations. With so many financial advantages, voluntary hospitals prospered. They embraced their tax designation and became known as nonprofits. They catered toward those who could afford their fees. The result was a worsening class divide as more and more middle-class Americans visited the newer hospitals. Poor Americans, meanwhile, could only visit the neglected public hospitals.

"Houston, 1963, is a remnant of the Middle Ages as far as its charity hospital is concerned; and now yet another cut in its budget is proposed." Jan de Hartog's words appeared in an op-ed published by the *Houston Chronicle*. Having volunteered a full month in the city's lone public hospital, Jefferson Davis Hospital, the Quaker novelist had witnessed horror. What he had seen and heard at JD still boggled his mind:

Staph infections roiling through the maternity ward, killing dozens. Newborns in the nursery crying and crying for milk that wasn't there. Patients sitting in their own filth waiting days to see a doctor. A cockroach crawling into a child's tracheostomy tube. And now, funding for JD was caught in a standoff between the county and city governments that jointly funded the public hospital, each of which had plans to scale back their budget. "If the cut goes into effect," de Hartog continued, "Houston will soon boast the most expensive stadium and the most backward charity hospital in the civilized world . . . This is to govern a modern metropolis with the mentality of a colony of maggots, feeding on the suppurating wound of the illiterate, the damned."

The passage of Medicaid was supposed to help level the playing field between public hospitals and nonprofits. When the program first started in 1965, there was hope that within five years it would leave no person in America uncovered. "Unfortunately, many Americans live on the outskirts of hope," said President Lyndon Johnson on announcing the plan, "some because of their poverty, and some because of their color, and all too many because of both. Our task is to replace their despair with opportunity."

Having lived through poverty himself, President Johnson understood that a poor person in America might not feel something as vital as hospital care was accessible. Those who qualified for Medicaid—initially, this was limited to poor families with children—could visit any hospital that accepted this insurance, and most hospitals did. The idea, as Paul Starr notes, was to plug the poor into the mainstream of American medicine. By 1970, the percentage of people with low incomes who'd had a surgical procedure increased 40 percent from the pre-Medicaid days.

There was hope that Medicaid dollars would trickle down to public hospitals, too. As David Oshinsky recounts in *Bellevue*, the belief was "the chronic underfunding of municipal hospitals . . . will come to an end." But people with Medicaid generally chose to visit the best hospitals they could, which typically meant the freshly renovated nonprofit hospitals. Only those who did not qualify for Medicaid were left with no choice but to visit public hospitals.

Today, the tax breaks nonprofits receive every year are worth $11 million *per hospital*. Taken together, they amounted to more than $24 billion in 2011. While the majority of nonprofits demonstrate services to the community that outweigh their tax benefit, almost a third do not. They select patients with as much rigor as their voluntary antecedents, but their criteria have shifted from moral codes toward reimbursement rates. It should be no surprise, then, that the gleaming tower looming over Roxana's neighborhood belongs to one of Houston's most prominent nonprofit hospitals. It receives tax incentives to treat people like Roxana every year. Roxana, however, didn't feel she would receive the attention she needed there. And in all likelihood, she was right.

Clearly, the hospitals the US government had hoped would fill in the coverage gaps weren't able to provide this care, either because they were running low on funds or because they had prioritized profit. Roxana would need to find a different hospital, one with a mission focused on helping those who lacked insurance.

Safety-net hospitals aren't defined by their source of revenue. Rather, they're defined by their mission: to treat *all* patients, whether they have private health insurance or not. As I mentioned earlier, most safety-net hospitals are public hospitals, but some are nonprofits or even for-profits focusing on vulnerable populations. To achieve their mission, safety nets rely on multiple funding sources, including federal grants given to hospitals that care for the uninsured. Since many patients who visit safety-net hospitals are freshly uninsured—or are seeking healthcare for the first time—safety nets also actively identify those who qualify for Medicare and Medicaid.

For those who don't qualify for the governmental insurance programs, safety nets often offer sliding-scale payment schemes. Since many of these hospitals serve local needs, they receive local government funds. Top-tier trauma centers and burn units, which require highly trained personnel and specialized equipment too expensive for other hospitals to maintain, can often be found in safety-net hospitals. All this is to say, safety-net hospitals have evolved to serve the needs of their communities.

Ben Taub's history reflects this evolution. Weeks after the *Houston Chronicle* ran de Hartog's op-ed in May 1963, Ben Taub General Hospital opened its doors. A new public hospital had been planned even before de Hartog witnessed the atrocities that spurred his op-ed. Funds from the Hill-Burton Act made building one possible.

In his op-ed, de Hartog had pleaded with Houstonians not to allow Ben Taub to suffer the same fate as Jefferson Davis Hospital. Spurred by his words, volunteers streamed into the new public hospital, compensating for the shortage of nurses and doctors. A year later, de Hartog published a book, *The Hospital*, detailing his experiences at JD and Ben Taub. Again, his words had a galvanizing effect. Now the whole world knew the city's shame. "Houston's Zoo Air Conditioned, Charity Hospitals Are Not," read one international headline. Reporters called Houstonians heartless.

Pundits from across the country began to weigh in. De Hartog debated the county commissioner on national TV. The bickering started to sound like the same old, same old, one side calling the other bleeding hearts, only to be called compassionless in return. It could have ended there, but a civic leader took the bull by the horns. County Judge Bill Elliott, a Democrat and one of the most powerful politicians in 1964 Houston, decided "to do as a man what he could not do as a county judge." He trained himself and secretly volunteered as a nighttime orderly at JD. As other city leaders slept, he embedded himself within JD's walls, keeping an eye on how the hospital worked, who received care, and who was abandoned.

Judge Elliott verified all of de Hartog's reporting. He pushed for Houstonians to vote on the measure again, convinced the only solution was to set up a new local tax, one that directly financed the hospitals. A vote to create a hospital district—an organization like a school district that levies its own taxes from property owners in the county—would provide a new Ben Taub and a dilapidated JD with a steady stream of funds from which to hire nurses and doctors and give adequate care to the poor. It all came to a head in January 1965, when Houstonians voted a second time on the hospital district measure. Protesters against the measure came out in full force, not to be outdone by the hospital district proponents. De Hartog yelled until he was hoarse. It didn't matter. The measure was roundly defeated. Judge Elliot called it a "sad day for Houston and Harris County."

The politics seemed impossible. The city was divided. Both sides had dug their heels into the ground. One group wanted the poor to receive humane care, while their opponents painted them as wasteful and unrealistic. The other group believed in financial responsibility, including when it came to healthcare, and their opponents painted them as racists who opposed any benefit to African Americans. It was, by all appearances, another irreparable standstill, but Judge Elliott persisted. He managed to convince the Harris County Medical Society to support the hospital district. And in November 1965, Houstonians voted a third time, electing to support the hospital district through local taxes. Today, the district is named Harris Health.

The transition from a lone public hospital to a safety-net healthcare system transformed the city. Shortly after the formation of the hospital district in the 1960s, community health programs were opened in medical deserts. By the 1970s, primary care became available in working-class neighborhoods, much of it paid for by property taxes. In the 1980s, Harris Health opened the nation's first freestanding HIV clinic at the height of the AIDS crisis. In the nineties and in the new millennium, the system opened school-based clinics, an ambulatory surgical center, and pop-up clinics to attend to those displaced by Tropical Storm Allison and Hurricane Harvey. Out of the ashes of a dilapidated charity hospital rose a functioning system for Houstonians unable to afford healthcare.

Roxana wouldn't find help in the nonprofit hospital looming over her neighborhood because she didn't have private health insurance and couldn't qualify for any governmental insurance. Emergency Medicaid would only cover hospital fees for emergencies; her problem, however, was chronic. That left her with one option: she needed to visit a hospital not beholden to a board of business leaders or stockholders, one whose goal wasn't to bring in money. She needed a safety-net hospital, one capable of delivering on its lofty mission, and she found one: "Harris Health is a community-focused academic healthcare system dedicated to improving the health of those most in need in Harris County through quality care delivery, coordination of care, and education," read the safety-net hospital's mission statement.

She told the hospice nurse that she needed help and that she was going to Ben Taub. A friend from her *iglesia* knew the hospital well and confirmed she could probably receive healthcare there.

Though Houstonians recognize the name, Ben Taub usually isn't the first hospital people think of when they fall ill. Even healthcare workers often don't think to direct their uninsured patients to the safety-net system. This is likely a compound effect of multiple factors: poor advertising by Ben Taub, resulting in doctors' and patients' limited understanding of the resources available to them; and a systemic preference for private over public institutions. In either case, Roxana didn't know that Ben Taub existed, even as she was in need of its specific services.

Another friend from her *iglesia* drove ambulances, Roxana remembered, and so she told the nurse there was no need to dial 911. Once the hospice nurse left, Roxana asked Marí to dial this ambulance driver. He arrived within the hour, and soon Roxana was on a stretcher. The driver loaded her into the ambulance, turned on the ignition, and eased onto Gessner Road.

For a while, they were just another ambulance with the lights off in America's fourth-largest city. After passing beneath the I-10 overpass— twelve roaring lanes of traffic—he turned onto the access road, accelerated up the ramp, and merged onto the freeway heading east. Every subtle swerve made Roxana's stretcher sway a little, and there was no way for her to hold herself in place. She prayed and talked with the driver the whole ride.

Finally, a large building composed of yellow and gold bricks emerged over the tree line. Its base was boxy and stark, rising seven floors. Atop the structure lay a simple A-shaped roof. This was Ben Taub Hospital. At a little before 2:40 p.m., the driver pulled into the ambulance dock.

At the triage station, a nurse slid a blood pressure cuff over the live portion of Roxana's arm and took her vital signs. Then, swiftly, Roxana was taken to the holding area, where thirty stretchers were parked on one side of the wall, thirty on the other, with patients on them, always. In a central command center transecting the room, young doctors typed and talked and checked out the new portable ultrasound and waited for the Spanish translator. One of them would see Roxana shortly.

The question about what to do with Roxana—whether to admit her into one of the hospital wards or send her home—already hung in the air. For years, doctors, hospitals, and insurance companies had sparred over what admitting unfunded patients meant to their bottom line but also to their identity. For Roxana, the moment of truth was at hand.

Wards

In 1984, an eighteen-year-old arrived at Parkland Memorial Hospital in Dallas, Texas. We don't know *how* he arrived, if a taxi dropped him off or if he managed to stumble in, but we know he got there. His head hurt. He seemed delirious. He had a sky-high fever, the type that makes doctors nervous.

Unbeknownst to the doctors at Parkland, the boy had a note in his pocket written out on a prescription pad. In the space where words like "Valium" and "penicillin" would typically go, someone had written out instructions: "This patient is sick with meningitis, please treat him."

It turned out that the boy had visited a nonprofit hospital before arriving at Parkland. He didn't have insurance, but he felt hot and he knew he was sick, so he went to the closest place for help. The hospital had the means and the personnel to treat the boy, but since he had no insurance and the hospital was sure it would not receive payment for his care, the doctors chose to refer him to the safety-net hospital. At Ben Taub we call this a dump.

It was a classic case of bacterial meningitis, a fast-moving infection that can have disastrous effects if left untreated. In the time it took the doctors at the first hospital to write the note and send him on his way, the bacteria inside the boy's brain had multiplied, making their way through his temporal lobes and down his spinal cord and into his optic nerves. The boy didn't even make it to the holding area. He collapsed, dead, right on the floor of the emergency ward. As doctors attempted to revive him, they found the piece of paper sticking out of his pocket.

Things must have changed since then, we tell ourselves, right?

Yes and no.

At the time, dumping uninsured patients onto safety-net hospitals was a rampant practice, and not just in Texas. There was new literature popping up in all the big journals, like the *New England Journal of Medicine* and the *Journal of the American Medical Association*, describing how often doctors bore witness to this villainy. This was how the Parkland boy's story became known.

Some doctors began collecting data on the problem. Seventy-seven percent of the patients transferred from other hospitals to Parkland, for *any* reason, had no insurance. The vast majority of the patients transferred to Cook County Hospital in Chicago—the basis for the TV show *ER*—were Black or Hispanic (89 percent), unemployed (81 percent), or uninsured (87 percent). Only 6 percent of the patients transferred gave written consent for their transfer.

The problem wasn't necessarily that these poor and uninsured patients were being told to go to the safety-net hospitals—that's why these hospitals existed, to take care of the indigent—but *when* they were told. Boys sick with bacterial meningitis, women in labor, car-crash victims—the dumping occurred even at critical moments, when immediate medical intervention meant the difference between life and death.

Somebody had to take a stand. In the end, it was the most unlikely player who decided enough was enough. In 1986, Texas became the first state in the country to pass anti-dumping laws. Three years before, the state legislature had passed a law that made it a felony for doctors and hospitals to deny patients care for socioeconomic reasons. Now it was upping the ante. Patient dumping was expressly prohibited. Hospitals could only transfer emergency patients with their consent and if it was in the patient's best interest to do so.

Soon thereafter, the US Congress passed a statute: any hospital with an emergency room that accepts Medicare funding—which is virtually *all* hospitals—must treat all patients in the throes of an emergency, regardless of their ability to pay, until they are stable. EMTALA, or the Emergency Medical Treatment and Labor Act, became the law of the land. Now there were penalties for patient dumping. Now a hospital could lose accreditation if it didn't treat an undocumented person at risk of losing their life. Now a woman in active labor wouldn't be turned away from a hospital if she didn't have private insurance. But EMTALA said nothing about how the doctors caring for these uninsured patients and the hospitals where this care took place would be paid.

In 1986, the federal government assigned the responsibility of emergency care without guaranteeing income. It had decided that healthcare in critical moments wasn't earned; it was a right.

EMTALA's effect on healthcare was seismic, its results mixed. It changed the medical calculus of determining who is sick and who can return home. The law made terms like "uncompensated care" and "disproportionate share" part of a hospital's lingo. It also led to even further changes in the hospital architecture, as waiting rooms in the ER became more crowded than hospital lobbies. For people lacking insurance, a hospital's emergency room became their de facto doctor's office, a place to handle everything from too much earwax to heartburn to an inability to control urine. The financial instability EMTALA created, particularly for hospitals in rural and underserved areas, led to closures, if not survival tactics. Whole programs closed, and employees were made to perform jobs beyond their capabilities. Filing a yearly budget became an act of prayer, a shot in the dark. To remain profitable, nonprofit and for-profit hospitals have had to adapt to EMTALA. Safety nets, meanwhile, have found themselves overloaded. All of these changes to American healthcare are evident in a hospital's wards, where the most important and expensive healthcare decisions are made. Safety-net hospitals give doctors the right environment to make medical decisions in these wards, not financial ones.

For hospitals, EMTALA also upped the financial ante on what happens in the ER. If doctors in the ER decide an emergency is truly life-threatening, for instance, the resulting hospitalization and therapy to stabilize the patient's condition—which can include surgeries, procedures, the eyes of multiple specialists, etc.—will generate costs, which is acceptable if the patient has adequate insurance, and bothersome for the doctors and hospitals if the patient doesn't.

In the ER, the motivations of doctors, insurance companies, and hospitals converge. A risk-averse doctor might be inclined to treat and admit more than what the financial health of a hospital permits. On the other hand, a doctor thinking too much about finances might send a critically ill patient home too early and violate that person's right to emergency care. All of this on top of the fact that it's *already* extremely difficult to care for patients in an emergency. Thinking about insured versus uninsured only makes a tough job more difficult.

My father and I could always talk about medicine. I could text him at any time with questions like "Do you treat BV empirically?" In patient care, questions like this always pop up. He knew as well as anybody that when there was a patient in front of you with a problem, their life mattered most, nothing else. Within minutes, his response would buzz on my phone: "Gram stain in office."

What you do for a patient in front of you is one thing—my dad and I could agree on pretty much everything there—but how a patient arrives at the hospital and what happens when that patient leaves your sight is another. That's where our disagreements began. Politics divided us, and, correspondingly, the political implications of healthcare divided us, too.

My dad lauded Ronald Reagan's big Medicaid cut in the 1980s. I was too young at the time to know what that meant, but today I do, and he and I can't talk about it without getting heated. My dad blamed the Clintons for catering to insurance companies in the 1990s when the country was debating managed care. And he despised the idea of Obamacare, which again seemed to give more control of medicine to those who ran insurance. As his practice grew more lucrative throughout the years, he became more entrepreneurial with the money he earned seeing patients. He bought stocks and invested in real estate. He saw his practice as a mom-and-pop shop fighting its way forward in a world run by McDonald's. To him, the problems of healthcare could be solved by shoring up the private side—less government intervention—to make competition fair. He rejected the idea that healthcare should be controlled by the public.

Meanwhile, I went the opposite way. I attended a Jesuit high school and learned about social justice. I spent a summer in rural Brazil, living among those without basic sanitation. I attended a Jesuit university and minored in theology. These were all experiences afforded by the private world, since my mom and dad paid for my education. When I was admitted to medical school in my hometown, I celebrated, but it wasn't long before I decided to quit. I couldn't foresee myself working like my father had, thinking about insurance companies and co-pays. I deferred my admission for a year and then I took a leave of absence for another. I worked in New Delhi and Nairobi for organizations focusing on drug rehabilitation and HIV care, trying to find an alternative to medicine in America. I loved coming into contact with people I wouldn't have otherwise encountered. But I also saw how close to zero my bank account balance hovered. I was financially insecure. I decided to return to medical school for the same reason I had delayed it: money.

Ben Taub kept me in medicine. I didn't know what I would do with a medical degree, except that I still didn't want a life centered around private insurance claims. As a medical student on the Ben Taub wards,

I found an alternative: Here people seemed to receive good care, and doctors received paychecks. The hospital took in everybody. You came into contact with people from all over the world. There was no haggling with insurance. The focus was medicine.

Some of the attending doctors I met told me about moonlighting at private hospitals and how easy it was to bill. I wasn't sure I could handle the conflict. For me, it was easier to work for a paycheck and not deal with the temptation of more money and the compromises that might come with a financial incentive to do too much—or too little.

I decided Ben Taub would be my home. My dad liked what was happening inside the hospital, but as ever, politics crept in, little comments here and there on both sides. If he used the word "freeloader," I might mention how nonprofits "rip people off."

The healthcare talk blended with our family dramas the way we tossed English in with our Spanish. For a long time, it was just part of how we communicated. And then one evening over dinner, he mentioned Ben Taub.

"You owe us eighty million dollars," he said.

I don't remember if he said eighty or one hundred eighty or even two hundred eighty million, but it was in the tens of millions, and more than that, he'd used the words "you" and "us," which made me seethe. He reasoned that Harris Health owed the nonprofit hospital system where he worked many millions of dollars because the undocumented and uninsured used their emergency room, as mandated by EMTALA.

Somehow we remained civil through that night. We hugged briefly in the restaurant parking lot and walked to our respective cars. On my drive home, I thought about what he'd said. He had a point. One of the responsibilities of the public's safety-net system was to provide healthcare for the indigent. It was part of Ben Taub and Harris Health's mission statement. But for many years, the emergency wards where I worked had been overwhelmed to the point that some visitors avoided the hospital because of the long wait times.

Ben Taub is one of only two Level 1 trauma centers in Houston. This means that there is always an anesthesiologist, a surgeon, and an open OR primed to care for any patient who needs a potential life-saving surgery. It's the highest designation an ER can earn. When a community is growing the way Houston has over the past fifty years, the necessity for a trauma center increases. Experts estimate that a city should have one Level 1 trauma center for every million people. Apart from Ben Taub, Houston, with a metropolitan area of just over seven million, only has one other major trauma center, which happens to be right next door. Such are the consequences of poor city planning: the trauma needs of a ten-thousand-square-mile metropolitan area—larger than New Jersey—rest on two city blocks. It means that Ben Taub is doing the work of three or four trauma centers.

The wait time at Ben Taub's emergency ward is as legendary as the trauma care it provides. In 2019, the Centers for Medicare & Medicaid Services (CMS), the federal agency that runs these entitlement insurances, released its yearly hospital ratings. Hospitals were rated from one star to five based on quality metrics. The hospital where my dad spent his career received four stars. Harris Health, including Ben Taub, received one star. The low rating was due in large part to the numbers coming out of the emergency wards: the average time a patient spent in the emergency ward before being admitted to the hospital was eleven hours. Even when comparing this number to other large-volume ERs throughout the country, on average, patients at Ben Taub waited twice as long. Five percent of patients left without being seen—again, double the average. They likely got tired of waiting.

My dad wasn't wrong: many patients who should've gone to the safety-net hospital went to nonprofit and for-profit hospitals throughout the city, and they incurred debts. In many cases, these hospitals had to absorb some of the cost of this healthcare—regardless of how exorbitantly they may have priced it—making them even more apprehensive to provide care to other uninsured patients. This resulted in a vicious cycle.

When visiting Ben Taub, uninsured patients had to make a calculation: were they sick enough to endure the eleven-hour wait? Those who decided to stick it out had to make another decision: how much privacy am I willing to sacrifice to receive healthcare?

When Ebonie arrived at the Ben Taub ER, a nurse at the ambulance dock triaged her to OBI, or Obstetrics Intake, on the third floor. There, on the labor and delivery ward, nurses settled her stretcher into one of the seven slots surrounding a large central desk that served as a much smaller command center than the one in the holding area downstairs, where Roxana had been situated. Ebonie had green curtains that separated her from her new neighbors. They remained mostly closed. Sometimes the monitors to which she was connected beeped, announcing to the other soon-to-be mothers accelerations of her heart rate, as well as her baby's.

The tension between what is public and what is private is fundamental to the hospital. We arrive at our weakest and most vulnerable. We present ourselves before authority figures clad in scrubs and give our arm for a vital-sign check, our tongue to see if we have a fever, our insurance card, if we're lucky enough to have one. We give our words, the histories of our health, our rendition of the events that brought us there. And then we wait. We wait among others. We absorb things from these strangers, not their contagion, but their bodies' instrumentation of it. We hear wheezes, dry heaves, muffled sobs. We see yellow skin and black bruises and the spectacle of human organs in conflict with themselves. We smell the dehydration of others, the sweet ketones in their breath, their sweat and bile. And still we wait. From now until we are discharged, we are the hospital's wards. When, finally, it's our turn, we find ourselves led to a stretcher cordoned off by a sliding glass door, a wraparound curtain, perhaps even drywall and a door. We think we're better off like this. We believe this privacy constitutes more personal care, and we certainly pay more for it—but are we really better off? We are no longer with so many strangers, but we are no longer in view of the nurses and doctors, either.

How much privacy is appropriate in hospitals? Over the last one hundred years, the architecture of emergency rooms and medical wards has changed to make care more private. Originally, 100 percent of hospital beds were laid out in large wards, where patients lay side by side. But by 1910, that number had dwindled to 28 percent. As the care of the wealthy migrated from their homes to private rooms in hospitals, the large communal wards began to disappear.

Hospitals accommodated the middle class with semiprivate rooms, which offered some but not full privacy. The adoption of health insurance over the next decades reinforced the trend. Privacy, however, doesn't necessarily equate with better or even more personal healthcare. Private health insurance isn't always about health so much as the allure of privacy. Healthcare pricing in America reflects the drive toward privacy, and, more generally, toward the care of the individual instead of public health. As more money pours in, healthcare grows more private for more and more people to accommodate and retain those dollars. Indeed, some hospitals aim today toward providing fully "personalized medicine."

Correspondingly, hospital wards overloaded with patients because of high healthcare costs and the responsibilities incurred by EMTALA must cope with a lack of privacy. The largest section of the Ben Taub ER is an open ward, or what used to be called a Nightingale ward. While Ben Taub's ER has some bays with individual rooms, this open ward is very different from the rest of the ERs in the Texas Medical Center and certainly from any designed with insured patients in mind. Nightingale wards are filled with patients like Roxana, lying in rows with healthcare workers bustling between them. Not all safety-net hospitals have Nightingale wards, and not every emergency room of a safety-net hospital is organized into open wards. But these spaces are more common than you think and can be found in many of the large hospitals dedicated to the uninsured, especially those in big cities, and especially in emergency rooms.

You might think that lining up patients is unsafe and unsanitary, but actually, the open ward earned its place in history for proving the opposite.

In 1854, a young English nurse with a proclivity for statistics named Florence Nightingale visited a military hospital in Turkey during the Crimean War. What she saw appalled her. Not only were there too few medicines to treat the wounded soldiers, but mass infections were spreading through the overpacked wards. There wasn't a clear system to care for the sick soldiers. The numbers were daunting: any soldier admitted into the hospital stood a 42 percent chance of dying.

Nightingale published an op-ed in her hometown newspaper the *Times* of London pleading for the government to fix these deplorable conditions. Her article shocked the public so deeply that the British government prefabbed and shipped a new hospital to replace the decrepit structure she'd described. The design of the new hospital at Renkioi emphasized sanitation, spacing, and surveillance. The ward was long and narrow with a nurses' station in the middle and no more than thirty beds against each wall. Between all the hospital beds were tall windows, which provided ventilation. If a patient required immediate assistance—after vomiting, perhaps, or after a fit of coughing from fluid in the lungs—a nurse could easily identify the problem from the nurses' station in the middle of the room. The open ward kept patients safe.

Mortality at Renkioi plummeted to only 2 percent. The change impacted Nightingale so profoundly that after the war, she toured nearly every hospital in Europe. She collected statistics at each stop and thought about how a hospital's architecture impacted healthcare. Then she wrote a book, *Notes on Hospitals*, in which she told the story of how a change in spacing helped nurses help patients. She hadn't designed the wards, but she endorsed them wholeheartedly to the public. As a result, they became known as "Nightingale wards."

For many who've experienced only the labyrinthine layouts of modern ERs with their individual rooms or six-patient bays, coming into one of these wards can be a bit shocking. It's a little like walking the streets of Manhattan for the first time when all you've experienced is smaller cities—it's not just the density of people you feel but their purpose, everyone on task trying to survive.

Open wards give doctors and nurses constant contact with patients. They allow the staff to survey a patient's behavior before deciding whether that person should stay in the hospital or go home. They are also economical to construct, which is one of the reasons they're still part of the architecture of many safety-net hospitals.

I must acknowledge that my position on the open ward was a privileged one—this is true of all caretakers. Ben Taub's open ward allowed me to stand back and observe all of my patients' activities as if they were a TV show. I had only a small, protected role to play in the drama that unfolded in the Nightingale ward. If I were the one lying on the stretcher, connected to electrodes, waiting for CAT scan results, I have no clue how I'd handle myself amid the shouting and the retching and the flashes of nudity. On one hand, I suspect I'd want to make sure the medical staff had the best chance of assessing me; in that case, I might wait patiently in an open ward. On the other, I would probably want privacy if my illness made me feel vulnerable.

Some of my patients have told me that their time waiting in the Nightingale ward changed their lives. "God wanted me to see it," one patient said to me. She described herself as middle-class and lived in a wealthy suburb named Sugar Land. She'd never thought she'd come to Ben Taub as she'd had health insurance most of her life. But a divorce left her uncovered, and that was exactly when she got sick. All of her friends told her to come to Ben Taub. She waited in the ER for many hours, desperate to figure out why she was losing weight and feeling tired. As she waited, the drama of other lives unfolded in front of her. She saw prisoners and people in the throes of psychoses, all from different social classes, trying to cope with their own problems, and she found it transformative.

"Seeing that pushed me out of my bubble," she said.

Bubble, I thought when she said this. The word reminded me of a quote from philosopher John Stuart Mill that Paul Starr used in his book:

> One of the effects of civilization (not to say one of the ingredients of it) is, that the spectacle, and even the very idea of pain, is more and more kept out of the sight of those classes who enjoy in their fullness the benefits of civilization.

Patients tell me they commiserate in the Nightingale ward, that they build solidarity. Sometimes the best kind of healing happens there. Another patient told me she never wanted to wait the way she did in the holding area again. The only saving moment, she told me, was her conversation with the man next to her. He was recovering from a crack binge. He was sobbing at the state of everything, how his life was in ruins. The woman was a recovering crack addict and had been totally drug-free for going on ten years. She told me she sang a hymn with the man, tongue-lashed him a bit ("You the *only one* that can stop"), told him exactly what she'd done to quit, and prayed with him.

Without a doubt, none of us working at Ben Taub that day had been as helpful to the man as she had been.

Stephen's wife dropped him off at Ben Taub's ER very early the morning of April 15. It was just the previous evening that he'd been turned away from a nonprofit hospital in town for being underinsured. Like nearly all Houstonians, Stephen knew about Ben Taub's reputation for treating gunshot wounds, and so part of him expected chaos when he walked into the vestibule at the emergency room entrance. Instead, he saw order. He heard instructions.

"Can you please join the line against the wall, sir?" a security guard asked him.

Once Stephen had taken his place in the COVID screening line, the guard offered a friendly greeting: "How are you doing?"

There were not many patients in line at this time, just one, in fact: a middle-aged woman. As she spoke with one of the screeners, her voice shifted in volume. Why is she so loud? Stephen thought. Two plastic grocery bags, both overflowing, lay at her feet. Stephen wondered if these might have carried all of her possessions. He momentarily felt compelled to leave, but the restaurant manager in him, who had gutted out hard shifts with undesirable customers, focused on sticking through it and forging ahead. Soon enough, the woman picked up her bags and proceeded into the larger waiting area.

With Stephen, a screener marched through a questionnaire. He strapped a blood pressure cuff around Stephen's biceps, clipped a pulse oximeter onto a finger, and inserted a thermometer beneath his tongue. Stephen could see a kind expression through the screener's facial shield, in the sliver above his N95 mask. After some chitchat, Stephen advanced down a short hall into the waiting area.

With COVID spreading throughout the world and the city on lockdown, the lounge appeared less like a bustling trauma center and more like a snowed-in airport. The blankets were out, the news ran muted in the background (CNN on one TV, Fox on another, BET on a third), and people took advantage of the social distancing by draping their legs on the armrests between vinyl armchairs. Three desks aligned in a row signaled the end of the waiting area and the entry into the treatment zones of the ER. Atop each of these desks sat a computer and stacks of paper. At any other hospital, the people working at these desks might have been insurance verifiers, the business side of the hospital, but at Ben Taub, these were triage nurses.

The woman with the bags spoke loudly with a nurse at one of the desks. Stephen sat down in front of a nurse dressed in black, unsure where all this would lead.

To the question of why he'd come to the emergency room, Stephen initially said, "I have tonsil issues." Just as easily, he could have told the nurse, "I don't have health insurance."

The stability of Stephen's vital signs indicated he didn't require the constant oversight of the Nightingale ward. The nurse and Stephen began to chat, not just about how Stephen had gotten there but about how the world had changed. The kindness created an opportunity for Stephen to elaborate on why he'd come to this hospital.

"I think I have tonsil cancer," he said.

Within thirty minutes, he was telling his story to an ER doctor in one of the examination rooms. Not long afterward, he received a CAT scan of his face and neck, an examination by an ENT resident, and then another exam by an internal medicine doctor. Everyone agreed: Stephen needed to stay at the hospital overnight, and perhaps for some days, to plan out how to treat the cancer. There was no time to waste.

A transportation tech entered Stephen's exam room with a wheelchair. The two maneuvered through the emergency room and to the elevators, shooting the breeze the whole way. The hospital didn't look as dirty as Stephen had imagined, just a little scuffed up, like sneakers worn exclusively for racquetball. Black streaks along the walls indicated where stretchers had been parked. Here and there, an odd medley of framed prints brought color to the hallways: a zoom-in on God's and Adam's fingers touching from Michelangelo's masterpiece, a framed quote from Edith Wharton. Nothing looked fancy, but it didn't look run-down, either.

It wasn't until the transportation tech left him that Stephen realized he had yet to discuss money with anyone in the hospital. Financial counselors at Ben Taub visit patients to identify whether they have health insurance, but this only occurs after a patient is stabilized and has a medical treatment plan.

Stephen reflected a bit on how kind everyone had been to him and began settling into his new temporary home. He felt good that the focus didn't appear to be money as much as taking care of his problem.

By pure luck, he had been assigned one of Ben Taub's few private rooms.

Ebonie was bearing her pain out in public now, in the obstetric section of Ben Taub's Nightingale ward. After the first tests came back, however, her doctors decided that their next conversation should be held in private. They snapped the green curtains tightly against the wall as if to summon the hospital's confidentiality. A dark shadow fell on the stretcher.

The tests confirmed that she had lost at least two and a half liters of blood. An ultrasound showed that her nineteen-week-old fetus looked healthy, but it also revealed something ominous. The placenta, the large network of blood vessels that nourishes the fetus during pregnancy, was attached to the opening of Ebonie's birth canal, a condition known as complete placenta previa. When something so large blocks the birth canal, a normal birth is physically impossible. To make matters worse, the location of Ebonie's placenta put her at very high risk of losing even more blood, dangerous amounts, throughout her pregnancy. The boilerplate written by the radiologist, in this case, reflected real urgency and concern: "Continued surveillance is necessary."

Terminating the pregnancy, her doctors explained, would be the safest choice.* This would prevent any more life-threatening bleeding because it would remove the source, the placenta. It could be accomplished in one procedure, in which both the placenta and the fetus would be scraped away. By this point, Ebonie's blood volume was half of what it should have been, putting her vital organs at risk of not receiving enough

---

* SB 8, the Texas abortion law that went into effect after the Supreme Court overturned *Roe v. Wade* in June 2022, contains an exemption to save the life of a pregnant mother. However, a maternal-fetal medicine specialist told me that Ebonie's condition of placenta previa would not qualify for this exemption, as it is reserved for women very close to death or actively bleeding. All of which is to say that, if the same situation happened today, Ebonie would probably not be offered an abortion to save her life.

oxygen. There was no reason, no reason at all, to think the bleeding would stop. Her life was in danger.

Ebonie tried to piece together the words. Do you mean an abortion?

Yes, an abortion, the doctors replied. That's what we believe is most safe.

But Ebonie had never had an abortion. She couldn't imagine life without her four children. They gave her solace and stability, just as her siblings had when she was a young girl. Ebonie had grown up poor and, at times, homeless. She remembered nights when she would fall asleep on some California beach, wake up early to the sound of the surf, and use the public bathrooms to wash up. These weren't happy memories, but the presence of her brother and sister beside her during these tough times had created a bond she held as sacred. And when Ebonie began to have her own children, this new family became the most important part of her life.

Ebonie began to cry. She called her partner in California, who implored her not to end the pregnancy. She called her mother, and she talked with her sister Sharonna, who had accompanied her to Ben Taub.

What should I do? she asked. The fluorescent lighting pressed through the curtains. Sharonna's skin started to look like jade. Whatever you decide, we'll support you, Sharonna told her sister, the same thing their mother had said. No matter what.

Ebonie envisioned her own kids giving one another that same type of unconditional support, and she knew then and there what she would do—she'd have the baby. She had only just turned thirty-three and wasn't even halfway through her seventh pregnancy.

You have time to decide, the obstetricians told her. They ordered two bags of blood and admitted her into the hospital.

How long will I stay? Ebonie asked.

Possibly a day, possibly a week, the doctors told her. They wanted to make sure she wasn't bleeding for a full forty-eight hours before letting her go, for her own safety.

Ebonie was now a Ben Taub patient. Doctors admitted her into the labor and delivery ward, in case the bleeding became so significant that they'd have to wheel her into one of the ORs down the hallway and perform an emergency cesarean to save her life.

Roxana lay in one of the holding area slots of the Ben Taub ER, the back of her stretcher raised thirty degrees, her head inches from the wall. Wires of all sorts clung to different parts of her body. There were electrodes on her chest and shoulders connected to a heart monitor overhead. A blood pressure cuff on her upper arm automatically insufflated and deflated every thirty minutes. Taped to her earlobe, because it couldn't go on any of her fingers or toes, was a pulse oximeter, a gauge to measure how well her cells received oxygen. She was tapped into the hospital now. Any big changes in her body—for example, if bacteria from the gangrene leaked into her bloodstream, causing a spike in her temperature and an acceleration of her heart rate—would set off the alarm in the form of beeps and flashing numbers.

What had she gained by coming to Ben Taub? Nothing, yet. She was still an emergency patient receiving an emergency assessment, still waiting to see if doctors would admit her into the hospital. Any hospital that followed federal law would have done the same. Each time a doctor or a student walked in her vicinity, she prepared for bad news. *You have no insurance. You are undocumented.* In other words, *You don't deserve healthcare.* It frightened her to think she might have to go back home with these arms and legs.

She watched as, nearby, half a dozen or so doctors huddled into a small mob. En masse, they moved from stretcher to stretcher, pausing at the foot of each bed to deliberate. One of them talked while the others contemplated. Another manned a computer on wheels. They gave each other looks, some bored, some tormented, but what was the tenor of these discussions? Roxana couldn't make out what they were saying.

Some of her new neighbors were being wheeled away in their stretchers. To a CAT scan? Upstairs? Others started to dress themselves in street clothes. The nurse helped untangle them from the IVs and wires. She handed them papers, and just like that, they left the emergency room. A cleaning person arrived shortly afterward to wipe the stretcher, freshen the sheets, and lay out two folded hospital gowns. With that, a new neighbor would arrive, and the process would began anew. The cycle never ended.

This was the pressure the doctors in the Ben Taub ER worked against. Thirty people on stretchers in the holding area, each one expecting their medical decision—Discharge? Observe? Admit? Dozens more waited in the large room outside. Some had checked in more than ten hours ago. Each one was a ticking clock. On a flat-screen TV, each patient's name was listed, Roxana's among them. Beside Roxana's name and her location appeared the number of hours and minutes that she had waited since checking in at triage. Another TV displayed the capacity levels of emergency rooms across the city. The words "CRITICAL VOLUME" in red appeared beside many of the hospitals listed. It meant more ambulances were being routed to Ben Taub. The line was growing longer. More ticking clocks. Would this affect the decisions doctors made?

If the modern hospital is a body and each of its departments an organ, the whole must work better than the sum of the parts, since it's only in a functioning and cohesive organism, a system of systems, that sick patients receive good care. The OR is the liver, capable of metabolizing or dispatching illness with the nick of a scalpel. The ICU is the adrenal glands, secreting epinephrine, or the most urgent hospital resources, in times of peril. Hospital wards are the muscles, doing the brute work of administering to sickness. And the ER is the digestive system, taking in illness, roughly breaking it down, and distributing it to the other organs for processing.

When things work well, the organism of care *moves people*. The sick go to the right part of the hospital and the not-so-sick, after receiving proper attention, leave. But increasingly in the United States, things don't work that way. The ER has become the first stop for all medical ailments, large and small. The sheer volume of uninsured patients has disrupted the flow and changed the way this organ operates. ERs have become bloated with so many patients seeking basic healthcare that they can't function properly.

In 2002, a nonprofit named Save Our ERs conducted a study to see how overcrowding affected trauma care. Researchers found that the mortality rate doubled when Ben Taub and its neighboring Level I trauma center were overfilled and unable to accept any new patients. People died at an ill-equipped hospital that was desperately trying to arrange for a transfer, or perhaps at the site of the wreck, amid the static of the radio telling them that Ben Taub was filled to capacity, that it could no longer accept any more patients, no matter how sick they were. The ER doctors were not only serving the patients within Ben Taub's walls. *Keeping people moving* was a life-or-death challenge that impacted an entire city.

The gangrene on Roxana's arms looked wet, which wasn't a good sign. Would a surgeon be able to amputate them? The ER doctors didn't know, and so they consulted an orthopedic surgeon. It was a difficult job deciding if Roxana ought to stay in the hospital, but at least the doctors at Ben Taub could make the choice with a clear conscience and with a laser focus on medicine.

The group of ER doctors arrived at Roxana's stretcher. One of them spoke while the others listened. The orthopedic surgeon had examined Roxana and looked at all the results of the blood work. There was bad news. Taking Roxana to the operating room now for an amputation wasn't an option. There was evidence from the blood work to suggest that Roxana had an infection on her right arm, where the hospice nurse had discovered oozing. The tests also showed that Roxana's kidneys weren't working optimally; good kidney function is a precondition for amputation.

Roxana felt dismayed. She didn't want to go back to her apartment like this. What if the infection worsened? "What should I do ?" she asked, lifting up her arms.

And here we arrive at the most crucial moment of Roxana's journey. She knew it, and so did the ER doctors. But the moment extended beyond these bodies. In fact, this next decision crystallized a divide in our country. Is healthcare a right? Who should receive it? Who should pay for it? All of these questions were embedded in this next decision on whether to admit Roxana into the hospital wards or to discharge her.

Some say that healthcare is earned. That is one side of the fence. Healthcare is earned and paid for through the mechanism of private insurance. If you cannot afford it, the thought goes, then you cannot participate. America is a meritocracy, according to this view. If those with means would like to purchase privacy and extra healthcare, they should be able to through the market. This side believes suppliers of healthcare act in good faith. The market for healthcare isn't only fair; it's the only way healthcare should be provided.

Most hospitals in America operate by this principle in cases of non-emergent care. It's likely that elsewhere in Houston, perhaps at many of the gleaming nonprofits, the doctor in the ER would have taken another look at Roxana's arms, another look at the labs, a third look at whether or not she had health insurance, and told themself, "Well, she's not dying." Then they'd have written out a prescription for Bactrim or maybe clindamycin, unaware that for two weeks' worth it's at least a hundred bucks. They might even have made her an appointment at a primary care doctor's office, or the office of a doctor specializing in infectious disease, and called it a "follow-up," as if the assistants in those offices would open the exam room door when Roxana was unable to hand over an insurance card or cash up front. The ER doctor would then have clicked on the "Discharge" option on their computer screen and moved on.

The terrible part is that in doing this, they wouldn't have been wrong. Even though Roxana's arms showed signs of infection, her life wasn't in danger, at least not yet. Federal law states that a condition like Roxana's should be stabilized, but they could have argued that she was stable. They could have written a note to that effect that, again, wouldn't have been wrong.

This reasoning is a ruse, however, one I've seen hundreds of times.

One of the most prominent features of Medicine Inc. is that it is divisive. If healthcare became corporate in the 1980s, then it has been subsumed by politics in the 2000s. Healthcare today is as much a part of identity politics as any other issue, and yet, at its core, when it comes to the kind of care people like to receive from their doctors and hospitals, there is agreement.

Until we move on from Medicine Inc., we will be stuck in conflict with one another and with ourselves. The real reason an ER doctor at a nonprofit or corporate hospital would have discharged Roxana is because she lacked private insurance, not because they didn't want to help her. She couldn't pay for an admission into the hospital, and so this fact would have influenced their decision. This is the medical world that people without insurance must deal with. They are subject not to medical decisions but to decisions based on whether or not they can pay. The ER doctor wouldn't have been wrong, necessarily, but they wouldn't have been right.

At Ben Taub, people are admitted from the emergency room into the hospital wards based not on whether or not they've earned healthcare, but on the basis of one question: Sick or not sick?

Roxana was clearly sick. Admitting her into the hospital was a no-brainer. At Ben Taub, doctors are able to make decisions based on medical judgment. Whether or not someone has insurance doesn't figure into the equation.

One of the ER doctors told Roxana herself. She would be admitted into the hospital to receive IV antibiotics. Surgeons would examine her to see if an amputation would be possible once the kidneys recovered. An internal medicine doctor, the doctor in charge of making sure she received proper care, would be by shortly. She would, finally, be tended to.

Still, the question hung in the air. How would all of this be paid for? Admitting Roxana into the hospital was the correct medical decision, but it didn't solve the problem that she lacked insurance. No healthcare is free in America. Even safety nets must find ways to pay for it. It was very likely that Roxana would remain uninsured for the foreseeable future. But at least now she could take comfort in knowing that at Ben Taub, she wouldn't be damned for it.

PART TWO

Symptoms and Solutions

Assumptions

When I first started seeing patients as a medical student at Ben Taub, the senior resident on my team received notice from the emergency room that a patient needed to stay in the hospital wards overnight, to receive treatment. He wasn't the type to argue with other doctors over the phone, but it was clear by his questions—"So no fever? And she's totally hemodynamically stable?"—that he wasn't impressed by what the doctor in the ER was telling him. Immediately after hanging up, he grabbed a colored marker and wrote a name on the whiteboard hanging on a wall in our team room. In his North Carolina drawl, he spit out three letters that sent me on my way:

"UTI," he said, capping the marker.

Patients aren't usually hospitalized for urinary tract infections, which may have explained his questions.

Med students examine their patients every day and keep track of how their illnesses progress, but they don't write orders, not even for over-the-counter medicines like Tylenol. Even the patient histories they write must be rewritten by residents, who are above students and below licensed doctors in the medical school pecking order, since only doctor notes, and not student-doctor notes, can be used for billing. It's easy to feel useless in these circumstances. When you're the last in the pecking order, you desperately want to avoid looking bad in front of other doctors, which was why I hurried down to my new patient's stretcher armed with a book summarizing all of internal medicine in microscript—appropriately named *Pocket Medicine*—as well as a folded piece of paper pre-outlined with all the parts of the patient's story I didn't want to miss: "Past Medical History," "Review of Systems," "Allergies," etc.

I arrived to find the Ben Taub ER in full swing, the pace of healthcare—the nurses drawing blood, the techs gathering vital signs, the doctors migrating from stretcher to stretcher in small teams—frenetic. I followed the numbers posted above each stretcher until I landed on the one I was looking for. A young and fit Hispanic man in his thirties sat at the foot of my new patient's stretcher. I introduced myself briefly to him, explaining who I was, before unsheathing my paper and sliding past him to collect my new patient's history.

After a few questions with little response, I could see by the way she moved her eyes why the ER doctor had referred her to us. She was in her forties, broad shouldered and tall, with bushy black hair and wide pupils that drifted from me to a nearby noise or a passing nurse, then back to me, with a saccade, like a typewriter. I thought I must have had the wrong language, so I tried Spanish.

"Ella sólo habla inglés," said the man sitting beside her. *She only speaks English.*

Now it was his turn to field my questions. Instead of short, inattentive nods, I got descriptions, in Spanish, about how frequently the woman was urinating. It was happening so often that she had to wear diapers.

"Since when?" I asked, looking at her. Once more, her eyes drifted and then quickly returned before drifting again. I turned toward the man.

"Is everything okay with her?" I said.

His look—not toward me, but directed at her—said it all. "This is how she is now," he said. When they'd married a few years before, she'd been different. They'd lived the routine life of couples: working, eating together, dancing occasionally. But once the mental deterioration had started, it was relentless. The woman in the diapers sitting beside him was now someone he barely recognized. She looked much older than him, but in fact, they were similarly aged.

I asked him more questions, and soon enough, I'd built a hypothesis in my mind: This woman had early Alzheimer's. Or Lewy body dementia. Or Wilson's disease, where the copper we eat isn't properly processed, leading to buildup in the brain. I referred back to the neuro chapter in *Pocket Medicine* over and again. I couldn't believe that nobody before me had noted such an obvious cognitive problem in the chart. I planned to organize my history around this and not the urinary tract infection— maybe my upper level would feel better about keeping a patient with undiagnosed early Alzheimer's in the hospital.

As I returned to my team room, I happened to run into Dr. Robert Graham, one of Ben Taub's most recognized internal medicine professors. Some residents called him Cowboy Doctor because he was known to visit his ranch near the Hill Country on his weeks off and subsist on the animals he hunted and the tomatoes he farmed. Others were scared of him. Everyone knew that he'd once shot and killed a man who had broken into his home during the night. Not too infrequently, he shared stories of his boxing days as a white kid raised by a Mexican family in Houston's rough Third Ward.

But the real reason students and residents feared him had to do with how he presided over our daily "Morning Report" conference, where we discussed hospital updates and reviewed interesting medical cases. Graham sat with legs crossed in the front row and a Styrofoam coffee cup in his hand while someone presented a case, usually of a patient with puzzling symptoms. Whenever something interesting came up, Graham jotted down notes on the cup—that was always a good sign. More often, however, he interrupted presentations. If a vital sign or physical exam finding sounded incorrect to him, he grilled the presenter to make sure the audience of other students received accurate data. If someone cited a journal article, he pried into how the study had been conducted—"They enrolled only five patients?"—and whether we could derive any real meaning from it. Doctors, he believed, must admit when they're wrong, an insight he'd gained by reading Augustine's *Confessions*. He argued openly and vigorously with other professors, but always with the same calm, measured demeanor. I imagine he shot a rifle the same way. The biggest sin a resident could commit while presenting a case was to obscure findings on purpose for the sake of making a presentation more interesting. Graham cared about truth above all else. Anything less was a dog and pony show to him.

I retold him the history I'd just gathered from my new patient. "Something seems wrong," I said. I kept on repeating to him the part of the story that stood out to me most: "She's still young."

I mentioned the diapers, how her eyes couldn't keep still. I said that this was the first anybody had mentioned her cognitive problems, which grabbed Graham's interest.

"Let's go," he said, motioning quickly toward the computer. He never rushed through the hospital; rather, he pranced, his slender frame springing from the balls of his feet. He sat down and logged in to the system with two index fingers. Fans of eighties movies might have seen a similarity between Graham and Dabney Coleman from the movie *Cloak and Dagger*. That was his look: a cleanly shorn face pegged with a mustache, a polished dome wrapped by a thin rim of hair, and a face that switched between extremes of drama and comedy. I doubt anyone would have been able to guess he was a doctor when he wasn't wearing his white coat, and that was just how Graham liked it.

I gave him the patient's name and medical record number and he began scrolling through the numbers. We still used paper charts for notes, but all the results of blood draws and imaging could be found on the network.

"What's she in for?" Graham asked.

"UTI," I said.

He scrolled through the woman's latest head CT. Then he released the mouse and sank back in his chair.

"Well, I definitely don't think she has early-onset Alzheimer's or any of that other stuff you mentioned," he said.

I began to defend my reasoning, though not too aggressively. "But she's so young," I said. "She can hardly talk. She can't control her urine."

Graham's blue eyes lasered in on me. "This woman has untreated diabetes," he said. "It's caused her to have thousands of small strokes that have killed all these parts of her brain. That's what's causing her dementia."

All I could mutter was something so obvious that it revealed, to a professor, no less, how little I understood this illness. It had never occurred to me a patient would be allowed to get this sick with something so common and so (relatively) easily managed. It had never occurred to me to look up the symptoms of untreated diabetes. "I didn't know it could do that," I said.

For a student attempting to put the science of medicine together with its practice, the revelation was earthshaking. After that day, whenever I went back to *Pocket Medicine* and looked up therapies, an asterisk appeared in my brain with a phrase beside it: "If patient can afford."

That little book had been my Bible. It organized diseases by organ systems, and from there, into the ailments of individual components: hepatitis, pancreatitis, gallstones, etc. I had written myself little notes in the margins in different colors and underlined revelations. How beautiful: a blueprint for how to think and help sick human beings. Under "Change in Mental Status," the book relayed only those causes, like vitamin deficiencies or opiate intoxication, that its writers believed were a danger to a typical patient. There was no listing of "untreated diabetes." The book assumed the "typical patient" would have been treated for it.

Pocket Medicine didn't mention "a life without health insurance" as the cause for any illnesses. In retrospect, that's one of the things I loved about my little book: it described a world where diseases and scientific facts mattered, not policies. In the *Pocket Medicine* world, it didn't matter if you forgot your insurance card or found yourself between jobs. If you had a medical problem, there was a suitable description and there were potential solutions, not just for you, but for anyone who shared the same problems. Everyone was equal in this world.

In a world where everyone has coverage, there wouldn't be a disconnect between the illnesses I read about in *Pocket Medicine* and those I encountered during my training at Ben Taub. Graham told me untreated diabetes was the cause of the woman's dementia, which was true. But if diabetes caused her decline, so did lack of health insurance.

As I spent more time at Ben Taub, I began to see less and less of the world reflected in *Pocket Medicine*. A belief began to take shape in my mind: whether or not someone had insurance impacted their health as much as, or possibly more than, their genetics. As I was wrestling with this idea and the effect it had on so many people's lives, studies were attempting to elevate this very same belief to scientific fact.

In 2017, *Annals of Internal Medicine* published a review of eleven studies that examined the question of whether people are more likely to die if they lack health insurance. Most of the studies were observational, which is to say, scientists did not introduce an intervention: they simply looked at prior data to see how people with health insurance fared compared with the uninsured. These observational studies showed that insurance reduced premature death by as much as 6 percent, which is about as much as taking an aspirin will reduce the chance of dying from a heart attack.

Another study went a step further. It was a randomized control study where a group of people in Oregon were given Medicaid via a lottery. Scientists looked at how this group fared versus other Oregonians who remained on the Medicaid wait list in 2008. The study wasn't able to distinguish whether people died more readily without Medicaid than with it—too few people died during the year the study was conducted to draw any conclusions—but researchers gleaned some important information. Those who received coverage were far more likely to have diabetes diagnosed and managed than those who remained uninsured. The coverage also significantly reduced a patient's financial strain. It looked like insurance helped quell the fire of diabetes, while in the uninsured, the illness burned like wildfire.

Diabetes is a very expensive illness to treat even for people *with* health insurance. The cost of needles and syringes and extra doctor visits as well as work wages lost from visiting the hospital adds up to nearly $4,800 every year on average, according to researchers. For someone who makes the average US salary listed by the Bureau of Labor Statistics, that amounts to a little less than 10 percent of their income. Coverage helps diabetics obtain medications, but even then, the expenses go well beyond what you receive at the pharmacy. The uninsured have a much steeper mountain to climb, and they generally have less income with which to climb it.

According to a 2017 study estimating the economic costs of the illness, one out of every ten Americans is diabetic. Americans spent $327 billion that year on care for their diabetes, two-thirds of which came from government-sponsored insurance. Diabetes is responsible for more than half of all deaths from renal disease, as well as more than 20 percent of what Medicare spends each year on dialysis. Twelve percent of all patients who visit the ER are diabetics, and, even more distressing, 7.5 percent of all the hours spent in nursing homes are due to the effects of diabetes. That was what my fortysomething patient needed now: twenty-four-hour supervision offered by a nursing home. Of course, neither she nor her partner could afford such a cost. The young man, in his thirties, acted as her nursing home attendant, feeding her, bathing her, ensuring she didn't fall or burn herself on the stove. One factor the authors hadn't taken into account when compiling the cost of diabetes was the salary forsaken by family to care for their diabetic loved ones.

Not long after she entered the hospital, the woman with uncontrolled diabetes left. My supervising resident discharged her after starting antibiotics for a UTI we didn't think really existed, since the symptom of urinating on herself was more attributable to her dementia. Our team's most valuable action, apart from normalizing her blood sugar and giving her a prescription for insulin, was to consult the social worker to look for community resources that might provide her partner relief in his role as carer. I never learned if he was able to access that help or if she continued her decline. In fact, I never saw the woman or her husband again.

Over the years, I've reflected on patients like her quite a bit, envisioning how they might be living and getting through their days. I think about whether the woman's husband might be showing signs of age from the stress of providing care, for instance, or if he's even still with her. Where, in what little corner of our city, was she living? Was she dead? These imaginings can lead me to feel sad and useless, at which point I tell myself that Ben Taub can only do so much. A hospital is a hospital. It isn't, as my dad likes to say, the end of the rainbow. In my patient's case, with the advanced state of her disease, Ben Taub couldn't do much for her medically. No hospital could. This was why she didn't spend much time with us. The cells in her brain were already dead. What had once been a controllable, preventable medical problem was now mostly her and her young partner's problem. Because of the care she now required and her partner's lack of resources, this meant it was also society's problem.

I can imagine something different, though. I can rewind her life in my mind the way we used to rewind videotapes and stop at a critical moment. She is in her twenties. She is leaning against an exam table. A doctor stands before her. She isn't happy. Her eyes shift from the doctor to her flip phone. She has just been diagnosed with diabetes. It's pretty severe diabetes, too. Her blood sugar is consistently very high. The doctor tells her about diet and exercise. The scene pauses. What, now, can be done for her? How can we change the ending?

Giving her health insurance will help make sure she can receive insulin prescriptions and checkups. She will still need to afford an average of $4,800 in expenses every year. Will health insurance change the ending? It could.

Let's take it further. What if American assumptions about healthcare didn't apply? What if she were part of a real system, where government wasn't precluded from providing healthcare? In this version of our world, no person is deemed unworthy of healthcare. Here, most doctors make decisions based on medical necessity rather than insurance coverage. In this story, healthcare isn't so expensive, and it's individualized and accessible.

Would her outcome have been different? In all likelihood, the answer is yes.

The following year, I received a page about a patient whose blood sugar was too high for him to leave the hospital. After pricking his index finger and feeding the test strip into the glucometer, the ER staff thought there must have been some sort of malfunction. The machine read "> 499." A normal level is around 80. The patient's glucose level had broken past the upper limit of the scale. Another test confirmed his blood was nearly saturated with sugar. "He can't leave like this," the ER doctor told me over the phone. And so, I descended the stairs dutifully to the ER with a plan of care already brewing in my mind. I would lower my new patient's blood sugar sufficiently to get him home.

I was now a senior resident and Graham was my supervisor. Nothing from the patient's history or physical exam that I performed changed my plan of attack. After organizing the data and historical details into a cogent presentation, I called Graham so he could sign off on the plan. "Be right there," he said.

We met at the patient's bedside, at which point, I launched right in. "Thirty-eight-year-old male, history of uncontrolled diabetes, presents with dizziness and malaise," I started. The words rolled off my tongue. I made sure to take into account some of the nuances other residents might have missed—like the times when he administered insulin, the tribulations he faced having gained so much weight so fast, and his ability to pay for his medicines. I concluded with my assessment and plan: what this patient needed was an even larger dose of insulin than the sizable one he already took at home. I was just about to explain what dose I wanted to give when Graham stopped me.

"Ooh," he said to me like the boss in *9 to 5*. "I'm not sure I'd do that."

He rotated his torso so that he faced the patient in the stretcher, Sam, the thirty-eight-year-old who weighed over four hundred pounds. Now Graham led the conversation. He asked Sam some of the questions I had already asked, like what he ate, but he also asked him *when* he ate, *with whom* he ate, and if he ever found himself feeling extremely hungry after injecting insulin.

Sam's hair was so thick and black it looked like a Russian ushanka hat perched on top of his head. Now, however, he spoke. "I gotta eat," he said.

It was a vicious cycle, Graham explained. Higher doses of insulin pushed sugar into his cells, but they also had the effect of making him hungry, which caused him to eat, which caused his blood sugar to go up again, which resulted in another slug of insulin and more eating, and on and on. Sam nodded.

Graham asked him about his activity level too, not only if he exercised but also who he walked with, where he would go, if he had a bike at his house or a gym nearby.

"I need to find one," he said.

I had planned to keep Sam in the hospital for a few hours or, at most, a day, enough to document a normal glucometer reading. But Graham insisted on keeping Sam in the hospital for at least three days. He needed time to prove his point.

"Your diabetes is curable," he said. "Every hour, I want you to walk around the hospital three times." He turned to me. "No insulin."

I knew Graham delighted in making maverick moves like withholding insulin for a patient with a blood sugar that broke the scales. In retrospect,

I probably didn't argue with him in part because I doubted this plan would work. Sam took nearly one hundred units of insulin a day at home. An average diabetic patient might use ten or twenty units daily, some as many as fifty, but usually not much more. I explained our plan to the nurses.

"Just remind him to walk," I said, "and no insulin."

For two days, Sam walked around the hospital every hour, prodded by me, the physical therapists, the nurses, and Graham. He ate nothing but a low-carbohydrate diet. There was never a need for an emergency snack. And for two days, I documented blood sugars that never went above 110. My fears had been proven wrong. Insulin wasn't the solution. What Sam had needed was a whole new approach to his diabetes. Before he left the hospital, I told Sam to keep up the walking at home.

He smiled enthusiastically. Now it seemed a few strands had broken loose from his bonnet of hair. "I can't wait," he said.

But home might not have been conducive to exercise or a low-carb diet, and that was exactly the problem. If someone in Sam's family brought home fast food one day, could we really expect him to sit at the table and not eat it? In Sam's case, controlling diabetes had even more to do with his life than it did with the medications he received.

I never saw Sam in the emergency room again, and I never heard whether he kept up with this new approach to his diabetes. I never learned whether those three days at Ben Taub helped kick off a whole new ending on his life's videotape. But I witnessed a seemingly insurmountable problem like uncontrolled diabetes—one that routinely made me feel like I was kicking a can down the road—be helped. Graham understood the science of diabetes well enough to opt for a new method. He had challenged the assumptions made by all the other doctors who had treated Sam before him. He hadn't followed the conventions; instead, he had tailored a medical plan particularly for Sam.

To my inexperienced eyes, medicine was the product of three priorities coming together. Everything around me—the CAT scanners and the clean hallways and the glucometers and the armies of nurses and techs and doctors scuttling about—represented science. Science gave medicine its precision. It offered statistics and principles and data. Whenever Graham railed against residents and students for overembellishing symptoms, he was emphasizing the rigors of science.

I wasn't naïve enough to think that science came for free, which was why cost was the second factor. I knew that science wasn't cheap and that costs should keep science targeted and focused. Good doctors figured out the right balance between science and costs.

The third component of medicine was its most basic. I thought of it as people. People were the motivation behind my desire to become a doctor in the first place. Without human beings, there is no medicine, but "people" meant something different to me. I'm not talking about just "helping others," though that was definitely part of it. "People" meant connecting. It meant trying to understand your patient as a complex person, not as a set of symptoms. It meant communicating prognoses and treatment plans clearly, ensuring the patient received the personal service they deserved, and doing so with respect and compassion. In philosophical terms, if science represented the objective, people represented the subjective.

But "people" went beyond practice. How a doctor interacted with their patient was just as important in helping a sick person as the science and the cost, and so "people" includes that doctor's personal imprint, or style. Graham's style had pried out key information from Sam. It had allowed him to evaluate the diabetes with a more precise scientific lens. "People" was medicine's art.

I'd learned much about this from my dad. Once, he delivered a baby while wearing a tux. I was in line for hors d'oeuvres at a Houston Hispanic Chamber of Commerce gala he'd invited me to when I felt a tap on the shoulder. Before I could turn around, my dad was already walking away. "Be right back," he said.

We didn't see him again for almost an hour. My mother and my girlfriend—now my wife—speculated he was just telling his jokes as usual, but no, it turned out that the labor of one of his patients had gone on longer than expected. As he relayed the events to us, I imagined him hunched over like an umpire, wearing a loose gown over that tuxedo. I asked him what his patient thought. The man who loved his profession beyond anything except his family responded, "She liked it," before diving right back into the party.

I wasn't there, but I imagined his style accomplished much of what Graham's had with Sam. Could seeing the tux have relaxed the mother enough for her to push harder? I imagine the woman telling the story to her loved ones: "My doctor delivered my baby wearing a tux." This is why medicine isn't just science. There are always incalculable moments that could tip patient care one way or another. The way a doctor pronounces a word, the way they dress, their accent, the respect, kindness, and compassion a patient does or does not sense in each syllable, even the volume at which someone speaks, all could influence whether a patient decides to take a medication or participate in physical therapy or even undergo a procedure.

I knew that the doctors I admired had perfected the "people" part. A good doctor gave their patient confidence. A good doctor arrived at a diagnosis from taking a detailed history and used specific labs only to confirm their thoughts. A good doctor gave their patient what was needed at key moments, whether it was a hand on the shoulder, a statistic, or, as I learned from my dad, even a well-timed joke. I'd seen Graham connect with Sam as well as with a young Black man who grew up in his old neighborhood. Medicine was as much about how science's message was delivered as the science itself.

I could almost see it as a graph, medicine as the balance between science, costs, and people. Costs didn't matter in the world of *Pocket Medicine*. And they mattered less in countries that directly provided health services, like England, or that provided universal private health insurance, like Canada. In America, I thought, costs mattered as much as science and people:

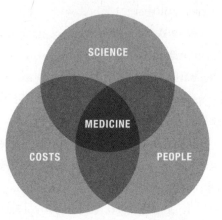

But the more I encountered patients without access to basic care, the more I realized that I had been naïve. In America, costs have become primary. The "people" part of medicine has been relegated to the back seat. *Pocket Medicine* doesn't matter as much as what a patient carries in their pocketbook. That was the problem with Medicine Inc.: it was all out of proportion.

These thoughts gathered steam, sometimes leading to extreme conclusions. Doctors didn't practice medicine anymore; they participated in the healthcare system that developed around them. Doctors didn't serve people; people served as income sources for doctors, hospitals, and middlemen. A new graph took shape in my mind.

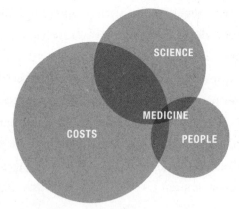

The graph for the uninsured looked different. EMTALA all but guaranteed that the uninsured received science-based treatments in cases of life-threatening emergencies. But for medical problems that weren't emergencies, the uninsured found little recourse. Who they were didn't matter as much as the fact that they couldn't pay. In the uninsured's graph, people had been almost entirely pushed out by costs. The result was that doctors didn't practice medicine on the uninsured so much as provide them healthcare:

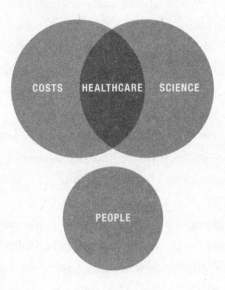

The precise and personal care Graham had given to Sam could only happen in an environment where profits weren't prioritized. It's very unlikely that a for-profit or nonprofit hospital would have allowed Sam to stay an extra two days just to test a method for controlling his blood sugar, especially once records showed normal glucose levels. Even with insurance, Sam would have likely been discharged quickly. Recognizing that insurance wouldn't reimburse the hospital for a diagnosis of "high blood sugar," a seasoned hospital administrator might have called a doctor with administrative and leadership capacities. This doctor, understanding the problem brought forth by the middleman, might then have called Graham. "Are you sure this patient needs to stay in the hospital?" the doctor-administrator would have asked. Graham likely would not have relented, explaining, "I want to control this diabetes long-term." He might, then, have received a page or a text or more phone calls every hour henceforth to check on his progress: "Are you sure this patient needs to stay in the hospital?" "Are you still sure?" And if Graham persisted despite these nudges, he might have received a very different phone call later in the day: "We think it's in this patient's best interest if a different doctor serves him." At which point Graham would have noticed Sam had disappeared from his list of patients. Shortly thereafter, in this scenario, Sam would have disappeared from the hospital: his new doctor would have discharged him. He would have left the grounds with a fleck of blood still coagulating on his fingertip and a new prescription for 120 units of insulin.

Some of my colleagues at Ben Taub who worked previously in nonprofit and for-profit hospitals have had patients usurped like this. They believed it happened because of money. It's one of the reasons they left.

Graham could practice medicine the way he wanted to at Ben Taub. Being there let him give precise and personal care. It allowed him to focus on science and people. Costs were still a factor, but at least they didn't determine his course of action. The safety-net system helped mitigate these costs, as well: the supplies to manage diabetes, which account for much of the $4,800 diabetics pay yearly, were given to patients at a fraction of the cost.

With Graham, Sam experienced the unique care available at a hospital not operating by Medicine Inc.'s principles. Graham had served as his doctor, not his healthcare processor. At a hospital funded by the local government, he had received precise and fair care. There were limits to what a safety-net hospital could provide, but Sam had been given the right measure of scientific and personal attention. In this circumstance, it looked like the circles of science and people and costs overlapped perfectly.

Unfortunately, this wasn't always the case.

Emma adored her only son, Geronimo. As I walked into the hospital room on Ben Taub's sixth floor, her love for him was as obvious to me as the yellow glow he gave off. The glow came from Geronimo's skin and the whites of his eyes. It radiated from the tube coming out of his nose and the canister attached to the wall receiving fluorescent fluid drained from his stomach. Geronimo had jaundice. Old red blood cells, instead of leaving his body, were leaking into his tissues and, in so doing, depositing the bright stain. When illness leaves physical signs like these on the body, marks visible to the world, doctors call it stigmata.

After ten years of working as a doctor at Ben Taub, I had seen plenty of stigmata. I'd seen them in all phases of my education, as a student and an intern, practicing on my own, and now as a teacher to internal medicine residents and medical students. My eye could distinguish different shades of yellow the way that mechanics diagnosed how worn-out a tire was by glancing at the tread. Of course, the jaundice grabbed my attention coming in, but so did Emma. She sat upright beside her son and attended to his every need. She rubbed his swollen feet and massaged the areas around where the morning needles went in. The two had already spent a week in the hospital, and there would be many days more.

She was familiar with Ben Taub and how things worked here, which was to say that she expected me to come by on rounds. Emma spoke no English, but she had been bringing her son here, to Ben Taub, since he was thirteen. Back then, it was for epilepsy. Now Geronimo was thirty-six and one of his major organs was shutting down. She had urgent questions, no doubt, but humility prevented her from speaking first.

"Tienes dolor?" I asked after introducing myself and the medical student accompanying me. *Any pain?*

Geronimo shook his head. It wasn't pain and it wasn't even vomiting. He was having a hard time breathing. That's what was tough. There was weakness, too. He hadn't been able to walk the whole time he'd been here at the hospital, but wasn't that related to his shortness of breath?

I think so, I said. There were so many things going on with Geronimo. The level of salt in his blood was dangerously low. There was fluid around one of his lungs, preventing it from expanding to take in sufficient oxygen. His bowels were paralyzed and his kidneys were slowing down. Every day, the yellow glow deepened, a fact borne out by the numbers. Lab tests showed the bilirubin in his blood trending higher and higher.

We already knew that Geronimo had hepatitis C, a virus that caused liver cirrhosis at rates that surpassed alcohol. Doctors at Ben Taub and its affiliated clinics had discovered it in his blood six years before, and since then, Geronimo had received a substantial amount of treatment. He saw specialists—experts who published regularly on these diseases—routinely in clinic. The safety-net system had provided him with access to liver doctors, evidence-proven medications, even procedures, all ordered in the hope of keeping Geronimo's cirrhosis controlled.

Treating the hepatitis C wasn't possible because of Geronimo's epilepsy medications. Liver doctors feared that if Geronimo added the hepatitis medication, it would put too high of a burden on his already damaged liver. Despite all the specialists' efforts, the illness had clearly gotten out of control.

I listened to the medical student relate these facts to me in a structured presentation—chief complaint followed by past medical history and then past surgeries, etc. It was a format burned into my brain, one I had learned and practiced many times at Ben Taub as a medical student. The history and physical were methodical assessments of events and facts culminating in the "A-P," the assessment and the plan: what do we think is going on, and what are we going to do about it?

Halfway into the medical student's presentation, I already *knew* what was going on. I had seen enough patients like him over my five years of teaching to know what the stigmata meant. Geronimo's liver was failing. In fact, he was dying of it.

As for what to do, I already had ideas. I recognized Geronimo's liver disease from descriptions in *Pocket Medicine*. But my quick judgment about what that liver disease meant came from elsewhere. It happened as I looked past the stigmata, past the yellow in his eyes and his bloated belly, to features I recognized in myself, his black hair, his tanned skin, the angle of his eyebrows, which looked Latino to me.

The majority of my patients at Ben Taub had been Latino. I connected with them every day through my accented Spanish. Despite this, I found myself slipping into stereotypes, particularly when costs made my job as a doctor difficult. Maybe that was why I rushed to judgment. Seeing Geronimo's features and his liver disease triggered a chain of assumptions in my mind: He's undocumented. He's uninsured, I thought. It wasn't long before a third idea occurred to me: We don't have the right treatment to help him at this hospital.

For many years, as I learned and practiced medicine at Ben Taub, I didn't know what the word "rationing" really meant. I had encountered the word in articles and op-ed pieces written about healthcare. I knew that during World War II, the government rationed food and other products, including tires, coffee, butter, canned meat, and gas—and, with it, travel. Americans at the time could only purchase these items on a first-come-first-served basis, or with the requisite coupons produced and distributed by the federal government. The Office of Price Administration, now defunct, determined what Americans could consume, how much, and when. It even had the power to tell Americans not to drive their cars for pleasure. The lines forming outside butcher shops and markets in New Jersey and Texas and Oregon started to look like what we imagined British and even Russian queues looked like. Black markets sprang up. Panics occurred. Mobs waiting for canned meats broke out into fistfights. Police stood inside shops and defused, sometimes violently, the tension of hungry crowds. Americans ate horse meat. These were extremely difficult times.

The idea that healthcare might be rationed like this stirs even deeper emotions. Imagine if a ventilator to supply your or my lungs and body with oxygen wasn't available to us even though we needed it. We might die. During the COVID pandemic, the idea of rationing took on urgent significance. Many doctors wrote articles about the moral distress of deciding to save one person over another.

But rationing, or controlling how scarce resources are allocated, happens all the time. It is an intrinsic feature of supply and demand. We assume that healthcare isn't rationed in this country, but that isn't the case. Healthcare doesn't use coupons or a points system the way the government did during wartime, but for the scarce resources it manages—like primary care and specialty doctor clinic appointments—it uses wait times. Each time we call to schedule an appointment and are subjected to long and winding automations—"Press or say two for billing questions"—we are feeling a tendril of rationing. When finally we schedule an appointment with our primary care doctor on the first available date, in three months, we feel rationing's full force. There simply aren't enough doctor slots to go around, and so we wait in line.

Rationing occurs more insidiously in Medicine Inc. as well. High co-payments for doctor visits and medications are a form of rationing. Insurance companies' denying payments to doctors is another, and so, too, are the low payments Medicaid provides doctors. Only if we are wealthy enough to have our own private doctor and hospital ready at our behest do we not feel the rationing of healthcare in some way.

All forms of healthcare delivery require some form of rationing. It is a necessary evil. The question isn't whether rationing happens but rather how we want it to occur. Do we prefer that corporations or government ration our healthcare? To date, the answer in this country has been, "Anything but government."

I wasn't necessarily surprised to find out that rationing happens at Ben Taub and Harris Health. It had to, especially for a healthcare system that depended on a budget provided by public funds. What surprised me was how that rationing—in other words, the limits of healthcare in the safety net—looked.

For example, consider the way I ordered antibiotics at Ben Taub. Unlike doctors at most nonprofit and for-profit hospitals in Houston and around the country, I don't have the authority at Ben Taub to order any antibiotic that I'd like. The hospital doesn't restrict me from ordering basic antibiotics, like a Z-Pak or Keflex or ceftriaxone. But many more expensive antibiotics require the approval of the infectious disease doctor, who is given authority by the hospital to restrict their use. In this instance, rationing occurs for two reasons: first, to ensure that antibiotics aren't used improperly, because improper antibiotic use can result in resistant infections that can spread to other patients; and second, to ensure that I don't make a wasteful decision and order an expensive antibiotic when a cheaper one would suffice.

The technical term for rationing antibiotics like this is "antibiotic stewardship." Many studies have shown that stewardship and rationing reduce the costs and consumption of the precious and scarce resource of antibiotics. Studies have also shown decreased spread of certain infections and, most important, no increased deaths.

Many therapies and diagnostic tests are rationed at Ben Taub in this way, with medical experts weighing in on the clinical value and financial experts weighing in on the monetary value of each service. Under noncrisis conditions, rationing should achieve the best bang for the buck. Determining what is that best bang, or best value, requires middlemen. At Ben Taub, most of the middlemen who determine that big bang deal directly with patients.

This utilitarianism means that pharmacies at Harris Health dispense mostly generic medications. Some newer medications not yet available in generic form are available, pending an expert opinion on their clinical value.

Most of the time, rationing in the safety-net system manifests through queues. Elective surgeries are rationed through wait lists, some of which can be lengthy, especially when temporizing measures are available that might alleviate a patient's symptoms without providing a cure. Diagnostic tests such as MRIs are rationed this way as well: with fewer machines to perform the tests, queues form. It can take a patient days to receive an MRI. Emergencies are always prioritized, and Ben Taub prioritizes trauma care, which is why many of my patients for whom I've ordered a study must wait.

It's rare that a necessary procedure or test isn't available *at all* within the safety-net system. Patients receive chemotherapies and cancer care deemed standard by the National Comprehensive Cancer Network, but bone marrow transplants, for instance, aren't performed at Harris Health. No transplants are performed. The costs of these procedures—which include the infrastructure and the staff to select, perform, and oversee these interventions' success—would make it too difficult to afford all of the other therapies the safety net offers.

A cruder way to put this is that transplants don't offer great value. This wasn't what I wanted to think when my new patient, at the young age of thirty-six, showed signs of liver failure. All utilitarianism fails when you come into contact with a person left behind by the formula.

And so it was with Geronimo and his mother, Emma. Harris Health offered so much to people in need, but we had reached the limits of the safety net.

Once the medical student finished with his presentation, I turned immediately toward Emma.

"Cómo lo ve?" I asked. *How does he look to you?*

Throughout the history, she had been preening her son, smoothing out his bedsheets, patting his lower back when he coughed. Now she stopped.

"God will protect him," she said, forcing a smile onto her face. She had long straight hair that hit the middle of her back, gray with streaks of black. As we spoke, she began to smooth her beautiful mane.

It was too much to take in at once. I don't mean emotionally, I mean medically. How do you talk about these symptoms? Do you start with the fluid around the lungs? The paralyzed gut? The yellow? I said we wanted to focus on her son's breathlessness for now. Maybe medications would help him pee out some of that fluid. Otherwise, we might have to consider inserting a needle into his back and draining the fluid.

"Bueno," said Emma.

We shook hands again, this time to say goodbye. I nodded toward Geronimo and he nodded back. In the hallway outside his room, the medical student and I spoke more pointedly.

"He's not a drinker?" I said. It was a necessary question. Alcohol is a leading cause of cirrhosis, and Geronimo was in his thirties. Hepatitis C causes liver cirrhosis, but only many years, if not decades, after the initial infection. Some other malady had to be helping the hep C wreak this level of damage on Geronimo's liver, and it seemed reasonable to suspect alcohol.* It would have been foolish to ignore the statistics. But I was also grasping for hope. If binge drinking had damaged his liver acutely, then maybe with sobriety and patience, it would improve.

This wasn't the case.

"I don't think so," said the student. "He says he doesn't drink, his mother says he doesn't, and the notes say it, too."

---

* Today, five years later, non-alcoholic steatohepatitis is recognized as the leading cause of cirrhosis and the most common reason for a liver transplant. We now think that Geronimo's diabetes wreaked as much damage on his liver as the hep C.

"He looks bad," I said. "The liver enzymes keep going up."

The medical student confirmed this with a quick glance at his notes. "Correct."

By a quick mental hopscotch I concluded he was going to die within the next thirty days. He needed a liver transplant, but Geronimo was poor and uninsured. I sighed loudly. If ever there was a therapy that absolutely required a patient to have health insurance, it was liver transplantation. Every transplant center in America utilizes financial officers to verify how patients intend to pay for the procedure. While some centers perform transplants on a charitable basis, these happen only rarely, and they only justify the rule: you cannot receive a liver transplant in the United States unless you are wealthy enough to pay the estimated half-a-million-dollar initial cost out of pocket, or if you have sufficient health insurance. Liver failure is one disease where health insurance determines life or death. People who receive a transplant have a 75 percent chance of survival after five years. Over the same time period, people with fulminant liver failure who don't receive a transplant have a 100 percent chance of death.

The meeting place on the Venn diagram of science and cost did not have room for Geronimo. It didn't matter who the person was in front of me; the problem seemed unsolvable. No insurance, no liver transplant, no life.

Resigned, I checked to make sure my facts were straight.

"I assume he's got no coverage?" I said.

The medical student peered down at me. He was tall with a soldier's haircut and always furrowed his brow while absorbing my questions.

"Correct," he said. "He used to have Medicaid."

"What?"

The notes stayed right at the medical student's side, no glancing this time, just another furrowed brow. "He had Medicaid for a month, then it was taken away," he said.

We reentered the room. It was just as we had left it, with Emma looking after her son and the canister slowly filling, the yellow glow.

"Señora," I said, "did he have Medicaid?"

"Antes," she said, *Before*. She sat down next to her son. "They took it away."

What Emma had just told us was vital for a couple of reasons. First, it confirmed that Medicaid had once deemed him eligible. This insurance had been taken away because he had earned too much. What if his earnings had decreased in the throes of illness? If Geronimo had been covered by Medicaid before, could he receive coverage again?

"We need to get in touch with the social worker ASAP," I said to the medical student. He started to write it down but then just nodded. "We need to see if he can qualify for Medicaid again."

Life was slipping through Geronimo's fingers, all on account of a few extra dollars on a disability check, it turned out. But the fact that he had once qualified for Medicaid brought the hope that maybe Geronimo's life could still be saved. The medical team set out on a journey to find our patient coverage.

Beliefs

In the late 1800s, a philosophy took root in America called the Scientific Charity Movement. The leaders of this movement intended to deal with poverty by applying numbers and statistical analysis. "The task of dealing with the poor and degraded," wrote Josephine Lowell, one of the movement's leaders, "has become a science, and has its well-defined principles."

The movement gathered data about the poor, including what caused 1,407 families in Buffalo, New York, to be destitute. They determined that at least 35 percent of the families were poor directly because of medical problems, including trauma, handicaps, and "insanity." They intended to help the poor in their own homes. Lowell had been raised as an abolitionist and cared deeply about the disparities faced by the poor. At the time, government wasn't able to offer as many expansive services—like disaster relief—as it does today, and Lowell believed that government should play a role only in extreme cases of poverty caused by mental illness severe enough to require institutionalization. Other than that, she felt the responsibility to care for the poor should fall on private charitable institutions.

To better study the poor, the movement classified families as "cases." It applied an accepted scientific principle, Darwin's theory of evolution, to statistics and used caseworkers to classify the poor in two different categories: those "deserving" of charity and those "undeserving." Statistical analysis, driven by social Darwinism, determined how they meted out care.

The result was disastrous. After many years, Reverend Gurteen, another of the movement's leaders, recognized how difficult distinguishing between worthy and unworthy cases could be. More than that, the movement took on extreme ideologies. They proposed castration for the poor so that their inferior genes would not propagate. They used asylums to hold "defective cases." One journalist at the time noted, "The workers in the new charity are active propagandists. They insist continually upon the evils of indiscriminate giving. They assail the public authorities with facts and figures, and the churches with biblical quotations."

The mission at the core of the movement—to help the poor help themselves—seemed innocuous enough. But the group had confused science with belief. They believed government only made poverty worse by helping the poor, and they convinced themselves this belief was scientific fact. The statistics only deepened their beliefs and obscured the moral incertitude of their actions.

The forced sterilization of sixty thousand poor men and women took place in America in large part because of this group's clout. Supreme Court justice Oliver Wendell Holmes, who wrote the decision that legalized the forced sterilizations, echoed the Scientific Charity Movement's ideas: "It is better for all the world if, instead of waiting to execute degenerate offspring for crime or to let them starve for their imbecility, society can prevent those who are manifestly unfit from continuing their kind. The principle that sustains compulsory vaccination is broad enough to cover cutting the Fallopian tubes."

Vestiges of the Scientific Charity Movement remain today. Demanding that patients work to receive healthcare, for instance, is today's way of saying, "Prove your worthiness." The eight states that have approved legislation requiring that patients work in order to receive Medicaid—including Ohio, Arizona, and Indiana—use justifications that hark back to the movement's principles. In 2018, the Trump administration noted that those Medicaid programs that incentivized people to work would help "families rise out of poverty and attain independence." The memo refers to multiple studies that correlate higher earnings with longer life span, giving the recommendation the guise of science. But, in fact, it is nothing more than the merging of two beliefs: that some people are not worthy of medical care, and that healthcare should not be provided by the government.

Healthcare workers in America may not share this belief, but whenever they request a patient's insurance information up front before seeing them, or tailor the therapies they offer according to the maximum an insurance company will pay, they play into it.

A few years after starting his private practice, my father began asking about insurance up front. He felt he had no choice: as his practice grew, and as insurance companies consolidated, the number of uninsured patients who knocked on his door also increased. After looking at the monthly ledgers, he began turning down patients to keep the business profitable. It wasn't something he enjoyed. In El Salvador, during the year he lived as the only doctor in a village, he saw every patient, no matter what, even if they could compensate him with only a few colones or tomorrow's eggs. In Kansas, sending patients away wasn't anything he had to worry about. The people working the front desk did that. But now, as the proprietor of a private practice, and with few employees, the distasteful task fell to him.

In time, he was able to hire people to perform the deed. Eventually he stopped hearing about the uninsured people they sent away. But even as he protected himself from this hard reality, a new issue arose. Aetna and Blue Cross and Cigna began challenging requests for payment: they denied claims on account of improper billing codes or services my dad performed they thought weren't necessary. In some cases, they flat-out refused to pay. Sometimes his staff would prevail after sending letter after letter, but the checks came late. As my dad saw it, the insurance companies were holding on to *his* money.

Billing issues like this started to spill out at the dinner table. One night while I was in high school, I asked him why he had sat down to eat with us still wearing his scrubs.

"There's a woman in labor," he said, the youth in his face momentarily drained. "Not my patient."

At his hospital, all the ob-gyns rotated taking the uninsured women who came into the ER in labor. Evidently, it was his night. Since these women had no access to prenatal care, and therefore no ob-gyn, he rarely received payment for serving as their doctor. His hospital could bill an emergency Medicaid fund, but that usually only covered the cost of their stay in the labor and delivery ward and not my father's work.

Maybe younger and more optimistic doctors considered these on-call nights to be the price of doing business. My dad wasn't there anymore; the losses were starting to show. The man who for years had insisted on wearing a full suit to the clinic when seeing patients had begun wearing scrubs more often. Our life was costly, no doubt. Both of my sisters and I attended private Catholic school through eighth grade and then prep school after that. With the expense of college on the horizon—and not just any university, but a private one with name recognition to help me get into medical school—my father worked more and more. By the time I graduated from college, he never wore anything to the office but scrubs.

"Se aprovechan," he said of the women in labor he met on his call nights. *They're taking advantage, Ricky.*

He could complain all he wanted to his family about these patients and his losses, but we all knew that the moment he walked through the doors of the labor and delivery room to the wails of a woman having contractions, the tension in the room—the pain, the fear—would disappear, and he'd act as her doctor. He'd reach out his hand to this woman respectfully but also casually, as if the two had been friends for years. "Muy buenas noches," he'd say. No doubt, he'd tell a small joke, one that would bring a smile to her face, before diving into the technical parts of his job, twisting the baby's skull a few degrees clockwise, wrenching the miniature shoulder loose and free, checking that the rhythm of the child's heart wasn't too slow or too fast. And after pulling the child from her, he'd announce proudly to the room, in the woman's native tongue, "It's a beautiful girl!" Only after he'd left would she realize how lucky she was to have had him as her doctor. What a nice and competent man, she'd think.

It was and remains my hope that he dropped the weight of business in front of his patients. But I've also experienced the knife of pressure and how it can jar loose words or behaviors that don't represent a person's full body of work, or even their beliefs. I've seen doctors, including some of my colleagues at Ben Taub, address patients with a tinge of resentment, knowing any extra work they poured into a patient would be given pro bono. I've emerged from patients' rooms feeling frustrated, only to realize that I'd let the pressure of efficiency and productivity get to me. Why couldn't you have just chilled? I've asked myself.

My dad is the definition of a people person. Put him in a room with people in it and watch him come alive. Nobody's too meek or too grand for my dad. If they're flesh and blood, then they're his kind.

He loved serving people, but still he detested the losses.

Perhaps he felt something was being stolen from him. Money. Respect, I guess, or opportunities. Who knows? Whatever it was, the feeling was powerful. The idea that he was losing something when he served the uninsured became a part of him. It made a people person rue having to help someone in need.

I don't know how he would've handled uninsured patients elsewhere, but in Houston, he had an out. As he accepted fewer and fewer uninsured patients, his staff began giving many of the women they turned away a piece of advice. They said, "Have you ever heard of a Gold Card?"

The Gold Card isn't health insurance. It isn't Medicaid, Medicare, or Blue Cross Blue Shield. It's not the card you take to your dentist's office or to

CVS. These days, it isn't even a physical card, though it used to be. The Gold Card is more of a concept—it is financial assistance provided by the Harris County community to subsidize healthcare for its residents who can't afford it.

But it's more than just financial help. It's also a gateway to a network of primary care doctors and specialists, many of whom treat insured patients. The Gold Card provides access to affordable healthcare for all Houstonians. It provides entry into a safety-net healthcare system.

Whereas Medicaid allows patients to access any private doctors and services that accept it, the safety-net system is self-contained. Patients can only access healthcare within Harris Health facilities. That is the trade-off: healthcare for all residents, regardless of ability to pay, in exchange for more limited choices.

Medicine Inc. runs according to the belief that the private sector should provide medical services and therapies. The Gold Card represents a different operating premise, that the neediest in the community deserve basic healthcare as much as anybody, and that healthcare is best coordinated by teams overseen by the local government.

In this system, the belief that everyone deserves equal access to healthcare is codified into policy. Everyone living in the county is eligible for the Gold Card. Proof of residency isn't even required, except to receive healthcare beyond emergency treatments. And residency is defined broadly, to admit as many people as possible. In the Harris Health System, a resident is anyone who "has a home or fixed place of habitation that is located in Harris County, Texas."

In other words, to have a Gold Card, one does not also need a green card. Undocumented immigrants like Roxana can receive healthcare at Ben Taub and Harris Health because they reside in Houston and because the funds to provide this care come from local property taxes, not from the federal government.

Texas law assigns county governments the responsibility of providing the indigent with basic health services. Some counties provide more generous services to the indigent than others. Counties are also free to define "indigent" using different poverty thresholds. The state offers guidance on what it considers to be indigent: a person can earn only 79 percent of the federal poverty level—less than $10,175 for a family of one—to qualify. Typically, the county indigent programs provide basic care in primary clinics and the hospital, but limited specialty care. Stricter counties follow this guidance. In 2019, 13.6 percent of the Texas population lived beneath the poverty line, or 394,000 people, only a small number of whom were considered "indigent" by the state's guidance. But Roxana lived in Harris County, which had its own definition of "indigent": Harris Health's program provided financial assistance on a sliding scale for a person earning up to 150 percent of the federal poverty level, or a $19,320 yearly salary for a single-person household.* The specialty care Harris Health provided was also robust.

Roxana hadn't been able to earn a salary for the five months since the surgery. Roxana was indigent, at least by the county's definition, and she had resided within Harris County for decades. She most definitely qualified for a Gold Card.

She greeted me with an outstretched hand, four carbonized fingertips peeking out of fresh gauze, when we met in her room on Ben Taub's sixth floor. After the emergency room doctor recommended a stay in the hospital to make sure the dead parts of Roxana's limbs didn't spread, a member of the internal medicine team wrote admit orders and observed her overnight. In the morning, I became the doctor responsible for her care. "Buenos días," I said, reaching out my hand.

Prior to the pandemic, I shook hands with all of my patients, unless there was a medical or cultural reason not to. In this case, as her doctor,

---

* In response to a budget crisis, Harris Health reduced the income threshold for financial assistance from 200 percent of the federal poverty level—or $24,120 for a single-person household—to 150 percent in 2017. It also enacted a program whereby the health system paid for the marketplace insurance premiums of select patients who no longer qualified under this threshold.

and with the oozing part of her wounds well wrapped, I found none. Her fingers felt like dried pepper husks, only weightier.

I explained who I was and that I had read through parts of her story—about the big surgery a few months back and the dry gangrene in her limbs—but that I wanted to go through it again, to make sure I had it right. She asked me how I knew Spanish.

"My parents are from El Salvador," I explained. "I grew up spending my summers with my grandparents in the hills outside the capital."

She took stock of my appearance and half-smiled. "Sit down," she said, motioning toward a space on her bed by her feet.

I can usually tell someone is Salvadoran a few sentences into our conversation. Beyond some telling colloquialisms—like using the word "*púchica*" to express dismay, delight, or intrigue, and to avoid using a highly recognizable curse word—Salvadorans pronounce consonants by striking the palate with the tip of their tongue a few millimeters behind the tooth line. Spaniards, on the other hand, tap the tips of their teeth with their tongues to create a lisp, while Mexicans press the backs of their teeth. The overall mechanics aren't too different from lighting a match. While some people press the match head against the strike strip with an index finger and drag a flame out, others prefer one swift dart-like motion against the matchbox. Salvadorans pick at their consonants—a few rapid touches on the palate before ripping a sonorous flame. The result, to my ears, is that Salvadoran Spanish sounds like singing. It's an accent I've developed an ear for, though it's not one I can easily reproduce. Some days lighting a fire seems easy. Other days, it feels like I'm running out of matches.

Roxana sounded like a Salvadoran. Listening to her, I could even distinguish that she had grown up in or near the capital. I knew a fair amount about her medical history after having read her chart, but hearing how she spoke opened a window into a deeper history. I asked her who might be helping her at home, the type of food she ate, how she got that food, and what kind of care she wanted at this hospital. I could have used that time to go through a checklist of items, to delineate a family history, for instance. In this case, it seemed like my time was better spent tracing how Roxana's life—the poverty she endured, her spotty access to healthcare, the stress she lived under before the surgery and now—connected to her illness, not her genes.

Roxana had cancer, one that sprang from a blood vessel in her back and eventually coursed into her heart and liver. The surgeons had extracted the visible portions. Nobody knew the cancer's status, but it had likely spread to other parts of her body. Roxana's specific type of cancer, which originated from her blood vessels, couldn't be cured. She would have to live with it for the rest of her life. Now the faithful from her *iglesia* came to cook for her, to spoon-feed her, to prop her torso up every hour or two so that bedsores wouldn't form, to stick a bedpan beneath her, to wash said bedpan, to wash her body, to change her clothes, to make sure she felt human. Of what use was it to Roxana for me to spend even a second asking about her (dead) parents and grandparents? Wasn't it more important to know whether her faithful caretakers were getting paid? Whether they had the energy to keep this up? Whether they were anywhere near giving up?

"I'm blessed," she said. "They help me with everything. I know they're tired, but they don't complain."

Using a stylus crammed between two fingers, Roxana showed me before and after pictures on her phone. Some documented how the death of her limbs had progressed from swollen deep purple to shrunken charcoal black. Others showed her standing at a coffee shop with some friends, her head wrapped in a scarf, her eyes bright.

"This was me," she said.

Over the next two days, as Roxana received antibiotics, and as we considered options for amputations, we talked about illness and faith and life in Houston. We talked about our families. Her daughter's visa would expire soon, she told me. All of the daily responsibilities to keep her alive would fall to the sisters from her *iglesia*. She hoped amputations would make her less dependent on them.

"Y tu familia?" she asked me.

My daughter wasn't yet two, so there was all that, I said.

"Y tus papás?" *And your parents?*

"They're divorced," I said.

The muscles on Roxana's forehead relaxed into a different pain. "I'm sorry," she said. She swung her dead arms in a pivot motion and scooted up in bed. "It's never easy."

During one of our final visits together, I told her I had bad news. While all the doctors were in agreement that there was no more gangrene, the surgeons had opted to postpone her operation for medical reasons. Thanks to the Gold Card, she would receive surgery, but she would have to be patient. They wanted to keep her on antibiotics for some weeks to cool off the infected areas and then see her in clinic. This meant she'd have to go home without the amputations.

Roxana understood the plan, that it made medical sense, though she wasn't necessarily happy about it. It was one thing to have an appointment with a doctor, but it was another thing altogether to pay for that visit.

"No tengo ni cinco," she said. *I don't even have five bucks.* How were the surgeons going to see her with so little money?

I explained that she had qualified for the Gold Card, that it allowed her to visit the safety-net system's clinics.

She nodded warily. "I trust you," she said.

"Patient very worried about not having many people to help care for her at home, and very much wanted surgery now," wrote one of the other doctors.

She returned to her apartment in the back of an ambulance. There, her sisters from *la iglesia* prepared a detailed care schedule—bathing, feeding, washing, changing. A nurse practitioner from Harris Health's house call service appeared at her door one morning to scrutinize Roxana's physical condition as well as her living situation. On the Palliative Performance Scale, a tool used to measure a patient's descent into incurable illness, she rated Roxana only a 10 out of 100 percent fitness, meaning that she required near-total care. On another performance scale named the ECOG, one used by oncologists, she rated Roxana a 4, which meant "Completely disabled, cannot carry on any selfcare." A rating of 5, the maximum on this scale, equaled "Dead."

In spite of this, Roxana made it to the clinic appointments. The new Gold Card allowed her to pay pennies on the dollar for healthcare. Based on her null income, she qualified for the highest level of support, Plan 1, which came with a co-payment schedule: $3 for a clinic visit, $25 for an ER visit, $50 for every day spent at Ben Taub. She paid $24 for a three-month supply of the pain medications that I prescribed. This might seem like a bargain, and it is, but for poor and infirm patients, especially those without income, these costs can mount quickly, which was why a disclaimer accompanied the Plan 1 co-payment schedule: "In the event you are unable to pay the requested co-payment, services will be provided." With the support of her friends from the *iglesia*, Roxana was able to cover her co-pays.

At Harris Health, the Gold Card offered three more levels of financial assistance on a sliding scale—the more you make, the more you pay. In working terms, this means that those earning the Texas minimum wage of $7.25 an hour, working forty hours every week, and living in a household of four qualify for Plan 1, the highest level of financial assistance, and the service is available whether the person is undocumented or not. Roxana's friend—her ambulance driver—had recommended Ben Taub for this reason.

Roxana was scheduled for two orthopedic surgery clinic visits in two weeks ($6 total in co-pays). She attended both of them, which signaled to the surgeons that she was healthy enough to withstand an amputation. They decided to start first with the legs. "Plan for bilateral BKAs [below-the-knee amputations] on next available surgery date," wrote one of the surgeons.

That was on May 20, 2017. She had surgery less than two months later, on July 3, 2017.

Though Roxana waited six weeks for her surgery, it could have been worse. Some patients wait months for elective and nonemergency procedures within the safety-net system. It's a problem with a limited number of solutions. Harris Health has attempted to outsource some of these surgeries to local private doctors, but wait lists continue to grow, especially for conditions considered less urgent, like gallstones. A team of doctors decides where a patient falls on the wait list. More urgent conditions—for instance, bone infections—get priority.

I could have called and argued on Roxana's behalf for the surgeons to push her up on the wait list. Maybe I should have. But I trusted the surgeons' judgment. They knew Roxana well and worked in the same system seeing the same patients as me. I believed they were making fair decisions based on the information available to them.

As Roxana waited, the safety-net system was under threat in Washington. Senators debated a Republican proposal to cut $610 billion from Medicaid in addition to the $839 billion proposed cut by the Republican-controlled House. The bill, the American Health Care Act, represented a repeal of President Obama's Affordable Care Act, passage of which would give President Trump the largest legislative victory of his presidency.

The Affordable Care Act, or Obamacare, attempted to extend private health insurance to more uninsured Americans. According to the law, Americans earning low incomes, or less than 138 percent of the federal poverty level, qualified for Medicaid. Those who earned more than this threshold but couldn't find health insurance through work could purchase private insurance through a marketplace established by the law. The federal government subsidized a portion of people's health insurance purchased through these marketplaces. States were also given the authority to run their own insurance marketplaces.

Safety-net hospitals initially foresaw receiving an influx of Medicaid dollars, but the law lost much of its force when the Supreme Court ruled that states didn't have to expand Medicaid; they could choose to do so or not. Texas chose against expanding the program.

The Affordable Care Act doubled down on the idea that private insurance should be the fundamental means by which Americans receive healthcare. I had supported its passing, in part, because it at least aimed to cover more Americans. I also didn't know any better. When the law passed, I was an internal medicine resident. I had seen quite clearly what lack of insurance and lack of safety-net hospitals did to patients. But I hadn't yet begun to appreciate that government could provide healthcare the way it did at Ben Taub. The Affordable Care Act proposed that government would purchase more people's health insurance, but the law explicitly excluded undocumented immigrants like Roxana. I supported it because I was clinging to the belief that the answer to our healthcare problems would come through private health insurance. I know better now.

Still, though it was flawed, that didn't mean I thought the Affordable Care Act should be repealed. The new Republican bill threatened to harm the people I care for in the safety-net system, and administrators at Ben Taub feared the worst. Though nearly half of the funding for our safety-net system came from local taxes, around a quarter came from Medicaid.

According to Harris Health's vice president of public policy and government relations, King Hillier, such a substantial Medicaid cut would not only have crippled Ben Taub; it would've also redistributed the cost of emergency care for displaced Ben Taub patients to every hospital, including the rich for-profits and nonprofits. In other words, nonprofit and for-profit hospitals depended on Ben Taub. "If we go, they go," said Hillier.

After a journey of six months that took her from one nonprofit hospital to hospice care at home and finally Ben Taub, Roxana entered the operating room right before the Independence Day holiday. She tried to imagine the charcoal-colored legs gone and, eventually, prosthetic limbs in their place to help her move. She took a breath of the anesthetic. The last time she had done so, she'd awakened with dead limbs. Now, as she drifted away, she hoped and believed she would never see those legs again.

The amputation, unfortunately, ended up being trickier than originally hoped.

"Given the extent of the dry gangrene involving the right lower extremity," wrote one of the surgeons in the operative report, "a through knee amputation had to be performed." The team had been hoping to preserve as much bone as possible.

Roxana woke up in her hospital bed to find her legs now ended in stumps. Surreal, bittersweet, joyful, frustrating, sad—the results of her long-awaited surgery were all of these things. Though she was happy to be rid of all the charcoal, it took her a while to get used to the stumps. Shortly after the surgery, problems started to spring up. It started with a fever of 101.4. Then Roxana began shivering. Soon her blood pressure plummeted. The surgeons consulted the internists, who examined the wounds and found yellow fluid draining from Roxana's right stump. "Probable sepsis," wrote one of Roxana's doctors.

It was the right call. Roxana returned to the OR six days after the first amputation, this time to drain away pus that had formed within both stumps. Infectious disease doctors started multiple antibiotics, concerned that the infection might spread throughout her body. But Roxana continued to spike fevers—100.9, 101.7, 102.9. The pain worsened to the point that when physical therapists came to help Roxana adjust to her new stumps, she sent them away—uncharacteristic behavior for a can-do person like her. Even the slightest motion caused her to squeal.

When I visited her in mid-July, I found her in limbo. The infectious disease doctors thought the surgeons needed to amputate more. The surgeons, meanwhile, argued they needed to salvage as much flesh as possible for future prostheses. Roxana was caught in the middle.

Despite this, Roxana maintained her sense of humor. When I removed her bedsheets to uncover the new legs, her left eyebrow shot up.

"Es mi 'new look,'" she said.

I never unwrapped the gauze around her stumps. That wasn't my responsibility. Roxana was under the care of other doctors now. My visits were only to check on her and see how she was holding up.

With other patients taking up my full attention, my visits became more sporadic. Sometimes I would peek my head inside the curtain to find her sleeping, still grimacing in pain. The fevers continued for another week, and the debate about how to proceed tipped toward the infectious disease doctors. New photographs uploaded into the chart showed two stumps that didn't look like knees at all. They were swollen, amorphous. The surgeons decided it was time to get rid of the infection definitively, even if this meant Roxana wouldn't be able to use her knees in the future. Surgeons always prefer for their patients to keep their joints, since it's much harder to walk without a knee. But if Roxana's infection spread up her leg, they might be required to amputate at the hip. "Plan on bilateral AKA's [above-the-knee amputations] on Monday," said the orthopedic surgery note. It was filed on a Friday.

Roxana prayed the entire weekend, as did her sisters from the *iglesia*. Sometimes during my visits, they would evangelize to me. Their method always took the form of explanation: we believe in one God, etc. Roxana expressed her belief much differently. She spoke openly about her faith, never veered away from it, but she never pressed me to explain my own beliefs, not even when things were at their most grim.

During one of my quick stops by her bedside to check in on her, she inquired about my home life.

"Have you visited your grandparents recently?" she asked.

"Not in a while."

Both of my grandparents had recently died, I told her, so there was that. But that didn't explain why I hadn't visited the rest of my family. The violence from the gangs in El Salvador had also grown out of control.

My daughter was one year old. Every year, I volunteered at a rural clinic and spent some weeks afterward hanging out with cousins and touring through my parents' homeland, the volcanoes, the highlands, the beach. Now dead bodies appeared in the roundabouts. I didn't want to expose my daughter to all that, and so I'd stopped going.

"Está muy feo," Roxana said wistfully. *It's really ugly down there.*

Twenty-six years ago, when she had come to Houston, the violence in El Salvador had been different. It was official: two sides, one communist supported, the other authoritarian, engaged in a civil war. Back then, there had been battle lines and territories. The violence today was even more brutal—the homicide rate had surpassed the rate of people dying from fighting in the war each year—and the divisions defied politics. It was barbaric. It was civilization versus the gangs. Roxana wasn't keen on talking about such things because her mother lived near the violence. She pivoted toward a subject she thought I might want to discuss, the op-ed I had written for the *New York Times'* "Sunday Review" section. Using Roxana's case as an example, I had spoken up against the proposed cuts to Medicaid.

"Did the article help?" she asked.

Healthcare was still on Americans' minds. The debate on the Obamacare repeal bill had intensified in the US Senate. While Roxana prayed in her room at Ben Taub, senators readied for a vote. The legislation would have left eighteen million more Americans without coverage. Whether it would pass or not was too close to call.

"I think so," I said. My instinct was to tell her no, that policies like these were determined by lobbyists. That was my belief, anyway. I told Roxana that I'd written the op-ed because it was hard to imagine there being no Ben Taub in Houston.

It would take the dramatic final vote of Senator John McCain to kill the bill—and to save coverage for millions of Americans and the hospitals that care for them. Ten days after Roxana's amputations, McCain had emergency surgery to remove a brain tumor. Still recovering, his left eye bruised, his surgical wound shuttered with Steri-Strips, he appeared on the Senate floor to cast his nay vote.

Was it possible his own healthcare experience compelled him to vote in favor of coverage? Had he felt what other Americans feel when they receive healthcare? Did his neurosurgeon keep him waiting in the ER to verify his coverage before moving him to the OR? Did he receive an $80,000 bill days after the surgery just because he happened not to be "in-network"? Did someone with a badge approach him to discuss deductibles in the moments preceding his life-extending surgery?

Probably not, but I'd like to think that *something* from his experience moved McCain enough to break party lines. Because that was the reality of it—our healthcare problem eclipsed politics. Democrats wanted to extend the government's role, while Republicans were wary of increasing governmental bureaucracy, particularly for people who might not work and, therefore, might not be "worthy" of healthcare. Democrats didn't offer any ways of cutting healthcare costs and making healthcare more affordable. Republicans offered the nuclear option of cutting funding from Medicaid. But didn't everyone agree on the basic idea that healthcare in America made people feel less like people and more like numbers on a spreadsheet?

I'd like to think that McCain realized how lucky he was to have coverage. Roxana was in pain, but she knew what coverage did: it put people in a position to receive help. McCain was a senator and former US presidential candidate, and Roxana was an undocumented Salvadoran woman, but the two shared something in those days and weeks beyond their cancer diagnoses. People had tended to them, thought about them, treated them like the sick and ailing patients that they were, and really, that made all the difference.

McCain died a year later on August 25, 2018. Before his death, he released a statement explaining his decision to forgo chemotherapies and further radiation to his brain. His medical options had evaporated.

Hospitals could no longer meaningfully help him. He died at his home under hospice care.

There were still plenty of ways Ben Taub could help Roxana, and that's what united us. The Gold Card gave her options. That was its power. Her lack of wealth or a green card was secondary to her right to good care. The Gold Card was an acknowledgment that she was a Houstonian. She was one of us.

I left her room fearing the surgeons might amputate her whole leg. I envisioned a bendable prosthesis on one leg, and on the other, a steel rod she would have to swing with each step. But on Monday, another decisive note appeared in her chart:

"Given improved appearance of stumps (decreased drainage, no frank pus) in the setting of lack of fevers in the last three days . . . will defer AKA [above-the-knee amputation] today."

Soon enough, the orthopedic surgeons canceled the operations. It had taken time, but the infection had cleared with antibiotics. Roxana was able to keep her knees. She improved quickly, and within another week, she left Ben Taub for her apartment. At a clinic visit, surgeons expressed even more optimism: "Stump sites healing well; no concern for infection at this time."

The surgeons could now turn their attention to other things: amputating her dead hands, even prostheses. Roxana visited the necessary clinics, every time relying on believers from her *iglesia* to prepare and transport her. Their faith allowed them to give Roxana charity, but I wondered how long it could endure. The rehabilitation doctor referred her to Harris Health's prosthesis maker for new legs, and surgeons scheduled her for a bilateral hand amputation.

Things appeared to be moving.

Stephen settled into his bed at the public hospital. After his nurse gave him the rundown for the night, he picked up the control connected to his bed and began fiddling with it, easing the head of the mattress up and down, checking the lights, clicking through the channels on the small TV mounted in front of him. After a bit, he couldn't help but sigh. He wasn't lonely, per se. People came to check on him all the time, and Stephen, ever the restaurant manager, never missed an opportunity to chat. But this wasn't the burger joint. It was Ben Taub. He wouldn't have a personal surgeon checking in on him, but rather a trainee. His room was no-frills. Not that he was complaining. The bag of toiletries the hospital provided contained a short toothbrush. Hotels didn't even give you that.

All in all, he had to admit that things had gone smoothly so far. He'd made it through Ben Taub's emergency room without waiting too long and without seeing something that left him traumatized. Plus, his interactions with the doctors and the staff seemed fine, if not pretty good. There was the surgeon who hadn't minced words, for instance. Stephen liked that quality in people. He'd said the cancer treatment would likely be aggressive. Just like that: no beating around the bush, no pretending the big ball ballooning from the left side of his neck wasn't what it was, no tiptoeing around the C-word. The woman measuring his blood pressure had been kind, as well. The only downer had been that awful COVID test the nurse had administered. The plan was to wheel him to the OR once that was negative, take the biopsy, and then, finally, treatment. Stephen didn't quite understand why the doctors, and the world, for that matter, were so up in arms about this new virus. COVID, in his never-humble opinion, was a bit of a "fluke." In either case, he felt lucky to get this show on the road.

After watching his last show for the night and sending his last text, he clicked off the light. Immediately, hospital sounds crept into his room like fog rolling in beneath a bridge. He heard footsteps outside his door, machinery. He turned toward the window framing the night sky and turned back, over and again. It was going to be a long night. A question hung in the air: How did he get here?

He had always been healthy. Years back, his wife had made him visit a doctor after the sudden death of her brother made her newly wary. Stephen arrived at the doctor's office for a routine physical and the staff had to dig his records out of storage. That's how rarely he used his insurance.

He'd quit the smoking and the drinking. The gambling. It really felt like things were back on track. They had been for years.

The gambling. That was definitely one of the things that had landed him in here. Coming out of college, he'd joined the family business: dry cleaning. To teach his son responsibility and to help him develop a good business sense, Stephen's dad leased him a few stores. It was good money. He bought the family a house, himself a Land Cruiser, his wife a Sequoia. Every month, he would buy $300 worth of Texas Lottery scratch-offs and not think twice about it. But, man, would he bitch about the $700 a month that went to insurance, to the point where he dropped it completely, not just for him but his whole family. That was in the mid-1990s, when his son, Jamie, was just a child. If not for the pinch he eventually felt on his taxes after the Affordable Care Act passed—the government fining him for not having insurance—he would never have re-upped. Now, looking back, going so long without opting into insurance seemed insane and ignorant.

Tough love. That's what had gotten him through the last dark spot in his life, the tough love a parent shows a child. Stephen's dad had caught him red-handed. One puny little trip to Lake Charles had turned into a monthly trip, then every other week, then each Friday. It wasn't long before the casino set out markers at the roulette table, five thousand in chips, waiting there just for him. He couldn't walk away while he was up—that was the sad part. He was a good loser and a terrible winner. Getting up $15,000 early often meant that, by the end of the night, he'd played until he'd written a check for five thousand. Eventually, his dad caught Stephen taking deposit bags out of the safe at the dry cleaners.

"We can fix this," his dad insisted, after the emotions receded and the awareness of what this all meant—his son, a gambling addict—sank in. His dad did try. But addictions are stubborn. Bills didn't get paid. There was also the issue of grandchildren. Not even a year had passed since Stephen's second child was born. His parents had been forced to ask themselves: Are we enablers?

His dad took the leases to Stephen's dry-cleaning branches back. For six months, Stephen earned $800 per week from his father to help these businesses transition to a new owner. When it was all over and the businesses were safely in another's hands, Stephen's dad spoke frankly to him: "You need to find a job."

Tough love made him ask for a job at Cicis Pizza. Tough love kept him plugging away, day after day, until he began managing the burger joint. Tough love had saved him before. Could tough love help him get through his cancer?

He wasn't a fan of the idea that government was subsidizing his care at this hospital. He still believed in capitalism. If a hospital in Beverly Hills charged people $20,000 a visit, and people paid it, who was he to interfere? Let the market decide. But that same market had recently decided that Stephen was no longer of use as a restaurant manager. He hadn't been able to work there for nearly a month due to his illness. When the burger joint furloughed him, Stephen asked his dad for advice. He didn't want to take a handout, but he also needed money, and he was sick.

"You need to find someone on disability," Stephen's dad told him. Get the inside scoop, he meant, learn how to milk that system. In the meantime, Stephen gained access to a different handout. It all had happened so fast, over the last month, since the beginning of all this COVID pandemonium in March 2020. He had already started to collect an unemployment benefit of $520 every week.

Now he was here at this public hospital, waiting to have his tonsil biopsied. Rock bottom, so far, hadn't been as bad as he'd initially thought. People had been kind to him. No one had stopped him in the emergency room and told him to go elsewhere for his care, like they had at the nonprofit hospital. It felt like he was on track for a diagnosis and treatment. He didn't like the idea that the government was providing his healthcare, but at the moment, he would take what he could get.

I've heard variations of Stephen's old belief over the years. How if we extricated government from healthcare, the market would resolve the problem of expensive medical care in America. How government not only shouldn't provide healthcare; it should divest itself altogether from it and desist most, if not all, regulation of hospitals and insurance and pharmaceutical companies. Government, the thought goes, causes more problems in healthcare than it solves.

In a way, it makes sense. There are certainly examples of specific governmental actions that led to healthcare's becoming less, not more, affordable. The federal government's decision to adopt fee-for-service within the Medicare and Medicaid programs is one. Another is the "noninterference clause" that prevents the federal government from negotiating the price of prescription drugs for Medicare recipients.* Just taking into account these two rather large failures, it would be tempting—though not necessarily logical—to conclude that government has no place in healthcare and that Americans should obtain healthcare through a barely regulated market.

However, examples of the federal government providing healthcare adequately and efficiently do exist. For instance, in 2018, researchers compared the quality of care at Veterans Affairs hospitals, which are funded by the federal government, versus similar commercial hospitals, including for-profit and nonprofit. The researchers compiled hospitals' Patient Safety Indicators, which are statistics showing how a hospital performed in key circumstances. These include rates at which patients develop pressure ulcers or infections from catheters, or even the rate at which patients die when they're not supposed to ("Death Rate in Low Mortality Diagnosis Related Group"). The data, published in the *Journal*

---

* The Inflation Reduction Act of 2022 will allow Medicare to negotiate the price of ten high cost drugs in 2026, and as many as twenty in 2029.

of General Internal Medicine, showed that staying at a VA hospital was just as safe as or even safer than staying at a commercial hospital. A lower percentage of patients with a diagnosis of heart attack, heart failure, or pneumonia were readmitted within a month to VA hospitals compared to non-VA hospitals. Furthermore, the safety measures showed a lower percentage of patients who died from heart failure at VA hospitals. Finally, the study showed how VA clinics met safety metrics in the care of diabetics and people with high blood pressure better than clinics relying on private insurance, including Medicare. The study seemed to indicate that the government could adequately provide healthcare.

Two other things stood out from the study. First, the VA hospitals performed significantly worse in patient experiences as compared to the hospitals running on health insurance. In particular, patients at the VA felt the management of their pain wasn't adequate. And second, the quality of hospital care and patient experience varied widely across the different VA hospitals in the study. This seemed to dispel the notion of one standard monolithic governmental healthcare practice. According to the data, each VA hospital operated nearly as differently from others of its kind as it did from private hospitals.

And they certainly cost less. One study performed by the Congressional Budget Office in 2014 found that the full range of services performed at VA hospitals would have cost 21 percent more at private hospitals if hospitals and doctors billed Medicare. The cost would have been far higher for patients with private insurance.

Right now, Stephen didn't mind the experience. He needed healthcare. He needed treatment. He needed to get back on his feet. He had been stuck in the quagmire of the insurance racket, but now things appeared to be moving. If only he could settle down and sleep. Was it possible that the public hospital—that the government—could help him help himself?

Financial counselors visited Stephen in his hospital room while he waited for the surgeons to perform a biopsy. He presented all the necessary paperwork to prove he was a Harris County resident, including a valid photo ID, a utility bill showing his name and address, and his gross income for the last thirty days. Since he had been furloughed, Stephen's income didn't amount to much. Harris Health also used his assets—including the house he owned—to determine whether he qualified for financial assistance.

The tally of Stephen's assets with his unemployment benefit put him beyond the threshold for assistance. After the biopsy, he could continue to receive care at Harris Health clinics, including with the surgeons who operated on him, the financial counselors said. But he would have to commit to pay out of pocket, full price, for his care.

He was released home two days later, after surgeons removed both tonsils. Both were found to have cancer. A CAT scan after the operation showed surrounding lymph nodes with some remnant cancer. The ENT doctors presented Stephen's case in a meeting at Ben Taub attended by oncologists and radiologists and other cancer specialists. Everyone agreed that the proper treatment for Stephen's synchronous cancer of the tonsils that had spread to his lymph nodes was a mixture of chemotherapy and radiation. A few of his teeth would need to be extracted by dental surgeons as well in order to avoid an infection. Doctors spelled out this plan to Stephen a week after the biopsy results had been finalized. They were ready to begin treatment, but one item remained: payment.

For the second time, a financial counselor spoke with Stephen at the clinic. She had put together a very rough estimate of the cost. Considering the price of radiation therapy, chemotherapy, and doctor visits, the total figured to be at least $15,000, an amount much lower than what other hospitals charged. Could Stephen make a down payment of $5,000 now?

Stephen touched the rubbery ball beneath the skin of his neck. Here, again, was tough love. It was a jolting figure. Some people might wonder why anyone in this country would have to pay so much for treatment. But Stephen understood it differently. He didn't mind paying, so long as he wasn't being ripped off. He had received a biopsy, a diagnosis, and a thorough plan for how to treat the cancer on his tonsil before anyone had asked him for money. Now the chickens had come home to roost. He logged into his savings account. The balance made him laugh: $5,200. Was this a sign from God?

He resolved to pay the balance in full. After transferring the down payment, Stephen started himself on a plan to pay Harris Health $500 each month—a sizable amount, but one that, to Stephen, seemed fair. Every doctor visit would add $95 to that total, which he didn't mind, as long as the monthly payment amount stayed the same. Other costs would be added to the total as well, including the insertion of a feeding tube, which was necessary after the radiation made it too painful for Stephen to swallow.

There were complications, too. Stephen developed an infection on the left side of his neck, for which he received antibiotics for a week at Ben Taub. Due to the recurrent infections, oncologists weren't able to give the full dose of chemotherapy. The pain grew so unbearable that he began seeing pain specialists, who treated him with tablets of morphine and Norco. Despite the antibiotics and the radiation and the chemotherapy, the rubbery ball on his neck kept growing. In August, four months after starting treatment, doctors decided something more radical might be necessary: a surgery to remove all remnants of the cancer.

At the same time, Stephen received some bad news. The burger joint had converted his furlough into termination. With his cancer at such a stage, he couldn't work, and so he decided to apply for disability, something unimaginable to him just six months before.

Through it all, at least the safety-net system made him feel worthy of the treatment it offered. It had calculated what he owed according to how much he could pay. It was a public hospital, funded by the government, yet it seemed personable. So far, this public hospital had exceeded his expectations. A big surgery, however, awaited.

— 9 —

Misperceptions

Christian wasn't sure what he'd gotten himself into. He sat in the waiting area of what looked like a fancy clinic in Monterrey, Mexico. Everything was white: the stucco walls, the porcelain-tiled floors, the nurses, too. They wore white scrubs, white lab coats, white tennis shoes, white masks, white gloves. Sometimes while waiting for his name to be called, it seemed like he was back home in America. Many of the people sitting with him were white.

The clinic might have been upscale—visitors were encouraged to use the private pool outside—but the people inside were sick. There were teenagers without a trace of hair on their scalp or above their eyes. There was inconsolable crying. There were wheelchairs. Christian rubbed his knees. It was one of the benefits of wearing khaki shorts, putting warm hands directly on achy parts. A man dressed in a suit came in. He shook hands with some of the doctors and left. Was he a politician? Christian sat patiently, hoping the knee pain wouldn't flare up again. This place looks like a science lab, he thought. I don't know if I belong here.

Where did he belong, then? He had already left Houston in search of a diagnosis. He hoped his money would go further in Mexico and would buy him more attention and personalized care. The doctors in Tampico, however, had told him they couldn't help him with his kidney disease because it was chronic and he wasn't a resident of Mexico. When Christian reported this back to his mother, Norma, she reached out to family members for advice. She combed through the internet. She didn't have a doctor to consult. She considered previously unaffordable options. Why not send her son to the Mayo Clinic? If there was any-one who could tell her why he was having such terrible knee pain and kidney problems, it would be someone at Mayo. She read about clinics in Europe. The family took inventory of what they could spend. The Garzas weren't rich, but it didn't matter. Norma and Christian's stepfather would just have to work harder.

Christian's nephrologist in Tampico mentioned a clinic nearby in Monterrey where he could pay out of pocket for the service he received. This seemed to be the best option, since Norma had family there. Plus, people on Facebook seemed to love the place. The clinic's website offered packages that included medical care, doctors' fees, and transportation to and from the airport, but also a nice two-bedroom apartment while patients were in the city and excursions to local points of interest. We don't need any of that, Norma thought. She negotiated the most afford-able package—medical care and doctors' fees—and told Christian to get on a bus.

The seven-hour trip was hard on his knees, but Christian arrived in Monterrey with renewed hope. The very next day, he made his way to the Hematology Outpatient Services clinic—that's its name, no Span-ish original—in the southwest part of the city, near the Los Doctores neighborhood. He registered at the front desk, took his seat among the sick, and waited for his turn.

"Garza, Christian?"

Christian knew the clinic offered stem cell treatments, but he learned much more through the process. "The injections were in the butt," he later told me. They happened once, maybe twice each visit. Each therapy also included an extraction, which meant another needle inserted into the gluteal region. "What he took out looked like apple juice."

Nobody promised him a cure. The doctors were very clear with him. The stem cells were intended to slow down the kidney disease, that's all. Christian wasn't sure what they told the other people in the waiting area—those with cerebral palsy and autism and chemo-resistant leukemia—but the doctors didn't pretend the therapy would do anything for his knee pain. He appreciated the time and attention the doctors gave him.

What could he do? At a weekly cost of 3,500 pesos, or $400, and compared to the endless phone calls with the doctors and insurance companies he'd experienced back home—all so that doctors could do little more than brush over his symptoms—it seemed like the logical next step.

"We're willing to take the risk," said Norma.

The Garza family was looking for relief for their son. Like many who visit stem cell clinics, the problem they were experiencing had overtaken their lives. They wanted to make sense of Christian's knee pains, pains that hadn't been explained or treated by the routine care they'd found at home. The stem cell clinics offered hope when they felt they had few other options.

A 2018 article in the *Journal of the American Medical Association* identified 408 crowdfunded campaigns from the months of August to December of the preceding year that requested a total of almost $7.5 million specifically for stem cell therapies. (GoFundMe doesn't publicly share how many health-related campaigns it hosts, but YouCaring reported more than 62,000 at the time of the study.) What Norma and Christian knew about stem cells—that maybe miracles could happen—wasn't any more or less than what most people knew. They didn't buy into them as a God-given panacea, but they weren't totally skeptical either.

Nobody knows how many stem cell clinics there are in the United States, let alone in the world, since there is no authority overseeing these clinics, no registry, and no regulating body. The Food and Drug Administration hasn't yet approved stem cell treatment and likely won't for many years, if ever. There is simply no evidence that stem cell therapy works.* There is no evidence that it's safe. The potential to cure some of our most distressing illnesses with these cells remains theoretical, the way that a world run solely on renewable energy is something to strive for but not yet possible today. This hasn't stopped doctor-entrepreneurs around the world from opening clinics and charging patients cash for harvesting and injecting stem cells.

What will become of stem cell therapies—whether they'll prove to be a legitimate treatment or modern-day snake oil—remains to be seen. The surge in the number of these clinics, however, tells us something about how people like Christian and others feel about healthcare in America. These clinics fill a need. Stem cell clinics don't deal in cures as much as they do in hope.

"They cater to people whose needs reach beyond the powers of current medicine—people who want to believe in the almost mythic powers of stem cells, who feel corporate health and science have forsaken them," writes Erin Allday, a journalist for the *San Francisco Chronicle* who investigated public funding for stem cells and the for-profit clinics that administer them throughout California, including in Beverly Hills.

Stem cell clinics are only one example of how those who feel forsaken often seek alternative and unproven therapies that can be harmful. According to a study in the *New England Journal of Medicine*, at least 24 percent of Americans were hesitant to accept the COVID vaccine during the pandemic. Many demanded unproven therapies like ivermectin and hydroxychloroquine to prevent or even treat the virus. How these therapies were presented, and by whom, made a difference in whether patients wanted them. One study found that more than 40 percent of Latinos, and more than 50 percent of African Americans, preferred to receive the vaccine in their primary care doctor's office as opposed to

---

* Stem cell transplants have long been used to treat leukemia. But use of stem cells for purposes other than creating new bone marrow hasn't been proven to be effective.

places like pharmacies, which may explain some people's hesitancy. Anecdotally, many primary care doctors who refused to prescribe ivermectin noted far less animosity with patients they had built a relationship with as compared to those they'd just met in a drop-in clinic.

What this tells us is that without trusted doctors to guide them, patients are left rudderless in an ocean of high-tech remedies. Science is a language, one that can be difficult to understand. Doctors should serve as science's translator. But for those without good private insurance, and therefore without consistent access to a doctor with whom they can build trust, this important role isn't always valued: doctors are reimbursed for the services they perform, not the advice they give. The result is that patients often must interpret science by themselves. As a result, they can make misguided choices.

There wasn't a doctor in Houston willing to help Christian puzzle through the mystery of his knee pain. His rheumatologist focused on her own specialty and missed Christian's kidney disease. When she ordered a test that could have helped with the diagnosis, insurance companies interceded. He traveled to Mexico because care was more affordable there, but also because it was more direct and personal. Unaware of how science could and couldn't help him, he drifted until he happened to slip into the hands of an attentive snake-oil salesman—into a stem cell clinic.

A few weeks into the therapy, Christian felt like his overall health was improving. He felt happy for the first time in years. He couldn't really tell how his kidneys were doing, other than to say that he was peeing and didn't feel nauseous or swollen. The knee pains hadn't returned. Sometimes he allowed himself to think that maybe he had turned the corner. But the payments took a toll. After a month, Christian and his family decided it was time to come home, and so a few days before Halloween, he boarded a plane from Monterrey to Houston. The ninety minutes in the air weren't as tough on his knees as they were on his sense of security. Christian had felt comfortable in Mexico. He'd found doctors who listened to him and treated him with respect. Sure, his butt hurt from the injections, but he'd found some relief. What would happen back home?

Christian thought about going back to work. He had been on sick leave throughout his treatment. Even though he had health coverage at his current job, his coverage wasn't enough to address his problems. He'd already been down that road. He needed better health insurance, but more than that, he needed a doctor willing to interpret the science for him.

Two weeks after he arrived home from Mexico, "the shit hit the fan," as Christian later put it. The knee pains came back with a fury. His job let him go. He lost his health coverage. When the pain became unbearable, Christian started visiting emergency rooms and urgent-care centers again. Each time, he felt more like a product being processed than like a patient. The bills mounted, only this time, they were higher than the ones from the stem cell clinic. The Garza family thought Christian would qualify for COBRA, which is a health insurance program that allows people who've lost their job to continue their old plan, so long as the person covers the portion of the monthly payment that their old employer had previously paid. The insurance company balked. By law, they weren't supposed to: the Affordable Care Act precluded insurers from denying patients coverage due to preexisting conditions. Some people have claimed they've been denied coverage illegally, which is to say that the insurers have found work-arounds. In Christian's case, the insurance simply stopped returning Norma's calls. When she at last found someone to speak to, they explained he was no longer within the time window. Norma felt they had run out the clock on Christian's application.

Christian applied for Obamacare. He and Norma got all the paperwork together and started to work with a navigator, a counselor paid by the federal government to help uninsured citizens find healthcare plans. While the Garzas waited for the paperwork to clear, he kept visiting doctors in ERs and urgent-care centers. Most observed him for a few hours and sent him home. Very few talked with him about his kidney illness.

One doctor at an urgent-care center, however, was worried enough by the results of Christian's blood tests that he admitted him into a local nonprofit hospital. There, doctors performed a kidney biopsy. Christian was released before receiving the results.

The navigator struggled to find the Garzas a health plan. For some reason, none of the insurance companies offering Obamacare plans wanted to take Christian on. Norma felt that they were denying him coverage based on Christian's preexisting condition. Finally, the navigator advised Norma to negotiate with Blue Cross Blue Shield directly for coverage. Norma spoke with a representative and filed all the necessary paperwork. Again, she and her son waited. Weeks turned into a month.

The results of the kidney biopsy only made the Garzas more desperate for coverage. The doctor who had admitted Christian to the hospital confirmed that the kidney looked severely damaged underneath the microscope. What should have appeared like a cross section of pipes, with the mouth of each tube nice and round and distinctly organized, now looked like a smear of salmon-flavored cream cheese. The walls of the tubes had collapsed. Filtration depends on flow and flow depends on steady, unfettered movement. It was obvious looking at Christian's kidneys that very little of his blood was being filtered.

Christian's kidneys had started to fail. When the doctors looked at the piece of Christian's kidney with an electron microscope, they saw something that shouldn't have been there. Little round discs that looked like zebras appeared inside the kidney cells ("lamellar bodies" is the technical term). The doctors saw plenty of biopsies of kidneys wrecked by high blood pressure and diabetes and lupus. Zebras, however, were rare. They were so rare that the doctors wondered if these zebras could be the key to unlocking the mystery of Christian's knee pains.

"I think you might have Fabry disease," the doctor told Christian over the phone. It had taken just shy of seventy months and a voyage to Mexico to arrive at this diagnosis. Even with health insurance, Christian had to bounce through hospitals like a Ping-Pong ball before finding a doctor willing to give his odd symptoms the time and attention they demanded. After all, time is money in American medicine.

Fabry disease is a rare sickness, occurring in one out of every forty thousand men. Little recycling bins inside cells called lysozymes need a molecule called alpha-galactosidase to help sift through old proteins and repair damaged cell structures. In Fabry disease, this molecule doesn't work well, leading to a buildup of fat. This fat—or lipid—sticks on blood vessels in layers, giving them black-and-white stripes. The zebra stripes corrode blood vessels in the kidneys; they can also damage nerves, leading to the type of burning pain that Christian so often felt. The condition is caused by a genetic defect located on the X chromosome, meaning that Christian had likely inherited the illness from Norma.* Sometimes, medicines can be given to replace the faulty molecule. "You should see a geneticist," the doctor advised.

As difficult as it was to diagnose Fabry disease, this had been the easy part. Now the Garzas had to deal with the next difficult step: they had to visit a specialist without coverage.

Norma knew what to expect. They were back to paying cash, just like at the stem cell clinic in Mexico, only this time, cash only got them so far. The genetics clinic wanted $600 just to step in the door. Norma paid it. The two went to the clinic, and again, they were unable to see a doctor despite having paid the fee. A nurse practitioner explained that the tests they needed cost a minimum of $2,000 apiece. She recommended that Christian wait until he received coverage. "Unless you can afford it," she said.

Another $600 down the drain, thought Norma. She particularly didn't like the attitude she received. "Unless you can afford it." Who in the real world can afford prices like that?

---

* Since men have one X and one Y chromosome, X-linked genetic disorders affect men more than they do women. Norma didn't have Fabry disease because she had another X chromosome to balance out the one with the defective gene. Presumably, she passed the one with the faulty gene to Christian.

Norma called the health insurance company. What was the holdup? she asked. Why were they taking so long to review her son's case? She got the runaround. Finally, toward the end of the year, an insurance agent gave her the news. The company wouldn't be offering Christian coverage. "We'll try again next year," said the insurance agent. She made it sound so simple.

Christian and Norma felt like they had tried almost everything. They had one option left, but they hesitated. They didn't think of themselves as the kind of people who took handouts. That was for others, for poor people. Still, what other options did they have?

"What about Ben Taub?" Norma asked her son.

Ping-ponging back and forth from doctor to doctor, hospital to hospital, insurance to insurance, as an illness goes untreated happens all too often to patients in Medicine Inc. To receive good medical care that is streamlined and straightforward, multiple factors must come together. Depending on how someone receives insurance, a patient has to make sure their job remains steady, or has to stay married, or has to make sure they earn enough for co-pays and treatment. Any disruption of this delicate order can result in the illness's running rampant. To make things worse, this tightrope walk often happens at a time of great bodily upheaval, when the person is at their most vulnerable.

Doctors can help us navigate toward a diagnosis and the right treatment, and many do, but the American system incentivizes them to look away as soon as a patient falls off the insurance tightrope. As a result, some doctors can disregard their patients' needs.

Nearly a week into her hospitalization, in May 2017, I met Ebonie in her labor and delivery room at Ben Taub. Things were still touch-and-go. Even though the bleeding had slowed down considerably, she continued to spot. Additionally, Ebonie was having early contractions, a sign she might have been close to delivering. At nineteen weeks into the pregnancy, however, the fetus had a very low chance of surviving outside her body. Ebonie was determined to see the pregnancy through. Her obstetricians at Ben Taub wanted to make sure she could go forty-eight hours straight without any bleeding before releasing her from the hospital.

When I knocked on her door and introduced myself, she opened her eyes slowly, possibly an effect of the magnesium dripping into her veins to slow down the contractions.

"Would you like me to come back later?" I asked.

"No, I'm good," she said.

I sat in a chair beside her hospital bed and immediately took note of Ebonie's appearance. She had a nose ring and numerous tattoos on her arms and neck. Her standard-issue hospital gown bulged in different areas of her belly where electrode pucks captured the heartbeat within. The heartbeat monitors hung in unusual parts of the room, emitting blips at a different pitch than I was used to.

Labor and delivery wasn't a section of the hospital I visited too often. Working as a hospitalist over the previous seven years had taken me to Ben Taub's far corners, from the ER to the cancer ward to the dialysis unit and back again, but never to labor and delivery. Obstetricians cared for patients there, not internists. But Ben Taub had become my first window into the big healthcare problems of the day, maternal mortality being one of them. With so much attention on the spike in maternal deaths, I had reached out to one of my colleagues, Carey Eppes, the chief of obstetrics at Ben Taub, to see what she knew about the problem. "I have a patient I'm really worried about right now," Carey told me. "Let me ask her if she'd be willing to talk with you."

I also had personal reasons to look into the maternal mortality spike. Six months prior, right before Christmas, my wife had given birth to our first child. While we'd considered using Ben Taub for the delivery, my wife and I decided that our presence, as minimal as it might have been, would add extra stress to an already strained safety-net hospital.

How would our whims affect someone in line behind us without any-where else to go? We didn't want a fancy hospital, and so we selected a nonprofit safety-net hospital. My wife and I walked into it like so many first-timers, with a mixture of nerves and glee, totally naïve to what lay ahead. It all changed when the obstetricians administered Pitocin to ramp up my wife's contractions. Not only could I see pain in her eyes, but I also saw the fear that pain caused.

After an epidural and fifteen hours of labor, my wife gave birth to our daughter. Immediately, we doted on this new wonder. We listened to her tiny gurgles and cooed and rocked her back and forth in our arms. So enraptured were we that nobody noticed the monitor beeping. This wasn't the fetal monitor, whose electrode pucks and wires lay in a pile on the floor. This was the monitor connected to my wife.

"I feel a little dizzy," she said. Her blood pressure had dropped sig-nificantly, and her pulse was climbing. Her first instinct had been to attribute the feeling of light-headedness to the new ecstasy of mother-hood. But then a full thirty minutes after the birth, she grabbed her chest. She couldn't breathe. Darkness closed in on her. "I can't see!" she said.

I had resolved to check my medical impulses at the door during my child's birth. I didn't want to be the doctor dad looking over the obstetrician's shoulder. But I couldn't turn a blind eye to the frightening numbers blinking at me: 72/40, 138. I took the Call Nurse button from her fingers and hit it over and again. Then I went into the hallway. "We need a doctor in here now," I told the first person in scrubs I saw.

"What seems to be the problem?" said the covering ob-gyn.

I went straight into doctor talk.

"She needs a bolus, probably two," I said, pointing at the blood pres-sure reading. "Normal saline, LR, whatever you got, she needs it, now."

The doctor returned with a nurse, who immediately rushed a bag of saline into her veins. Over the next minutes, she regained her vision and began breathing normally again. The shock of delivering the placenta had caused her blood pressure drop, her doctor later decided, in what's called a vasovagal reaction.

Thankfully my wife recovered fully. Later that night we stayed up, the first of many nights with our daughter, tending to her loud wails, soothing her (my wife more than me, of course). But this moment of peril stuck with me. It was only a moment, and how lucky we were for that, but it remained a part of me like the drop of a roller coaster. I couldn't help but deconstruct it all. What if I hadn't been a doctor? What if my wife had been alone? Was it possible she could have been shouting and shouting with no one to answer her? What if she had been African American? What if, instead of my wife's being *doubly* insured that day, she'd had Medicaid? Or no coverage at all? Was there anything in my wife's recent experience that could clue me into why the maternal mortality rate was going up in our state?

Ebonie was no stranger to terror during pregnancy. In 2002, when she was nineteen, her then-boyfriend strangled her until she lost consciousness, and her body began to shake uncontrollably. The next day she awoke in a hospital, and doctors told her that she had epilepsy. A week later a urine test taken at a follow-up visit showed she was two months pregnant.

She had another seizure a year later, after the birth of that child, when, in the midst of another argument, Ebonie's boyfriend grabbed her again by the neck. Four years later, she had another child with the same man and finally ended the relationship. Her third pregnancy, with her current boyfriend, ended in a miscarriage, as did the fifth. The fourth required a cesarean section after the fetal monitor showed a dangerously low heart rate. Ebonie felt so fortunate that both she and her new daughter had survived such a harrowing experience that she named her Blessn. She commemorated what she felt was a miracle with a tattoo—"Blessn 4-26-12"—on her neck.

"With all my pregnancies, they used to give me the runaround," she told me, describing how she visited *too many* doctors in California, including obstetricians, neurologists, and even psychologists. "I had to go through plenty of doctors to find the right doctors."

So far, she'd experienced the opposite extreme here in Houston. With no regular doctor visits, she was bouncing from ER to ER.

"I've never felt that weak," she said, recalling her last ER experience, when doctors had to transfuse her with multiple bags of blood and urged that she establish care here in Houston.

Ebonie had come from the state with the lowest maternal mortality rate in the country. Medi-Cal, or California's Medicaid program, made her doctor appointments possible, but there was another explanation for how the state had succeeded in bringing its maternal mortality rate down. In fact, the reason interrupted our conversation. Ebonie was sitting on it.

During a quick exam, Ebonie's nurse slid a blood pressure cuff around her arm and recorded the reading. She told Ebonie to lie still while she strapped the two sonar pucks around her belly and recorded the fetal heart rate. Then she asked Ebonie to rank her pain on a scale of one to ten. All of this constituted standard practice for a labor and delivery nurse. But then Ebonie's nurse did something that L & D nurses in Texas didn't normally do but that the vast majority in California did. After asking Ebonie to lift up her hips and removing the bloody pad from beneath her, the nurse weighed the pad on a scale. Then the nurse documented this number—the weight of the blood Ebonie had lost in the last eight hours—in the chart.

Ben Taub was one of the only hospitals in Houston (and in Texas, for that matter) to use a system for preventing obstetric bleeding. The system involved teams of doctors and nurses working together to quantify *exactly* how much blood Ebonie was losing. It was part of the new standard way of caring for hemorrhaging soon-to-be mothers, one developed and put into practice by researchers in California and implemented at Ben Taub by Carey Eppes.

Previously, nurses and doctors at Ben Taub glanced at each pad before disposing of it and described the blood loss in the chart as "mild," "moderate," or "severe." Most hospitals in Texas and nationwide continue to do the same. But this practice of eyeballing was fraught with potential errors. What's moderate to one person may look mild to the next. Plus, pregnant patients don't bleed in a consistent, predictable way. How does one interpret one moderate loss followed by two mild losses? Couldn't a doctor be lulled into thinking a patient was safe when she had actually lost a dangerous amount of blood?

When Carey started working at Ben Taub, the practice of eyeballing bothered her. Even from an early age, she seemed naturally predisposed toward a career involving numbers and measurements. She grew up in Maryland, where her father worked as a computer software engineer. And so quite naturally, in pursuing a career in medicine, she veered toward statistic-heavy sciences, earning degrees in both molecular biology and psychology from UT Austin. In medical school, she found herself drifting toward neurosurgery, a profession that offered hands-on precision, not to mention a slew of research possibilities. It seemed like Carey's career was headed toward the technical end of medicine.

But then something happened. During her OB rotation in medical school, one of Carey's patients arrived late to her clinic appointment. The woman's pregnancy was considered high-risk: she had kidney failure and received dialysis three times every week. After the woman finally checked in, she told Carey that she hadn't made it to her last scheduled dialysis session. Later, on rounds, Carey described the woman's situation to the supervising doctors. That was when she used a term that even today makes her cringe. She called the woman "noncompliant."

Describing someone as "noncompliant" can't fairly be called a rookie mistake, since doctors at all levels of their careers use the term. It's a part of the medical jargon. Most medical people will use the term and not think anything of it, but something changed for Carey after the woman apologized to her for being late. The woman explained that she took four buses to get to work. And sometimes buses ran late.

The revelation opened Carey's eyes. What other misperceptions did she have about people's lives? Did these presumptions conflict with her numbers-driven analyses? Was she less likely to recommend a proven therapy to someone she regarded as "noncompliant"? Did the studies that influenced her to prescribe one medication or another take people's difficult circumstances into account?

Carey realized that the patient-doctor relationship was so complex that it required connecting with people at multiple levels that went beyond science. People's circumstances—like how a bus schedule might govern their lives—could make as much of a difference in a therapy's effectiveness as the therapy itself. Science didn't easily allow for those considerations of context. Science's rigidity, in fact, made it easy for doctors to judge and label patients. Having heard and read other doctors use the word "noncompliant" had already changed Carey's idea of the woman before her. What if she hadn't delved into that woman's life? Would she have given up on the patient? If you didn't know the difficulties people had in getting from point A to point B, could you give them honest and thorough advice?

She needed to expand her learning beyond the technical, and so she earned a master's in public health during her maternal-fetal medicine fellowship at Northwestern University. This helped deepen her understanding of the social factors that played into sickness. How did trust in their doctor figure into why pregnant women didn't receive the flu shot? Did HIV medications affect postpartum hemorrhage? She found herself attracted to the complexities that other doctors avoided. Whenever there was an ethical dilemma, she ran toward it, the way ER doctors run toward emergencies.

So captivated was she by these complexities that Carey decided to become a maternal-fetal medicine doctor—now she had two patients to consider, rather than one. After training, she took a job at Ben Taub, where she could engage the complexity she craved while connecting to people who needed help. The safety-net environment wasn't about covering up problems; it was about putting people like her in positions to figure them out.

"It makes me so much of a better doctor to hear when something goes wrong," she said.

Many students and residents I've met over the years enter medicine the way Carey did. They're driven by the desire to engage in complex problem-solving and their good intentions to help their patients. Few, however, experience an epiphany as meaningful as Carey's. Perhaps this is due to how mechanized and corporate the practice of medicine has become. Medicine today is often about checking off what an illness *isn't*, especially when doctors follow diagnostic checklists generated by algorithms. Fee-for-service incentivizes this "rule out" game. Someone coming into the ER with chest pain is often told what they don't have—a heart attack or a pulmonary embolism or an aneurysm of the aorta—rather than given a specific diagnosis. Similarly, determining costs requires checklists in the form of billing codes. Billing specialists working for hospitals and doctors can extract the highest payment for a patient's visit by adding information that isn't necessarily germane, like a patient's nutrition level, or an old and obscure diagnosis, even their weight. The way a doctor decides on a diagnosis and documents it in the chart, in other words, is intricately tied to how payments are generated. There's not much room for reflection. The checklists can crowd out the crucial personal details, like a bus running late. Many young doctors can check off a box marked "noncompliant" and be rewarded for a job well done.

Carey had learned that checkboxes couldn't reveal everything about the people she encountered. She'd seen the obstacles her patients faced. Some didn't take the medications she prescribed or follow her suggested course of care because these obstacles were overwhelming. So, instead of fitting people into the science of medicine, she applied scientific thoughts to people.

Before Carey became the chief of obstetrics, she was the director of OB quality care at Ben Taub, a title she jokes was "made up" by administrators to appease her proclivity for statistics. Soon enough, however, her titles became more formal. She was recruited by the CDC to serve as a key national researcher on the Zika virus. She serves as the chair of the Texas Collaborative for Healthy Mothers and Babies, an expert panel of scientists, healthcare providers, hospitals, advocates, and insurers trying to improve childbirth in the state. Jobs like these have helped her stay up to date at Ben Taub and have reinforced a culture of statistical analysis to accompany bedside care.

"We track everything," she said, scrolling through Excel spreadsheets depicting the obstetric ward's latest numbers on transfusions and unplanned ICU admissions.

Once she was promoted to chief of obstetrics at Ben Taub, her attention shifted to blood loss and how to keep women like Ebonie from bleeding to death. Carey knew she didn't have to reinvent the wheel.

Often in healthcare, the challenge isn't in finding answers but in implementing them. Researchers in California had already developed an evidence-proven system to recognize bleeding early and accurately that relied on weighing the blood lost. Carey didn't have to develop a whole new system, but she did have to change how doctors and nurses worked in labor and delivery. She had to use her powers of persuasion to change the healthcare culture.

Her first order of business was to sit down with her team of nurses and techs in one of the L & D conference rooms. On a daily basis, these rooms hosted the most gut-wrenching and the most joyous conversations imaginable. *The heart rate has decelerated. We think she has a genetic mutation. She's going to be okay.* Now the team discussed how to help women like Ebonie deliver babies more safely.

Carey explained why she thought the culture had to change and for what objective. Yes, she admitted, the system would add work, especially to the nurses, there was no way around it.

There were plenty of questions. *What if I'm busy giving Pitocin to another patient? What if the patient doesn't want to have her pads changed?*

In her signature style, Carey pursed her lips and tilted her head forward—gestures that served her well with her two young daughters—in a way that said, You have my full attention.

Everyone agreed it would be best to run a pilot study to see how much time weighing the pads added to an L & D nurse's responsibilities. Ten nurses volunteered. In the end, it was clear that the weighing added five to eight minutes of work to the nurses' load per pad. It seemed like a lot, but participating in the study had shown the nurses the importance of accuracy and how easily someone could misjudge the amount of blood on a pad. The right decision seemed clear.

"It was a unit decision, doctors and nurses together," said Suzanne Lundeen, the nursing chief of L & D. "We decided we wanted to decrease our patients' bleeding, and weighing the pads helped."

In Texas, adopting systems like this is up to doctor leaders and administrators, and most hospitals have elected not to change their practices. Which is ironic. In Houston, some birthing hospitals offer women spa-like amenities with ads for massages. Perhaps these offerings spring from overconfidence, from a misperception that the United States has overwhelmingly safe maternal care.

Meanwhile, the team at Ben Taub has adopted more evidence-based protocols for soon-to-be mothers with very high blood pressure (preeclampsia) as well as a Maternal Early Warning System to prevent complications for those who undergo surgery. When I heard about all of these safety systems, I thought that my wife should have delivered our daughter there, at the hospital where I work. Carey had done just that. She'd delivered her third daughter right there at Ben Taub.

What's good enough for doctors should be the medical standard for a community. Ben Taub's L & D ward proves that good care is not a matter of expense but of making a commitment to how things should be done and to following a system. Ebonie had only recently become a Houstonian, but she was receiving the same level of care—even without insurance—that she had received in her hospitals in California, where the maternal mortality rate was better controlled.

Here in Houston, Ebonie was trying to make a better life for her young family. The cost of living was far less, especially when sharing an apartment with her sister Sharonna. She'd have done anything to avoid living homeless again. But was keeping the baby worth the risk to her own life?

As we spoke in her room, Ebonie paused.

"I feel a little hot," she said.

I asked her if I could get her ice water. She closed her eyes and lost track of our conversation. "I feel another seizure coming on," she said.

Immediately, her eyes started to flutter. The heart monitor showed a rapid pulse, and the muscles of her face and neck twitched. She began to shake violently. I pushed the Call Nurse button. "It looks like she's having a seizure," I said into the speaker.

I made sure to tilt Ebonie's head to the left as the obstetricians entered the room. A person in the throes of a seizure has no control over their airway, and the shaking can sometimes cause them to vomit. This is the real danger of seizures: a blocked airway that doesn't allow the person to breathe.

Thankfully, Ebonie continued to breathe normally. As the obstetricians gathered around her bed, I slipped away, careful not to interfere with their care. Later that afternoon, neurologists performed an EEG and changed her medications.

The seizures stopped over the next four days, as did the bleeding. Carey and the obstetricians felt Ebonie was ready for discharge. But there was still the problem of what Ebonie would do outside Ben Taub. If she had no coverage, how would she see the right doctors?

At safety-net hospitals, making contingency plans like this is part of the job. A financial counselor helped Ebonie file her application for Medicaid. This was important for two reasons. First, it provided an added level of security. It was true that if Ebonie bled again, then federal law protected her, meaning that any hospital she visited would have to assess and, if necessary, stabilize her. Carey and her team knew this, but they also knew how things worked in the real world. Uninsured patients had a knack for looking "stable" more often than insured patients. Medicaid, with all its flaws, gave Ebonie a fighting chance.

Second, if Ebonie qualified for Medicaid, it meant that Harris Health, Houston's safety-net-for-all system, could bill the state and receive payment. Carey didn't have anything to gain from this, but the system, and all the other patients, did. Medicaid didn't pay much, but it paid something.

The criteria to qualify were extremely narrow, but it looked like Ebonie was one of the lucky few—she only had to make sure to get all the right paperwork in, and the counselor helped her with this, too. "Make sure to check your mail," she advised Ebonie.

With this in mind, Carey and her team devised a plan for the next bleed—Ebonie's brother (who also lived in Houston) and sister would drive her the eleven miles to Ben Taub. She could take seizure pills at home. They also scheduled an appointment for her eight days later with a high-risk obstetrician at one of Ben Taub's clinics. "We are prepared," the nurse manager, Suzie Lundeen, told Ebonie.

Ebonie went home on the last day of May, determined to stay vigilant and wait. As it turned out, she didn't have to wait long.

In the middle of June, a little more than two weeks after leaving Ben Taub, she awoke early one morning to find that her bed was wet again. She awakened her son, who had been sleeping with her. "Get up," she said. He jumped out of bed. His pajamas were soaked. Ebonie could see by the color, though, that it wasn't blood.

Ebonie called for her sister. "I don't know what the hell is going on, but I got fluids coming out," she said. Her sister rushed into her room, touched the bed, and looked at her fingers.

"Do you think your water broke?" she asked.

"I don't know," Ebonie said.

Her lower belly started to cramp in five-minute cycles. They felt like contractions to Ebonie, only stronger. Carey and the obstetrics team had told her to come immediately to Ben Taub if she started bleeding or if her water broke. The wait had ended. She had to go now. She was only a little more than twenty-three weeks pregnant, too early to deliver, but with the placenta blocking the birth canal, her life was in danger.

The ambulance arrived. The EMTs loaded Ebonie into the back. She told them she wanted to go to Ben Taub. But the driver didn't seem to be listening. "I'm high-risk," she insisted to the EMT, "and I want to deliver my baby there." Amid all the turmoil, she wanted a level of control. She had seen firsthand how the teams at Ben Taub gave her as much.

But before Ebonie knew it, the ambulance had dropped her off in the emergency room of a different hospital, a nonprofit in the Texas Medical Center. The L & D department's careful planning was for naught. As she waited for treatment, all she could do was hope—pray—for the best.

— 10 —

Miscalculations

I met Aqueria in September 2016 in one of the Ben Taub ER's isolation rooms. It was my turn for an admission, and a text message flashed over my pager: "Diarrhea, Weight Loss."

I noticed two things upon entering her room. First, Aqueria wore a thick sweatshirt atop multiple long-sleeved shirts and a ball cap that wobbled according to how animatedly she spoke. Second, there appeared to be another human being curled up in the stretcher with her, beneath the thin white hospital sheets. This person, I later learned, was Trachelle.

Aqueria and Trachelle were both twenty-one, though Aqueria looked younger. Whenever Aqueria said something during our conversation that Trachelle didn't fully agree with, a segment of the bedsheets would shake abruptly. Sometimes the sheets emitted an "Uh-uh" or "You know that's not how it is," to which Aqueria responded with loving eye rolls.

Physically, that was about all she could do. At the time we met, she was incredibly thin. The weight had dropped off over the past six months. It was a case of simple math: too few calories in, too much fluid out. Anything she ate felt like it got stuck in the middle of her chest while going down and came right back up. The diarrhea never went away. And so her clothes began to sag off her body, she no longer had the energy to walk very far ("It's like walking through sand"), and her core temperature had decreased. Aqueria had weighed 129 pounds. Now she weighed 79. She'd lost one-third of her body weight. "You're gonna turn to dust," Trachelle told her.

Aqueria knew exactly what was wrong with her. "I need my HIV medications," she told me shortly after we met, the ball cap on her head bobbing again. She'd said the same to the doctors at all four of the ERs she'd visited before coming to Ben Taub, and they had each responded in kind: "You need insurance."

This was true, and it wasn't. Aqueria had what doctors call "wasting syndrome." This was what AIDS looked like in the 1980s and early '90s, a body vanquished by a virus. At the time, medications only partially treated AIDS. We solved the problem with HAART—highly active anti-retroviral treatment—which keeps the virus at bay, in many cases reducing it to undetectable levels. Today, thanks to these medications, more than seventeen million people worldwide have near-normal, if not fully normal, lives with HIV. This breakthrough may very well be the biggest medical marvel since the polio vaccine.

HAART may have solved the problem immunologically, but getting the medications into people's hands, especially the hands of those who can't afford them, has proven to be a bigger quandary.

At one time, Aqueria had access. She *had* been insured, on Medicaid, all of her life, in fact. Medicaid had helped her stay healthy. With that health, Aqueria's life opened up: she consumed more, and not just nutritionally. She wanted more than just what a person living on welfare can earn, including better living conditions, better food, better experiences, all of which required more money. But there was an inherent problem with the way Aqueria received healthcare: she couldn't afford to *stay* on Medicaid.

About a year before coming to Ben Taub, Aqueria was working at a Family Dollar as a cashier and attendant. ("And a stocker," said Trachelle.) During a typical week, she worked eight hours a day, four days per week, and made $8 an hour. She actively avoided work some weeks for an important reason: if she earned too much, she wouldn't qualify for Medicaid. But if she earned too little, she wouldn't have enough to survive. For Aqueria, with her HIV, it didn't seem like much of a choice. Since Aqueria was an adult, the only way for her to keep Medicaid was by maintaining herself on Supplemental Security Income (SSI). This was a federal program that helped the blind, disabled, or elderly with cash, and it's more commonly known as welfare. But she was dangerously close to the income limit for SSI. No SSI, no Medicaid. No Medicaid, no meds.

Things changed when she met Trachelle. She found love, and love demanded more shared experiences, more eating out, more going out, all of which required more money. The price of this love was her welfare and her healthcare.

They met on Facebook in November 2015, nine months before we met at Ben Taub. Beside her relationship status, Aqueria posted a plea. "I need someone that's gonna stick by my side, stick it out through thick and thin," she wrote. Moved by what she had read, Trachelle DM'd her and a conversation—indeed, a courtship—ensued. After two weeks, Aqueria decided that if this blossoming relationship was going to work, she had to be more direct with Trachelle about who she was.

The problem was she didn't know how to reveal she had HIV. Aqueria didn't want to scare Trachelle off. How could she cleave those three letters away from her identity? She had been born with it, the virus having been passed to her during childbirth, in 1995. That year, AZT—a component of HAART—was already being used to prevent mother-to-child transmission. Pregnant women receiving prenatal care at Ben Taub and other safety-net hospitals in the area receive the drug, but unfortunately, Aqueria's mother didn't. Why she didn't was a source of despair for Aqueria. Neither of Aqueria's younger siblings had HIV. Her mother had received AZT at LBJ Hospital—another Harris Health safety-net hospital—during both childbirths. Aqueria was uniquely unlucky in this regard. She had heard conflicting reports over the years about how her mother had been raped, how she'd been a prostitute. What nobody questioned was that Aqueria's mother was addicted to crack. It seemed that prenatal care and saving her child from the transmission of HIV got lost in the blur of her addiction.

Aqueria heard her share of crack-baby jokes growing up. Few people knew about the HIV. The circle of trust included the infectious disease doctors at Texas Children's Hospital, one of the top pediatric centers in the world. In Texas, an HIV infection so early in life used to count as a disability. Multiple funds are available for HIV-infected children, including Ryan White funds, but Aqueria's path to HAART medications came through claiming disability, which ultimately earned her Medicaid and a welfare check. The medications were hers—she took them religiously throughout childhood—but the money wasn't. Aqueria said the aunt who raised her kept the welfare checks. The math was easy growing up because her aunt earned very little income otherwise. She gained custody when Aqueria was nine. She gave her niece food and clothes and made sure she took her medicines but didn't do much more.

There was discipline, though, which Aqueria said her aunt provided with belts, extension cords, anything she had on hand. Once, in order to escape her aunt's hanger, Aqueria shut herself in a bathroom by inserting a bobby pin into the lock. "They called them whoopings back then," she said. Aqueria couldn't help but tell me how she currently views them. "Nowadays they'd call it child abuse."

When Aqueria was a teenager, Texas Children's Hospital not only managed her HAART, it created a community for her, too. Every summer, Aqueria and other Texas Children's patients, including other congenitally infected children, visited Camp YOLO for two weeks in the Texas Hill Country. One summer, Aqueria got to see Beyoncé at a private concert (she was more a member of Destiny's Child back then than *Beyoncé*, Trachelle noted). Some of Aqueria's friends at the camp were white and wealthy. Some were middle-class. Some were Arab, Latino,

Nigerian, eastern European. All were very sick with cancer or premature organ failure or HIV, but they were very happy for those two weeks, and they were together.

Were there any risks to exposing a teenager like Aqueria—poor and chronically ill—to such a utopia? Could Camp YOLO and affordable HAART have given Aqueria a false notion of what life would be like as an adult? Was it possible that coverage during childhood gave her the idea that life didn't have to be about poverty? That there could be moments of joy and peace, that it wasn't just about the struggle? Was that why she eventually jumped toward love and messed up the math?

When Aqueria turned nineteen in 2014, she didn't know what to do, whether to live a life on disability or improve her livelihood by working and earning more. Her HIV doctor, Dr. Mary Paul, couldn't help but mention this struggle in her note:

"She has been in and out of care due to social difficulties but when she is in care persistently, she is adherent to medication. No AIDS defining illness," she wrote.

Meanwhile, there was another math problem at play in Aqueria's body. If Aqueria's CD4 count dropped below 200, she was at risk for an opportunistic infection. CD4+ T cells defend our bodies from bacteria and fungi and other infections. They also keep certain cancers from forming. A normal count is anywhere from 500 to 1,500 (cells/microliter of blood). When the CD4 count drops below 200, it means that the defenses are so weak and porous that infections that would be vanquished easily by a properly functioning immune system can thrive. This is what we call AIDS, or acquired immunodeficiency syndrome.

Dr. Paul had known and treated Aqueria since she was nine. She was concerned that her patient was slipping and not taking her medications. Worse, she worried that Aqueria might be forsaking coverage altogether. To keep her HAART medications, Aqueria needed to stay on Medicaid. To keep her Medicaid, she needed to stay on SSI. To keep her SSI, she needed to stay poor.

The whole medical team—nurses, social workers, case managers, Dr. Paul, everyone who knew her at the Texas Children's Hospital Pediatric AIDS and Retrovirology Clinic—wanted Aqueria to keep her coverage. They were emotionally and medically invested in her care. Even though Aqueria was an adult, Dr. Paul implored her to keep coming back to the children's AIDS clinic. It's not uncommon for patients who have established a rapport with pediatricians from an early age to continue with them into adulthood, which makes the point of handoff to adult doctors tricky. It was a critical moment in Aqueria's illness, so Dr. Paul asked Aqueria to keep coming back. She knew asking Aqueria to hang on to the Medicaid would be more difficult.

Life, inevitably, invariably, made the choice. In November 2015, right after Aqueria turned twenty, after she met Trachelle, she stopped seeing Dr. Paul. Frustrated by the financial tightrope she had to walk to keep her coverage, Aqueria behaved in a way that her difficult life had never allowed: she acted her age, like a teenager, and grew dejected. She gave up. She didn't see any doctor for a year. She didn't take her medicines, and her body experienced the consequences.

It was the two of them, Aqueria and Trachelle, against the world. After their initial encounter on Facebook, Aqueria moved into Trachelle's duplex. Trachelle worked as a cashier at Fiesta, a local supermarket chain. Since she had no restrictions on what she could make, Trachelle provided the food, and they split the cost of gas ($100/month), electricity ($50), and housing ($500). When they couldn't make the monthly payment on their duplex, they checked into a cheap hotel that offered long-term rates. Anything extra, Trachelle picked up. Aqueria still remembered that first treat Trachelle had given her—a game system. She'd never had one growing up.

It took them two months to consummate the union. Aqueria had a hard time disclosing her illness. "Something inside of my head was giving me excuses," she said.

Trachelle sensed something was wrong. "Trust and believe," she told Aqueria. "I won't leave your side."

Aqueria was good with words. She'd proven as much, earning As and Bs throughout high school (one C+, in math). But revealing this part of herself was hard. Finally, she decided to take a chance.

It didn't scare Trachelle off. Rather, it increased her concern for Aqueria. She learned more about HIV infections and HAART and CD4 counts. She started paying more attention to her numbers, their budget, the various delicate calculations. When Aqueria told her that she'd started working more hours at the Family Dollar, Trachelle knew what that meant: No more SSI. No more Medicaid. No more HAART.

Dr. Paul's office had continued reaching out to Aqueria for a follow-up visit. As the weight began to trickle off, Trachelle pleaded with Aqueria.

"Can I take off work today to go to the doctor with you?" she said.

But how? Her coverage was long gone. Dr. Paul was willing to see her in the office for free, but Aqueria felt ashamed. Eventually her body forced her to swallow her pride. The symptoms had decimated her.

"For the last 4–5 months has had weight loss, intermittent abdominal pain, loose stools without blood, weakness. Cannot complete a meal due to the chest pain," wrote Dr. Paul in a note dated August 31, 2016. "I am very concerned that this profound weight loss is AIDS wasting syndrome."

The social worker went into more depth about why this was happening. "Patient expressed frustration with the SSI process and states she stopped receiving benefits about a year ago," she wrote. "Patient's partner is employed and they use the check to pay for weekly hotels."

As Aqueria's body wasted away, so did her relationship. She and Trachelle fought. Aqueria grew angry at Trachelle for possibly flirting with someone else. They separated for a little and got back together again. Aqueria started to pile on layers of clothes to make up for the flesh she lacked. Work grew physically impossible. They started visiting emergency rooms. Doctors told them, "You need insurance."

They ended up here. When I met her, Aqueria's numbers looked terrible. Her CD4 count was 18, about as low as you could get (at Ben Taub, the lowest CD4 count I've seen is 1). She had descended into full-blown AIDS. What prevented her from eating was probably a fungus growing along the surface of her esophagus. Or the cytomegalovirus. Or both. That was the thing about AIDS: it opened the floodgates. AIDS doesn't kill people, not by itself. It is the OIs, the opportunistic infections, that wreak the damage. AIDS merely allows these infections to infiltrate.

Now Aqueria was susceptible to *everything*: histoplasmosis, cytomegalovirus, herpes, PJP, even cancers of the bone marrow and muscle and skin. This is what happens when you don't take HAART. This is what happens when the numbers fall out of balance. This is what happens when you don't have coverage.

The idea of fairness is so ingrained in the American DNA that we feel the need to express it in numbers. We conduct studies and devise complex tables and eligibility charts to determine precise levels of fairness, which is how we come up with numbers like $8,796 yearly and 138 percent of the federal poverty level to help us assign health coverage. We have it right down to the dollar.

We use these numbers to determine how best to deploy limited resources. We don't have all the money in the world, we say, so we have to prioritize, and numbers help us do that. Which is true—hard decisions always have to be made when it comes to scarce resources. But when we defer to these numbers to decide what is fair, we risk falling prey to presumptions. First, we presume that our numbers are accurate. We believe that the scientists and mathematicians are plugging the best numbers into formulas, and that these formulas are the right ones to determine fairness. But what if these formulas, and the numbers we plug into them, are biased? What if the people who collect these numbers and devise these charts have blind spots that make the calculations inaccurate and unfair? What if numbers merely promulgate the American notion that some people are worthy of healthcare while some people aren't?

A study in the October 2019 issue of the journal *Science* showed how seemingly small decisions made by statisticians at health insurance companies can snowball into unfair and even racist treatment by doctors. Maybe this shouldn't come as a surprise, since we've seen how the Scientific Charity Movement used statistics to push a social Darwinist agenda. But what worried me about the study in *Science* is that none of the doctors or scientists in the study *intended* to do harm. In our modern age, good people trying to do good things can unwittingly make medicine more unfair.

Whenever a doctor diagnoses a patient with an illness or notices a previously diagnosed illness has changed, they typically use a reference tool to help decide the next step. Previously, doctors consulted textbooks written by experts, like *Harrison's Principles of Internal Medicine*, which lists Dr. Anthony Fauci as an author, or even *Pocket Medicine*. The technological boom brought shortcuts: instead of textbooks and journals, doctors began using online tools and apps that let them type specific numbers taken from a patient's blood work into blanks, hit Return, and voilà, the answer for what to do next appeared instantaneously on the screen. Doctors trust that the answer abides by the rigors of science and that the computer program's algorithm or formula is based on proven studies. But researchers are starting to discover how these shortcuts can make healthcare less fair.

Ziad Obermeyer, a doctor and public health scientist, decided to take a closer look at an algorithm. He and his team focused on one that reminded doctors to refer patients for high-risk programs. If a patient had a high blood pressure reading, for instance, as well as a certain level of kidney damage and elevated sugars, the algorithm sent the doctor a reminder that the patient qualified to see nurses and specialists and educators. The reminder was part of an intensive effort to control the patient's health problems before it got too late. Multiple hospitals and healthcare systems across the United States used this algorithm. Obermeyer's study measured its effect on more than fifty thousand patients.

Obermeyer and his team found that the algorithm accurately predicted who was sick, but that it failed to refer all sick patients to the intensive care program. The problem, Obermeyer discovered, was that the algorithm also weighed the predicted cost of treatment. Algorithm designers had made a presumption when designing the formula. They decided that those who would be expensive for the hospital or health system in the future were the sickest. And so they plugged in the variable of future predicted cost.

At first glance, this seems reasonable—why not try to figure out who's sick early and send them to an intensive program to prevent costs in the future? The intention was good. But the algorithm's creators had made a leap of faith. They believed that cost equaled need. In fact, many of the sickest African American patients cost far less than their sick white counterparts. Black patients visited primary care and specialty doctors less. They were more likely to be poor and therefore had more problems getting child care, time off from work, and transportation from their apartments to their doctors' offices on the other side of town. Though Black patients cost less because they utilized fewer services, they still had the same medical needs; in many cases, they had greater medical needs. What this meant was that future predicted costs didn't necessarily equate to need. When Obermeyer and his team changed these predicted costs to another variable—for instance, one that predicted chronic conditions instead of cost—it made an enormous difference, with twice the original number of Black patients now being referred to the high-risk program.

"This mechanism of bias is particularly pernicious because it can arise from reasonable choices," wrote Obermeyer. The team reached out to the algorithm writers and informed them of its bias. After many simulations and tests, the writers found that the researchers were right. Both groups are now trying to work together to develop more precise and less racially biased algorithms.

"Algorithms can do terrible things, or algorithms can do wonderful things," Obermeyer said in an interview after his study made national headlines. "We make so many choices when we train an algorithm that feel technical and small. But these choices make the difference between an algorithm that's good or bad, biased or unbiased."

What this teaches us is that we have to be careful about the presumptions built into any algorithm or statistical analysis we use to determine who gets healthcare and who doesn't. For example: What presumptions do we make when we designate income limits for the disabled to qualify for Medicaid? A lot. For one, we presume that the people using statistics to figure out the income limits are trying to cover people who need it most. But it's very possible they want to cover the least number of people, and that they've arrived at $8,796 per year—which to most people seems ridiculously low—through complex but tainted math.

In her book *Automating Inequality*, Virginia Eubanks argues that algorithms and predictive models are being used by insurance companies, state health agencies, and governments around the country to reduce the number of poor people covered by health insurance. She offers the example of Medicaid in Indiana. In 2006, administrators decided to cut costs by shifting to an automated application system instead of a caseworker-based one. The shift was supposed to save the state millions of dollars by improving efficiency and "help clients reduce dependency on welfare assistance and transition into a paid work setting." Proponents of the new system argued that caseworkers would be able to repurpose the time saved toward applicants. But it turned out that the automated application system had, at best, committed an error (at worst, it was rigged). People insured by Medicaid started receiving the same message: "Your MEDICAID benefits will be discontinued due to the following reason: FAILURE TO COOPERATE IN ESTABLISHING ELIGIBILITY." The new system wasn't registering important paperwork turned in by applicants, even though the receiving office had stamped them as "Received." Needy people were left uncovered, unable to access care, and responsible for thousands of dollars in medical bills.

"The automation's impacts were devastating for poor and working class Hoosiers," wrote Eubanks. "Between 2006 and 2008, the state of Indiana denied more than a million applications for food stamps, Medicaid, and cash benefits, a 54% increase compared to the three years prior to automation."

Even when patients appealed the Medicaid office's decision, insisting that their documents had been stamped "Received," caseworkers gave them an ominous, if not chilling, reminder of the power of technology: "The judge will simply look in the computer, see this, and deny you."

Pressure mounted on politicians after so many people found themselves knocked off Medicaid.* Eventually, the state of Indiana sued IBM, the company in charge of automating and processing applications, for nearly half a billion dollars, insisting that their procedures had harmed people and led to health benefit denials. IBM countersued and won $52 million from the state, in part because it was so clear that the state government had been misguided from the beginning in its attempts to cut costs.

"Automated decision-making shatters the society safety net," Eubanks wrote. "It reframes shared social decisions about who we are and who we want to be as systems engineering problems."

For many years, I took these automated decisions as gospel. It was only when I investigated one of these decisions myself that I realized how much these algorithms impact people's lives and how I needed to think beyond numbers to help my patients.

Geronimo, my thirtysomething patient with liver failure, was born in Mexico City, raised in the state of Michoacán, and brought to Houston

---

* There's no official number of Medicaid applications denied during the automation, but one Medicaid lawyer in Indiana estimates that 95 percent of applications he handled during this time resulted in eligibility determination errors.

illegally when he was nine. His father had largely abandoned the family when Geronimo was a toddler, leaving Emma in Mexico to raise the children by herself. Emma and her children crossed the border in 1990 and quickly looked to establish a foothold in their new home.

For four years, Emma and her children lived the life that so many families lead in this city, Emma trying to nudge things forward for the next generation. In Michoacán, getting a better, more secure life was tough. If you didn't have an education, there weren't many ways to earn money. You could tend to someone's livestock. You could join Los Zetas and become a foot solider in the drug trade.

Here in Houston, it was different. There was work. You could clean dishes. You could vacuum offices at night. You could refill people's cups with ice water. The pay was decent relative to what she could earn in Mexico. Little Geronimo and his younger sister attended school. Things seemed poised to improve for the next generation.

But things in Houston were still tough. Emma started off as a florist, but soon, she took on a night job cleaning up a big sports bar and entertainment hall. The family was already living close to the edge when, at age thirteen, Geronimo started having seizures at school. His mother took him to Ben Taub, where neurologists diagnosed him with epilepsy. The medications they prescribed brought the convulsions under control, but the new health problems broke the fragile family's back. His father—never completely out of the picture, but rarely present—interceded. He believed that Geronimo would receive better medical treatment in Mexico, and so he demanded that he be sent back—alone—to live with his grandparents.

Emma knew not to cross her ex-husband, no matter how nonsensical his demands sounded. She had endured his beatings during their marriage, and it scared her to think the abuse might start again. And so, Emma saw her only son, a teenager now, leave for Michoacán. Immediately afterward, she regretted the decision and felt ashamed she couldn't have been stronger for him and their family.

In Mexico, Geronimo's grandparents put him to work tending their livestock. For seven years, he wrote letters to his mother and called her regularly. Then, when he was twenty, his father surprised him with something precious: a green card. It had taken years, but his papers had been fixed. Geronimo was now a permanent resident of the United States and could enter the country freely. He boarded a bus heading north and crossed the border without any hindrance.

When he arrived, however, there was the problem of income. To live in the United States is to pay *los billes*. Geronimo had only a sixth-grade education. His work experience was limited. But Geronimo had something going for him: he was bilingual, perfectly so, with no accent. To learn basic work skills, he joined the Job Corps, a career-training program funded by the federal government. The experience proved helpful, as Geronimo found work immediately afterward. With a little income, Geronimo moved into a two-bedroom apartment right off the freeway on Houston's southwest side. Emma was his roommate.

The two were back together again. A new equilibrium, it seemed, had been established, but it went deeper than that. Geronimo and his mother were more than just mother and son. They began working together after Geronimo found a job washing dishes at Emma's sports bar. They performed errands together, they ate together (though never at work), and since Geronimo couldn't drive on account of his epilepsy, they rode the bus together. Geronimo knew it was a special relationship, and it was more than just making up for lost time. He felt like he could tell his mother anything. Life wasn't easy, but they got by, together. The only jobs Geronimo could find paid little more than minimum wage, if that. He worked as a dishwasher, as a cook, and at a gas station. A portion of every paycheck he received, as with most Americans, went to Medicare and Social Security.

None of Geronimo's jobs provided him with health insurance. Since they didn't make enough to afford their own healthcare, Emma helped her son obtain a Gold Card. With this in hand, he visited the People's

Clinic, one of Ben Taub's feeder clinics, where he received checkups and access to prescriptions. A few health issues popped up—his primary care doctor diagnosed him with diabetes, for instance—but none was significant enough to keep Geronimo from working.

In December 2010, his primary doctor noticed early signs of liver damage on routine blood work. Further tests showed a hepatitis C infection as the cause. The hep C virus is usually transmitted through contact with infected blood, or, more rarely, through unprotected sex, and is one of the most common causes of liver disease worldwide. Geronimo confided to Emma he'd contracted it through unprotected sex.

For nearly four years, he received regular care at the People's Clinic and Ben Taub. Then, disaster struck.

On June 9, 2014, Geronimo started his night shift at the gas station feeling a little tired. As people filed in and out to buy cigarettes and six-packs, he felt weaker and weaker. A few hours passed. Suddenly, a wave of nausea spread through his body, and blood began to pour from his mouth. Geronimo dropped to his knees and then to the floor, unconscious beside the four pints of blood he'd just vomited. One of the gas station's customers called 911.

An ambulance brought him to Ben Taub. Geronimo was quickly admitted to the ICU and given a blood transfusion and medications through an IV to help shunt the flow of blood away from his digestive organs and toward the main circulatory system. He had regained consciousness a few minutes after the vomiting, but doctors sedated him to perform an endoscopy. As the snakelike camera slithered down his mouth and into his esophagus, the reason for the bleeding became clear: blood vessels inside his gullet had burst. His liver was so scarred by hep C that large amounts of blood preferentially coursed through his esophagus.

Geronimo recovered from his esophageal bleed. With Emma beside him, he listened to the liver specialist's assessment: His cirrhosis was now considered decompensated. It had progressed so quickly that his life was in danger at every moment henceforth. They would add medicines to help control some symptoms, like confusion and swelling of his legs and belly, but there was no curing the damage to his liver. At the age of thirty-four, Geronimo learned that only a transplant could save his life.

The Gold Card covered only the care given at Ben Taub and within the rest of the safety net. Ben Taub didn't offer transplants; only private hospitals did. Geronimo would have to find good health insurance if he wanted to save his life.

All of his doctors agreed that Geronimo's liver was so damaged that he qualified as disabled. This gave Geronimo hope. People who receive disability payments through SSI automatically receive coverage through Medicaid. There were at least five hospitals that performed liver transplants in Houston, and most of them accepted Medicaid for payment. Geronimo had an active green card, too. He fit all of the qualifications. All he had to do was to apply for SSI.

After doctors discharged him from Ben Taub in late June 2014, Geronimo visited the Social Security office with Emma. Over the next weeks, the two collected all of the appropriate documents. And in September 2014, Geronimo received a new Medicaid card in the mail. A liver transplant was within sight. He waited for his next appointment with his liver specialist at Ben Taub, who would be able to refer him to a transplant center.

Except that Geronimo never received the referral. Two months after his Medicaid card arrived in the mail, another letter from the state of Texas arrived. It was an automatically generated letter, informing him that his health benefits had been terminated. Geronimo's Medicaid had been revoked on account of his earning too much money.

How was it possible that someone so sick, who no longer worked, earned too much money? It was the result of a simple twist of fate—that, and a policy decision made by the Texas Legislature. When Geronimo and Emma initially went to the Social Security Administration office, whoever attended to them noticed that he had paid Social Security taxes. What happened afterward isn't clear. Was Geronimo's attendant simply doing his job and trying to get him a little more money? Or was there a different calculus involved? That day, Geronimo had left the Social Security Administration building feeling good because, in addition to qualifying for Medicaid, he'd learned he would start receiving a check. The check would be issued by Social Security Disability Insurance, to which he had contributed with his paychecks. Geronimo started to receive the $912 per month. Since disability payments count as income in Texas, the amount put Geronimo over the threshold to qualify for Medicaid.

It had already been a long shot for him to receive this coverage. Childless adults in Texas could only receive Medicaid coverage if they were A) disabled and B) earned less than $733 per month. Geronimo had managed to squeeze through the eye of a needle in qualifying.

He had also worked despite having epilepsy. He'd had to. No one could claim Geronimo was trying to take advantage of the system. If anything, he was trying not to be a burden. But working had cost him. Geronimo's paying into Social Security, in other words, made him ineligible for social healthcare.

Seventeen months later, there I was, sitting at the nurses' station of Ben Taub's step-down unit—an intermediate stage between intensive care and the hospital wards—and attempting to absorb this information. Geronimo was dying. The numbers in his chart were daunting. Low sodium level, high bilirubin, poor kidney and clotting function. But even now, the most vital number was 179. An extra 179 dollars every month on his disability check had disqualified him from Medicaid, and therefore, from candidacy for a liver transplant.

Had Geronimo lived in any other state, his Medicaid wouldn't have been taken away from him. States like West Virginia had adopted the Medicaid expansion as part of the Affordable Care Act. As a West Virginian, Geronimo would have easily qualified for Medicaid. His disability check from Social Security wouldn't have been considered income, but even if it had, his gross income wasn't even close to their cutoff of $16,141 per year—nearly double the annual income that Texas allowed.

Even in other states that didn't expand Medicaid, Geronimo might have had hope for a liver transplant. States like North Carolina and Missouri offer "medically needy" pathways, or "spend-down" programs, whereby patients can meet the Medicaid limit by deducting certain items, including unpaid medical bills, from their income. Texas has such a plan for children and pregnant women, but not for the disabled. When I told this to a social worker at a liver-transplant center in Missouri, she sighed over the phone. "Texas sounds tough," she said.

I respected my home state for many reasons, including the economic opportunities it's capable of creating. I paid $6,500 *per year* in tuition—the lowest in the country—for a private medical school education, in large part because of the state's subsidies. Beyond this, there seemed to be jobs available for everyone in Texas. Some of my patients at Ben Taub were homeowners. They had come from nothing in East Texas or El Salvador to purchase a house in Houston. It meant something to give people the ability to do this, and you had to give some credit to legislators for keeping the Texas economic engine moving. Would the cost of caring for the state's most vulnerable and sick impede the economy? Legislators seemed to think so. I wasn't convinced.

The team of residents and students and I visited Geronimo and Emma every day. We spoke with kidney and lung and liver specialists, trying to figure out how to curtail these latest bouts of illness. For the first forty-eight hours with him, it was as though we were watching a tidal wave in the distance slowly moving toward our patient, and us.

And then three days after taking over Geronimo's care, our team ran into the social worker in the hallway. The conversation started with a cordial, if not superficial, tone—"How's it going? Tough cases, eh?"—but very quickly, we began to lament the situation to her. The more questions we asked, the more it sounded like we were accusing her of backing the state's policies and not simply doing her best to work within them.

Would the Social Security office lower Geronimo's disability check to $733 a month so that he could requalify for Medicaid? No, administratively this wasn't possible. Would the nearest transplant center consider performing the procedure as charity? We'd have to ask each individual transplant center, but probably not. So all we could do was sit and do nothing and watch him die?

The social worker didn't respond to our last question. She looked away and started flipping through some papers she held in her hands. We took this as a sign that the conversation was over. We began to collect ourselves. Time to get back to it. There were other patients on our list to see, after all, and not so many hours in which to see them.

People with liver disease often find themselves in a confused state called hepatic encephalopathy. A toxic mist grips them, fueled by the urea the liver fails to metabolize. A medicine called lactulose helps the body clear this mist quickly, not unlike the loud snapping of two fingers. The improvement can be drastic—I've seen this medicine awaken people with cirrhosis who I mistakenly thought had dementia. What the social worker said next had a similar effect on our team as a slug of lactulose.

"Sometimes we write to congressmen about these cases," she said.

The social worker hadn't been trying to shake us off. She'd been going through her papers to find Geronimo's address, specifically, his zip code. Who represented Geronimo?

Geronimo lived in Texas District Seven of the US House of Representatives, a hook-shaped district that extends westward into the Houston suburbs, bends northward toward Cypress, and then curves ever so slightly toward downtown, ending at a point in a neighborhood called Jersey Village. Politicos know and covet the Seventh for the hook's hilt, which lies inside the city. Some of the country's wealthiest people live in these tiny villages: CEOs, doctors, lawyers, even the descendants of oil barons. Tourists drive up and down the avenues in these enclaves to catch a glimpse of sprawling manors like the ones you'd find in the eighties TV show *Dallas*. The names of these neighborhoods connote wealth: River

Oaks, West University Place, Tanglewood, not to mention Piney Point, the neighborhood my dad had aspired to live in since moving to Houston and where our family secured a home while I was in high school. With a median income of $77,300, the Seventh is the wealthiest district in Texas, but not because of people like Geronimo. On the district map, Geronimo's neighborhood of Gulfton, along US Route 59, looked like a piece of putty stuck on as an afterthought. And so it was that the elected official who represented Geronimo also represented some of America's elite.

Republican John Culberson had kept such a stranglehold on the Seventh during his (then) fifteen-year tenure that he often ran unopposed in primaries and even in the general election. He was as much a Texas Republican as Ted Cruz, opposing abortion rights and tax increases, advocating for gun rights, rejecting the notion that human beings were responsible for climate change. He was a card-carrying member of the Tea Party, so it came as no surprise that he vehemently opposed Obamacare. Before voting to delay the legislation, he famously said, "Like 9/11, let's roll!" Fighting against the healthcare bill, to Culberson, was more than just politics: it was a moral duty.

We confirmed and then reconfirmed Geronimo's address. There was no way around it. If we wanted Geronimo's Medicaid case to be reopened, we would have to write to Representative Culberson.

The social worker gathered her papers into a neat stack and shot us a decisive look.

"So do you want me to write to the congressman?" she said.

We all had other patients on our lists, other problems to solve, other notes to write. The temptation to let her handle this case and focus instead on things we felt more comfortable with was certainly there. But what about *this* patient? Would the social worker be able to convey what liver failure—especially in a thirty-six-year-old—looked and felt like to a caretaker? What was the best way to help Geronimo?

What if *I* contacted the congressman?

Algorithmania

After finishing my residency in 2010, I took a job as a primary care doctor at a Harris Health clinic on Houston's southeast side. Every day during my commute, I passed places I remembered from my youth. I'd gone to high school in this part of town, but not to the same schools as the patients visiting my clinic. The Jesuit prep school I attended was an island amid a growing sea of Chinese, Vietnamese, Mexican, and Central American immigrants. We ate cheap Chinese food in the strip centers off Bellaire Boulevard. We ran cross-country routes along Gessner and once got so lost that cops had to drive us back to campus. It never got old revisiting these memories while alone on my way to work. My favorite band, Arcade Fire, had just released an album named *The Suburbs*, which was based on the lead singer Win Butler's childhood in Houston. And so, on an average day, I'd pull into the tin-roofed carport in the People's Clinic's heavily potholed parking lot, belting out lyrics about the strangeness of growing up in this part of the world: "Sometimes I can't believe it, I'm moving past the feeling." I'd turn off the ignition, put on my white coat, and walk into the People's Clinic.

I was always slated to see twenty-four patients a day, a standard number, though there were always no-shows. The majority of the no-shows were follow-ups, people recently discharged from Ben Taub, people who, for some reason or another—transportation problems, family issues, already back in the hospital—were unable to make it back to the clinic.

They called it "primary care," but it was more like problem care. Blood pressures in the two hundreds, blood sugars in the three hundreds, headaches, boils, all that you'd expect at a clinic for people with limited healthcare access. There were also less urgent problems, cancer screenings and heart disease tune-ups and yearly physicals. Gynecological complaints usually compelled me to shoot off a quick text to my dad: "What dose norethindrone do u use for heavy bleeding?" It didn't take long for me to realize that I was the safety-net system's person on the front line. Months before, I had been seeing patients in worse shape with very similar diagnoses on the Ben Taub wards. Now it was my job to exercise foresight and to practice good preventive medicine. It was my job to keep these people out of Ben Taub.

In America, checklists make up an essential part of primary care. With those checklists come numbers: HDL of 40, bring the A1c down below 7, colon cancer screening at age fifty, etc. One of the most famous and influential books written by a doctor seemed to support this approach. *The Checklist Manifesto* by Atul Gawande argued that programming reminders into everyday practice, like with a checklist, could help avoid mistakes. By using these lists, surgeons had seen some complication rates go down by as much 35 percent. Why not apply this to primary care, then? Why not use checklists to track cholesterol and blood pressure targets?

As much as I admired Gawande and how he utilized checklists, my time as a resident at Ben Taub had made me wary of them. An extreme manifestation of this philosophy was something I called algorithmania. Algorithmania is the unexamined use of clinical road maps. These road maps can be literal, like the decision trees found in *Pocket Medicine* used to diagnose an ailment, or they can be intellectual, like a doctor's mental hopscotch. Algorithmania, then, is the compulsion to force patients onto a step-by-step decision tree when complexities in the illness or person's life ought to keep them off. An algorithmaniac puts the doctor's desire to give a quick and uncomplicated answer above the patient's need for help.

You know algorithmania when you see it. Consider this hypothetical but very common scenario: A woman with diabetes comes in for a routine check of her sugars. After jotting down the lows ("120") and the highs ("200, 250"), the doctor asks a series of routine questions: Have you had any fainting spells? Nausea? Vomiting? What about chest pain?

The patient pauses long enough for the doctor to perk up. He notices there's a conflicted look on the patient's face and that she is holding her hand squarely at her sternum. In Spanish, she says it's pressure.

The doctor attempts to characterize this pain: when did it start, where does it go, what alleviates it, etc.

Yesterday, the woman says. She's had the pain before. It's everywhere in her chest.

The doctor asks if shortness of breath accompanies the pain. The patient takes a short breath in. "Sí," she says.

Before long, the woman finds herself hooked to an EKG machine. The doctor tells her that an ambulance is en route to take her to the emergency room.

There, once the EMTs have checked her in, once another EKG has been performed, once a nurse has drawn her blood, a doctor asks some of the same questions about the chest pain: When did it start? Did you take an aspirin? Have you ever had it before?

Some hours later, a staff member informs the lady she will be admitted into the hospital for chest pain. Unless someone has taken the time to explain each decision, she is left thinking that her life may have been in danger.

As far back as the sixteenth century, doctors have used algorithms to organize a patient's clinical information. The first known algorithms depicted a common symptom with multiple branches flowing from it. Organizing associations like this helped to describe complex syndromes. With the advent of computers in the 1960s through the '80s, healthcare workers started to use algorithms in their protocols when treating emergencies and chronic illnesses. Some doctors expressed doubt about these new tools, fearing they had sapped medicine of its art. By 2007, the year I started residency, algorithms had become an essential part of assessing and treating a variety of illnesses.

This algorithm (*opposite*), published by the Institute for Clinical Systems Improvement, is fairly typical of the type I used as a resident to evaluate chest pain.

My problem with this sort of chart and the doctoring it produces can be summed up in one question: Who is the protagonist in this decision tree?

By reducing medicine to a set of ones and zeroes, algorithmania puts medicine's focus on the doctor, not the patient; the doctor becomes the protagonist. If a doctor satisfies the road map, then in their own mind, they have satisfied the patient. Diagnosis and treatment come down to how a doctor follows a road map rather than the report the patient gives. Ultimately, algorithmania pushes people out in the name of science and costs. It makes medicine more of a technical job rather than a vocation.

That's not to say that doctors shouldn't use decision trees. As complex as they may look, algorithms can be very helpful, if not essential. We've seen that algorithms can do terrible things, like ignore sick Black people in need of a health program, but they can help doctors pick the right tests and medicines at the right time. Researchers initially developed the chest pain algorithm to make sure that one of America's biggest killers, heart disease, is treated as quickly and as thoroughly as possible. But statistics show that heart attacks and heart damage from coronary disease are decreasing. Meanwhile, the number of visits to the ER for chest pain has skyrocketed.

At the People's Clinic, it seemed that algorithmania had led some primary care doctors to send more patients to the Ben Taub ER unnecessarily. The practice seemed to be part of a larger trend: Instead of using the algorithm as a tool, the algorithm became the care. Instead of trying

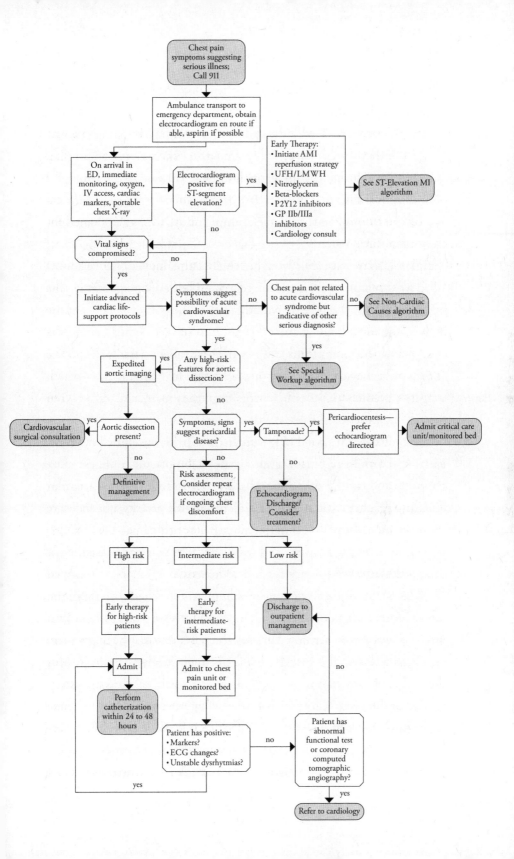

to solve the problem of what ails a patient, doctors jumped at putting patients on an algorithm.

The decisions made with the chest pain algorithm weren't necessarily *wrong*, but they weren't necessarily right either. There's a reason for that. When we use the chest pain algorithm, we're making two meaningful presumptions. Our first is that chest pain is the patient's most important, or chief, complaint. Take the example of the woman evaluated for chest pain during a check of her diabetes. Chest pain is not her chief complaint. In fact, we *don't know* her chief complaint because we haven't asked what symptom ails her most. She could be developing asthma. The high blood sugar could be dehydrating her to the point where her entire body aches, including her chest ("I shouldn't tell the doctor I *don't* have chest pain," she might think). Without these salient details, she arrives at the emergency room as a person transferred for "chest pain"—which triggers a predictable set of behaviors from the emergency team—even though she never used these words.

In some cases, it's good to prioritize chest pain, but not all the time. Fatigue, shortness of breath, even hiccups can portend an illness more ominous and deadly than heart disease, depending on the situation. Focusing on chest pain might help identify heart attacks, but focusing *too much* on chest pain—thinking like an algorithmaniac—will necessarily lead to wrong answers, and wrong answers will lead to higher use of unnecessary medical services and added costs.

Which leads to the second big presumption. The chest pain algorithm rules a heart attack in or rules it out; it doesn't satisfy a patient's complaint unless it is applied correctly. Let's say the patient wasn't having a heart attack after all—in this case, have doctors made headway in diagnosing the problem? Not really. The cause of the chest pain remains a mystery. Instead of thinking, Why is *this person* having chest pain?, doctors under algorithmania's spell might think, I need to rule out a heart attack. The result is that hundreds of thousands, if not millions, of people visit the ER every year and, after a blood draw and EKGs and tests, are let go without a solution to the problem they came in with. How many of these people will come back to the ER the next time? How many of these visits are wasted opportunities to find the right diagnosis?

At its worst, algorithmania can drive doctors to change their patients' words in order to fit them into the algorithm. It's common to see "I'm short of breath" converted to "chest pain" so that the doctor can use the chest pain algorithm and arrive more quickly at an end point. This is faulty logic because healthcare complaints are only rarely so cut-and-dried. A little chest pain can accompany a dangerous amount of shortness of breath, for instance. All symptoms must be graded and sussed out. For this to happen, there needs to be communication.

Working as a primary care doctor at the People's Clinic exposed me to a different rhythm than I'd experienced at Ben Taub. The major forks in each decision tree came over weeks and not minutes. But I was still making smaller decisions on the spot for more than twenty patients every day. If the blood pressure is above 140, what do the clinical guidelines say I should do next? For a patient with a headache, should I order an MRI or is my neurological exam enough? Proceeding down treatment algorithms often conflicted with what the patients at the People's Clinic needed in the moment. Of course they wanted to make sure their blood sugars and blood pressures were okay, but more than anything, they wanted someone to listen—to how the numbness or headaches impacted their lives.

Over time, I found I missed the immediacy of my work treating acute illness at Ben Taub. Its energy kept me moving and kept my attention on my patients. There, I'd figured out how to incorporate listening into practicing medicine. Now, with so much adherence to protocols, it didn't feel as possible to do the same.

* * *

A year and a half before I started to work at the People's Clinic, my grandmother asked me to give her medical advice. I didn't hesitate. I was past my internship and well into my second year of residency. I had passed the toughest parts of my training. More than anything, I spent days in clinic seeing people *just like* my sweet grandmother, people not accustomed to the complexities of healthcare in the United States, people who only spoke Spanish, people who didn't have much money and weren't looking for anything fancy, just a little bit of good, honest advice. If anything, I thought I might be the perfect person to give this to her. After all, how many other doctors could spot algorithmania and how it affected the experience of healthcare?

There were two problems that she needed advice on. Getting these out of her, however, proved difficult. For better or worse, Abuelita never spoke up. Her voice was soft and silvery, and often vanished during dinner conversations and family discussions. My grandmother had spent the majority of her life deferring to my grandfather and, when he wasn't in the room, to my mother or other self-assured talkers (of which my family had too many). One night, I managed to get it out of her while the rest of my family argued: she felt dizzy at times, she said. In fact, her doctors in El Salvador were treating her for an abnormal heart rhythm. She'd never fainted, which was why she hesitated to bother anyone, but she wanted to make sure she was on the right dose of her medication. She asked this of me sheepishly, as if the feelings of her doctors back home were on the line.

I took her hand and patted it. "I think they're using the exact dose that I would use," I told her, and I meant it. I had even brought my stethoscope to my parents' house to listen to her heart. Her atrial fibrillation seemed well taken care of.

Then she mentioned the second problem.

"No puedo tragar," she said in her soprano. *I can't swallow my food.* She wore a short-sleeved button-down untucked over khakis, as always. When she told me, the corners of her mouth hiked up her face into the smallest of smiles, as if to say that she felt silly even saying it.

But her grandson didn't take the dysphagia lightly at all. I asked about weight loss, belly pain, what her stools looked like. I asked whether she ate ice or dirt, trying to unearth an underlying iron-deficiency anemia. I asked about early satiety, the feeling of fullness after eating just a tiny little bit. I felt like I was onto something.

"How much longer are you here?" I asked.

"Only a few days," she told me. I knew any workup in the United States would have to be paid for out of pocket, since my grandmother had no health insurance in this country. It didn't matter. She had us, her loving family. We were going to do the right thing. We weren't going to throw money at the problem, necessarily, but money wasn't an impediment, either. We were going to follow the science. We would investigate the guidelines. We were going to use the dysphagia algorithm.

The algorithm pointed me to a test called a barium swallow, which would show anything obstructing the passage of the liquid into the stomach. My family was wary, but I was hopeful. To me, the scariest thing about the test was its name. I'd taken many chemistry classes over the years and had a decent memory of the periodic table of elements, but I still had no idea what barium was. The thought that X-rays couldn't get through it, allowing it to reveal the shadowy shape of whatever it doused, creeped me out a bit, but I'd never lost sleep over it. My grandmother dutifully swallowed her barium while a fluoroscopy tech shot X-rays. She came home from the test and less than twenty-four hours later, we had the results.

Normal.

The next I heard about her condition was six months later, after I had already started my final year of training. I got the news all at once. My *abuelita* had returned home to El Salvador and continued to struggle with swallowing, so much so that she started having chest pain. Her doctors recommended a different test, an esophagogastroduodenoscopy, or an EGD, to inspect the area from her mouth to her small intestine. A doctor who performed the test found an area that looked clearly cancerous. He took biopsies that confirmed she had esophageal cancer and referred my grandmother to a private surgeon in San Salvador, who, in turn, recommended a wide excision of the esophagus, the sooner, the better. The aunt who lived with my grandmother called my mother, who called me. The whole family wanted to know if I thought my *abuelita* should go ahead with the surgery.

Or rather, they wanted to know and they didn't want to know. It was a big decision, so of course it made sense to get the opinion of a doctor. In theory, that's what I was to them. But I'd also just missed a big diagnosis. Nobody said so out loud—not yet, anyway—but the family felt that I'd let my *abuelita* down. How could they really trust me with a decision like this? Botching the workup rendered fancy titles like "professor of medicine" and "doctor at a safety-net clinic" meaningless. I was back to being the Ricky they'd all known from the day I was born.

I got on the line with my grandmother. Her voice remained silvery and sweet as she described how well she was doing with her atrial fibrillation. She thanked me for the advice I'd given her.

"I'm so sorry, Abuelita," I said.

This is just so silly, she seemed to be saying, why should anyone feel bad? True to her nature, my grandmother wasn't in denial about her cancer, she simply didn't want anybody she loved to feel burdened by it.

She passed the phone to my grandfather, and I offered the same apology, "Lo siento," I said again.

"Bueno," he said. *Well . . .*

When my aunt came on the line, she got straight to business. What about the surgery? Should we proceed?

We didn't reach a consensus over the phone. The debate bled into our family discussions. For two days, it was all anyone could talk about. I didn't think she should have the surgery, not yet, at least. We still didn't know if the cancer had spread. Since the diagnosis, I had plotted my grandmother on a new algorithm, the esophageal cancer algorithm. The next fork on this algorithm wasn't surgery but rather another test, an endoscopic ultrasound. This would tell us if her cancer had metastasized or, at least, advanced to a point beyond where surgery could help. Operating on metastatic cancer carried the grave risk of causing unnecessary pain and suffering. Any surgery, especially a surgery to remove someone's entire esophagus, should be weighed carefully. And my grandmother was in her eighties, no less.

At the time, no doctor in El Salvador performed endoscopic ultrasounds. I insisted that we fly my grandmother back to Houston to receive the test. But I was outvoted.

My grandmother told me about the family's decision herself. She had been back to the surgeon for a preoperative consultation. "I feel good about it," she said. "With the love of God it'll go well."

The family had communicated my misgivings. The surgeon had reassured my grandmother that everything was going to be fine. His optimism spread to my aunts and grandfather. "Gracias, hijito," my *abuelita* told me. "I have a good feeling thanks to the grace of God."

I once got into a shouting match in the Ben Taub hallways with an oncologist. It happened a few years after my grandmother's diagnosis, when I was the head of an internal medicine team. One of our elderly patients was dying from metastatic cancer. After going through all the options, we recommended end-of-life care at a hospice. The patient's family agreed, as did the oncology team. Except that on the morning of the scheduled transfer, a new head oncologist took over. We received multiple pages from the patient's nurse after the new oncology team rounded on our patient.

"The family is very upset," the nurse said. "They want to speak with you."

We went directly to the bedside, where the patient's son awaited with a simple question: Why were we sending his father to hospice to die when the new cancer doctor said he had a 25 percent chance of surviving for two years?

We left the patient's room crestfallen. After many delicate conversations with the family about this man's cancer and the options, our relationship with the family had crumbled. It seemed we were sending a man with a chance at life to his death. When the oncology team emerged from a different patient's room, we confronted them. I asked the oncologist if the two of us could talk in the break room, where, immediately, an argument swelled.

"He thinks he has a twenty-five percent chance of living two years," I said. "You know there's no chance of that."

The oncologist said he was simply quoting the statistics. "I'm not responsible for what the patient hears."

We reached an impasse and parted ways. The two of us shook hands like twins made to apologize after a fistfight. I took the internal medicine team back to the bedside and apologized to the family for the poor communication they had witnessed but made sure to note we each had a different viewpoint. "It's a legitimate disagreement," I said.

Our debate highlighted two different roads, I explained. If they wanted to ensure the father didn't suffer any more and wouldn't be connected to a ventilator, hospice made the most sense. If the father wanted to try to live longer with this risk, chemotherapy made the most sense.

The family canceled the plans for hospice and decided to try chemotherapy. But his other ailments were too much. He died at Ben Taub within a week.

The oncologist and I remained miffed at each other, avoiding each other in the hallways, rarely saying hello. Our disagreement that day revealed a deep divide—a whole different way of looking at medicine and, perhaps, life. Afterward, it dawned on me that my job was to serve as a counterbalance to this type of algorithmania. Doctors employing this type of thinking used scoring systems and decision trees to make decisions. What couldn't be quantified, however, was a person's identity, and their desire to avoid suffering, and the circumstances of their lives. It didn't seem like a fair fight: these factors needed a voice. These people factors weren't the only ones that mattered, but they were often underrepresented in patients made vulnerable by poverty or race or an inability to speak English. At Ben Taub, I felt like I was doing my job by bringing these up routinely. I didn't shy away from debating my colleagues.

My grandmother could have used a similar debate. Instead, she was the recipient of her grandson's algorithmania and that of a surgeon, anxious to wield his knife.

The next time I saw her was in the ICU of a government hospital. She hadn't started out there. The surgeon had excised her esophagus in a private hospital on the outskirts of the capital. My family paid him three thousand US dollars in cash before the operation. The surgeon emerged from the OR with good news and bad news. He had removed her esophagus, as planned. That was the good news. The bad news was that during the operation, he'd discovered that the cancer had spread to her liver and possibly—probably—her spleen.

The costs in the private hospital mounted as my grandmother struggled to recover. My family kept saying over the phone that she was having "complications," but I knew what it was. It had been a butchery. The stitches the surgeon left inside her had started to leak. The surgeon collected his final payment before recommending a transfer to the government hospital. The surgeon and the private hospital had their own algorithmic thinking, it seemed, and they were now at a critical fork: once the family's well dries up, dump the patient on the government hospital, it said. And that's what they did.

I flew to San Salvador two months later, when things seemed close to the end. But that was the problem—in situations like my grandmother's, there is no end. Just the withering of a maimed and helpless body. Only one adult could visit her at a time, they told me at the front desk. Also, the nurses had to "prepare" her before I could enter the ICU. What did that even mean? I thought, dutifully taking my seat. Shouldn't she *always* look cared for, even if she's slowly dying?

It's the great mystery, whether or not someone who's sedated, unconscious, and connected to a respirator can feel you hovering above her, holding her hand, running your fingers through her hair, petting her as you would what's most precious. When I pressed my face close to hers, I could feel how much muscle had evaporated off her. I'd hoped that in her sedation she would look comfortable at least, but no, every breath pushed into her body only seemed to rankle her more and more.

"I'm sorry," I told her again.

She just breathed.

Tears welled up in my eyes. "I wish you were at Ben Taub," I said.

Nothing on this earth was going to vanquish the cancer or mend the cuts inside her. But I could imagine her doing better at Ben Taub. "Better" didn't mean free of disease. That was something Ben Taub had taught me. "Better" transcended the medical. "Better" meant "hopeful." I had seen a Guatemalan man flown back home by his own government to see his daughter one last time before dying. I had seen a child born to a teenager dying of liver cancer. I'd seen hope emerge through death. I'd seen people, and not the paycheck, motivate the doctors and nurses at Ben Taub. I'd worked alongside professionals who regarded medicine as a vocation, rather than merely a way of getting paid.

In America, the story goes that without a cure, there is no hope. That these two ideas twist around each other like the helices of a DNA molecule. Ben Taub taught me this linkage is an illusion. Hope is its own building block for life. Other hospitals aired ads about wiping out cancer and prolonging life. But this was disingenuous. This was advertising. This was false. In medicine, we have our algorithms, and sometimes those algorithms help deliver cures. But there are no algorithms for hope. There can be cures without hope, and hope without cures, but there are no medical miracles. Only human ones.

That's all I wanted for my *abuelita* in her suffering: not a cure, but the hope that she would retain her dignity through all this. That the people working toward a solution would also see her and treat her as a person. That hadn't happened at the government hospital in San Salvador or at the private hospital where she received the surgery. But I knew it could've happened at the county hospital in Houston.

She suffered for four full months in San Salvador. It was awful. She never got close to breathing by herself. She required a constant supply of medicines. Only the very rich received that in El Salvador. The government hospital lacked money; that much was clear. Every day, my aunt and mother had to buy medications from pharmacies outside and hand them to the nurses. The hospital looked clean enough, but the ventilation seemed poor. My *abuela*'s brow was always wet with sweat.

No doctor ever mentioned the possibility of palliative care. Not that my family wanted that. They kept buying medications for her, anything the doctors recommended. Finally one infection resisted all the medicines and overwhelmed her immune system. Or she developed an arrhythmia. Or her kidneys stopped filtering out the urea. Did it matter? When she died, I was happy. I didn't fly back for the funeral. I sent flowers and I meditated on who she had been as a person, a most gentle and kind woman.

I hadn't finished my job with her. She had asked me for advice, and I'd proceeded down an algorithm instead of sharing a moment with her and telling her the scope meant she didn't have longer to live, no two ways about it, and asking her if she might consider hospice services at her home in the hills instead of surgery. I don't think I killed her, but I blame myself for her suffering.

A few months later, after finishing my residency in June 2010, I volunteered to work as a doctor in Haiti. The earthquake that had rocked Port-au-Prince six months before I arrived had left the capital city—and its population of one million—with only two working hospitals. Afflictions like scurvy, kwashiorkor, outbreaks of cholera—the diseases of broken societies—descended on the Caribbean nation. Thousands of doctors from the United States and abroad decided it was their duty to help those beleaguered by the quake. I filled out the application, got my credentials in order, and was off to the Bernard Mevs Hospital, which housed the only intensive care unit in the country.

As I made arrangements for the journey, I reflected on the upheaval in my own life. Not only had my grandmother just died, but my marriage was on the rocks. My mom was preparing to file for divorce from my dad. Even my career seemed to have come unhinged. I'd only applied for one job after residency: to work as an attending doctor at Ben Taub.

My colleagues kept telling me I was a shoo-in for the position, but I had my doubts. Lots of people had applied, very qualified people. One had been an astronaut. In *space*. I only revealed how nervous I was about getting the job to a select few. "But you live and breathe this place," one of my friends said.

I had just finished a night call in the Ben Taub ICU when one of my friends told me to check my email, that the Department of Medicine leaders had decided who to hire on as hospitalists. And so, I snuck into the stairwell between the ICU and the step-down unit. Back then, we had to log in manually each time we checked our email. I entered my password and opened the email. The signature read "Dave," which was what the chief of the department asked his colleagues to call him, a good sign. I read on, from the top. In nice but direct language it became clear that Dave wasn't hiring me. I clicked my phone off. I walked back to the call room, where I'd tried to piece together some sleep the night before. I slammed the door shut. Who knows if any patients or any of the staff heard me. I wept. I hyperventilated. "What am I going to do?" I kept saying. I swore. I hated Ben Taub. I'd poured myself into it and the hospital had rejected me.

Two weeks on a beach or next to a pool might have served my body well after finishing my last shift as a resident at Ben Taub, but I feared having too much time to think. What a thrill it would be, I thought, to be working in Haiti, saving lives. It seemed like the logical next step.

On a layover in Miami, I received a phone call from one of the Haitian hospital's directors. Would I consider serving as the chief medical officer at Bernard Mevs during my two weeks? He explained that plenty of doctors and medical staff would be arriving with me—respiratory therapists, nurses, neurosurgeons—but they relied on a volunteer with the right experience to coordinate the care. The director noticed on my application that I had just finished an internal medicine residency at Ben Taub. "It would be a lot like that but a lot different," he said.

The director was right. Some of the skills I'd developed at Ben Taub definitely helped out those two weeks. During my second week as chief, two men carried a third into the area we used as an ER and laid him on the table. They said that the man had been assaulted, one big knock on the head with a cinder block. He lay there, arms and legs dangling, breathing. I saw no blood on his head or body, but what about a bleed inside his skull? That was the big fear, an intracerebral hemorrhage. There happened to be a neurosurgeon and an anesthesiologist volunteering at Bernard Mevs that week, which meant that if blood was indeed pooling inside of his head and compressing this man's brain, we had people with sufficient technical expertise to save his life.

The question was, how did we know if the cinder block had caused a bleed? In the United States and the developed world, anybody who suffers a severe blow to the head would likely receive a CAT scan to rule it out, the way I had after my concussion. But there were only two working CAT scanners in all of Haiti, the nearest a half-hour drive away. Additionally, the money for the exam had to be paid up front, $200.

My experiences at Ben Taub had taught me when to seek help beyond the hospital walls and when it was okay to use what you had on hand. I asked the neurosurgeon to examine the patient.

"Hello?" he said, shaking the man.

Nothing.

He rolled the man's eyelids back and flashed a penlight he carried with him into the man's pupils. The neurosurgeon then mounted the exam table, situating his knees on either side of the man so that he hulked above him. With all the force of his weight, he dug his knuckle into the man's sternum.

"HELLO," he yelled.

Slowly, through the deepest of fogs, the man picked up his head and moved his lips into a shape that looked sort of like a smile.

"SHOW ME TWO FINGERS."

The witnesses to the assault translated this command into Creole: "DE DW'ET, DE DW'ET!"

The man looked on either side of him as if realizing for the first time that he had two arms. Once the one on his right grabbed his attention, he gave us a peace sign.

The neurosurgeon dropped back to the floor, rubbed a dollop of Purell into his hands, and offered me a lesson on examining human anatomy that I've often thought back to. "Circuit's intact," he said. As I accompanied him from the ER to the cafeteria and back into the quiet, his message started to sink in: in medicine, you need to know *exactly* what you're looking for. In the case of this patient, we had everything we needed to determine whether blood was pooling inside the skull—we had our loud voices and we had knuckles. With these tools, we could rate the man's condition on the Glasgow Coma Scale, a recognized scoring system that predicts how patients recover from head trauma. In a lightning-fast test, the neurosurgeon had scored the man 13 out of 15. This meant he had a 99 percent chance of a full recovery.

"A CAT scan would be a waste of money right now," the neurosurgeon concluded. He recommended that we perform the same exam intermittently over the next few hours and keep a close eye on him over the next twenty-four.

"Call me if anything changes," he said.

Nothing did. We discharged the man the next day with a Ziploc full of Tylenol and ibuprofen. He walked home alone. "Merci," he said on his way out, his smile straightened.

I have no doubt that if this had happened in the United States or another wealthy country, we would have ordered a CAT scan. Not only because the test is readily available but also because we live under the fear that 99 percent isn't enough. We want certainty. Healthcare in America prices that certainty—the leap from 99 percent to as close to 100 percent as possible—at a premium. Algorithms suggest a route to 100 percent certainty, but in medicine, no such decisive path exists. It's up to doctors to weigh whether the leap above 99 percent certainty is worth the risk of the test—like extra radiation from X-rays—and the financial cost. In Medicine Inc., this has become a technical decision: doctors are trained to defer to the algorithm. But in my experience, better, more informed decisions come when algorithms are used as tools to complement, rather than usurp, physician judgment.

During my residency, Ben Taub had only two working MRI machines. Sometimes we waited days for a study. Sometimes we waited so long that in our wait, we decided the test really wasn't necessary at all. The most important studies—those that meant the difference between function and disability, life and death—were prioritized. Getting a study done fast depended on a doctor-to-doctor, human-to-human conversation with the radiologist. It depended on making a good argument for why our study needed to jump the line. It depended on our having thought not only about the MRI but also about alternatives. Sometimes we got our MRIs stat. The arguments always gave us an opportunity to hit the brakes and think harder. Most of the time, we realized we didn't need the MRIs.

Which might surprise some people. The idea that these powerful medical technologies with names so ingrained in our culture that they appear casually in our conversations could be overused might make us question the fundamentals of medicine. In the extremes of Medicine Inc., patients receive MRI after MRI without the touch of doctorly judgment to arrive at a diagnosis. Practicing medicine like this is like driving a car with an accelerator but no brakes.

But at least Ben Taub had MRI machines. The opposite extreme—the very little technology available in Haiti—also didn't work. Medicine in Haiti had brakes, but it had no accelerator. Doctors sharpened their clinical judgment under such conditions, but even the most astute diagnostician can miss a brain bleed that a CAT scan or an MRI can pick up.

Ben Taub hit a sweet spot in medicine. To me, it represented the right combination of technology and judgment, a car with both an accelerator and a good set of brakes. It wasn't a hospital focused on upselling and inflating the bill unnecessarily, but it wasn't Bernard Mevs, either. It was a place where doctors could work as doctors, where science and people and costs all overlapped. At Ben Taub, you could feel like you'd made progress, like you were actually helping to solve people's problems. Another patient in Haiti, a young man, had a bone tumor in his shin. The cancer was growing, slowly cutting off the blood supply to his lower leg. There was one option at Bernard Mevs, amputation, but the boy was only seventeen. He was an orphan. He only knew he wanted his leg. There was no way to find the boy radiation therapy or chemotherapy or to salvage his leg. We wrote letters to hospitals in the United States appealing for help, knowing it was just one of those things, that nothing would happen.

When I returned from my two weeks in Haiti, I knew I didn't have it in me to dedicate my career to an environment with so few resources. Were people's lives really improved by our visits or were these medical trips for our own well-being so that we could feel good about ourselves? What did we accomplish? In the best of circumstances, we diagnosed a problem and started treatment, but what happened when we left? That was the problem in Haiti. There was no standard and no sustainable organization—no system. There wasn't a drive toward excessive unnecessary care and excess billing like in Medicine Inc. There was just us. Doctors work better as professionals to provide personal care if they're supported by a system.

What my grandmother needed was two things: an organized health-care system and the right people. Without one, the other is helpless. I learned this lesson in Haiti, a country that, back in the day, had been wealthier than the United States, but whose infrastructure today made it one of the poorest countries in the world.

My grandmother could have used a sweet spot in medicine. She needed an accelerator when her diagnosis was in doubt, the scope when the swallow didn't suffice. She also needed someone to apply the brakes when it was clear her cancer was too far advanced. She could have used Ben Taub, where there's just enough and not too much, where the focus is on the person and not on the procedures. She needed algorithms *with* arguments, not just algorithms, and not just arguments.

Life as a primary care doctor at the People's Clinic settled me. Every day at five, I pulled out of the parking lot feeling tired and a little damp from the sweat produced by small movements, by typing into electronic charts and swiveling in my stool and placing my stethoscope on a person's back. Most days, I left work satisfied. I wasn't at Ben Taub, but I was with safety-net patients. I felt useful. I'd turn on the ignition and the lyrics would come over the stereo: "Sometimes I can't believe it, I'm moving past the feeling." Other days, my mind was boggled as I backed out over the potholes, shaken as much by cracks in the asphalt as by yet another shift full of mindless adherence to algorithms.

After nine months working at the People's Clinic, I reached out to Dave, the chief of internal medicine at Ben Taub, again, asking if there were any openings. I rewrote the email at least three times, editing away any sign of my bruised ego. I explained that I'd stayed in touch with many of Ben Taub's patients at the People's Clinic, but that I wanted to be closer to the action. I wanted to be part of the hospital's culture again.

I started to write essays about the lives of the people at Ben Taub. One of the essays, published in the *New England Journal of Medicine*, described the life of a patient with kidney failure named Santiago who had to visit the emergency room every three days to receive dialysis in order to survive. The US medical system didn't know what to do with Santiago. Across the country, different policies had been enacted to try to handle patients like him, people who needed dialysis but had no coverage for it. The dialysis problem was starting to spread nationwide. I wrote about what Santiago went through every time he came to the emergency room, how doctors decided when and if to help him, and the factors that had led Santiago to this life of just barely getting by.

The essay was enough for Dave to hire me on. I started back at Ben Taub, this time as a full-time faculty member. It didn't take long for me to sink back into the world I remembered from my residency. During my residency, I had devoted most of my attention to patients' medical histories; now, as I made a conscious effort to limit my algo-rithmania, people's everyday lives took on greater significance in my decision-making.

So much of why people ended up at Ben Taub had to do with costs. Healthcare was simply too expensive. Health insurance was too expen-sive. The reason universal coverage in America is still being debated isn't because most Americans oppose it in principle (though a few do). It's because Americans fear the costs. We are already paying so much for our own care; how much can we pay for someone else's care, too?

Some people think that to solve the problem of healthcare in America, we will have to spend an inordinate amount in overhauling what we have. But in fact, healthcare in America already has too much money. The excessive profits made by middlemen and corporations keep prices high. We don't need to spend more, we need to spend better.

To cover more people, we have to decrease healthcare costs across all of America. Perhaps in this regard, Ben Taub presents a model. It offers universal coverage to residents of Harris County and yet it manages to keep costs so low that it was listed by the *New York Times* as the second-least-expensive hospital in the United States. Is this an aberration? What problems arose from spending less on each patient? What good came from lower costs? I have witnessed both the downsides and the benefits for more than a decade, and I'd rather practice medicine in a system that stretches each dollar instead of one content to pass along exorbitant costs to patients. I'd rather practice in a system focused on people over profit. Whether or not the country is ready for such a shift requires us to explore the real price of unaffordable healthcare.

PART THREE

Costs

— 12 —

Excess

I don't remember how I first heard of Christian. Maybe I received a text that read, "CKD 5 and knee pain," as a handoff from a colleague. Maybe, one morning, I simply looked at my list of patients and found myself at his bedside a few hours later. Walking into his room, I knew that trust between us wouldn't come easily.

Christian had left his home country of the United States seeking an answer to why he was having knee pains. The health insurance he'd earned through his work in Houston hadn't helped him in this quest. He'd been denied coverage for major diagnostic tests. Christian's doctors cycled him through emergency rooms and the offices of specialists. Nobody had been able to put the facts together, and so Christian had left for Mexico, hoping he would get more personalized care there at a lower cost. The doctors in Mexico diagnosed his kidney disease, but since he lived in the United States and he didn't qualify for social healthcare in Mexico, they couldn't forge a long-term plan to treat him.

He'd tried a stem cell clinic, where he received attention and what amounted to a placebo. The knee pains recurred when he returned to Houston. Out of the dozens of doctors he had seen, only one organized a test that would give a definitive diagnosis, a kidney biopsy. The result showed Fabry disease, but Christian wasn't covered for the clinic

237

visits and genetic tests required to confirm the diagnosis. He was only twenty-four years old, but he felt like he was in his forties. He and his mother, Norma, were sick of receiving the same advice at emergency rooms and urgent cares when the pains struck. Now Christian and his mother wondered if the safety-net system—which, to their minds, only poor people visited—could help.

I didn't know this part of the history, not yet. What made me wary were the people accompanying my new patient. I couldn't help but notice one of the guests, a young man lying by Christian's side. He wore black Adidas Sambas and didn't look up from his phone when I entered the room.

"I'm Dr. Nuila," I said, "the internal medicine doctor."

Neither of the two young men stirred when I knocked on the wall or even as I approached the bed.

"Garza?" I said.

The guest turned toward me in the bed, but only partially. His features came into view. The stubble on his chin was blacker than mine. His entire neck was swallowed in tattoos, from the platysma he used to chew to his thick trapezius muscles, which gave him the look of a lean bulldog.

"We know English," he said.

"Gotcha," I replied, focusing now on my patient. Nothing was particularly noticeable about Christian's body: no tattoos, no inflammation. It even seemed like he might fall asleep mid-handshake, probably an effect of morphine administered to him for his knee pains.

The kidneys serve as a brake for natural hormones and many medications. It's not known where the word "*renes*"—the Latin root of "renal"—comes from, but it's thought to be related to the English word "reins," the straps attached to a horse's bit that keep the animal in check. That's exactly what kidneys do: they *rein in* opiates; they domesticate the drug, metabolize it. Since Christian's kidneys were in tatters, the reins had been slit. They were unable to control the excess salt and urea circulating through his body. Now morphine was galloping wildly through his system, making him drowsy.

Christian and I didn't talk about his pain, not yet, anyway. In those first moments with him, my attention was on split screen, shared between his drowsiness and the other people in the room. There was the weight lifter on the bed, but somebody else came into view on the foldout couch on the opposite side of the room, where daylight poured in. The woman had bleached blond hair. Her skin was tanned and she wore workout gear, not for yoga, but for an afternoon on Venice Beach.

"I'm the mother," she said, walking toward me and pausing on the other side of the bed. The cold streaming out of the vent didn't seem to bother her.

We shook hands over the body of her son. I introduced myself again and began to rehash some of the facts I thought I knew—that Christian's kidneys weren't working for reasons that were unclear and that he'd come to the hospital for the pain in his knees.

"It looks like they gave him morphine in the ER," I said.

"Yes, sir," she said.

"And he's been going in and out of hospitals for this knee pain?"

"Yes, sir."

"I read that you may have been diagnosed with Fabry?" I said.

"Yeah," he said, his attention perking up a bit. "The other doctors pronounced it differently."

"What did they call it?" I said.

"Fab-ray," he said.

"They called it Fab-ray," Norma reiterated. "Sir."

If my goal had been to simply "provide healthcare" instead of thinking about Christian's specific problem and trying to solve it with precision, the conversation would've ended there. Christian and Norma had confirmed the basic story line. To complete my job as a provider, all I had to do was lay my stethoscope on his body and walk away. I wouldn't even have had to say, "Have a good day." Then I could have gone to my desk and composed a note with information culled from the electronic chart, like the blood work showing Christian's kidneys no longer worked. I could then have submitted a bill and moved on to the subsequent patient.

But at a public hospital, the patient becomes the community's customer, and the doctor serves society. That's in the best of circumstances. In the worst of circumstances, when the hospital isn't resourced or set up to succeed, there are no customers. Like at Jefferson Davis, accountability is lost. The organizational structure at Ben Taub helped me see Christian and his family as my bosses.

In 2016, a group of researchers decided to survey the healthcare team members of a for-profit hospital in the United States to figure out if they could identify a "customer." Doctors, nurses, administrators, patients, patient family members, and anyone working at a hospital—including support staff and therapists—were asked, "Who is and is not a customer for the hospital, and what leads to customer satisfaction?"

The results, which appeared in the *Journal of Healthcare Management*, showed that neither patients nor doctors saw patients as a hospital's customers. Nearly everyone in the study thought that the hospital's customer was the doctor.

We shouldn't read too much into the study, though it's concerning. It's understandable that patients in the hospital don't feel as empowered as, say, a consumer buying a new couch. Without medical knowledge, they may not know what's best for them, and so they rely on their advocates, doctors, to guide them to purchase the right healthcare for themselves.

In most cases, the patient isn't the customer of their health insurance company, either. The patient's employer decides what healthcare benefits an employee will and will not have and signs a contract with the insurance company accordingly. Nearly half of all Americans, 156 million people, receive insurance through their employer, yet the insurance company considers the employer to be its customer, not the people with the plastic insurance cards in their wallets.

Patients aren't the customers if they participate in Medicaid, the government-funded insurance. Medicaid's low reimbursement rates make doctors and hospitals hesitant to take on Medicaid recipients, limiting their options significantly. The patient is often left feeling powerless.

As a doctor, it took me some years to figure out that Ben Taub's customer isn't me. The safety-net system doesn't coddle me or encourage me to order expensive studies. It also doesn't obstruct what I order, either; Harris Health simply provides me a dependable venue in which to practice, no more, no less. My salary is paid by the medical school, which it contracts to provide medical care for its patients. Because the hospital doesn't offer me financial incentives for increasing the number of services I order, the only incentive left is the people. Christian is my boss because the medical college holds me to patient-care standards. If I don't satisfy him, I fail in my contract with the medical college.

This mentality is more possible in a system without overt financial rewards. One of my colleagues who splits time between Ben Taub and private hospitals explained it to me like this: "The private system is set up to be overused." Working at nonprofit and for-profit hospitals introduced temptations he hadn't experienced at Ben Taub. He could call a colleague in during a surgery when he didn't really need an extra set of hands (and, likewise, expect to be called by that colleague). He felt incentivized to act lazily at times, letting other doctors perform the medicine he could handle well himself.

"Everyone is driven to some extent by the money attached to his/her job," he said. This applied in a lesser way at Ben Taub, too, where departments tracked productivity levels and assigned bonuses based on the number of patients seen. But in private hospitals, this drive seemed to be on steroids. It was easy to see how a doctor at one of these hospitals might come to believe that the medical system was designed to serve them.

I felt confident that the safety-net system would provide Christian with definitive therapies, despite his obscure diagnosis.

"I'd like to get him into the genetics clinic," I said, "but I'd like to focus on his kidneys while he's here in the hospital."

Norma was skeptical. The last genetics clinic they'd visited had required $600 just to walk in the door. "We've been down that road before, sir."

"The difference now is that he's got the Gold Card," I said, "ma'am."

Christian was a resident of Harris County and qualified for the in-network care provided by the Harris Health System. Now it was up to me to guide Christian through the next steps of therapy.

We'd get to the Fab-ray disease, I said, but we had to focus first on the kidneys. Christian should start on dialysis. That was okay, I said. People lived on dialysis, most people even felt better, but there were different kinds of dialysis. Some people could go to a clinic three times every week. Some people performed their own dialysis at home. And some others—*many* others, unfortunately—had to wait until their lungs were filled with fluid or their hearts started beating irregularly before they could receive treatment. Early intervention was the difference between a manageable life and a pretty awful one, spent going in and out of the emergency room.

The weight lifter sat up in bed and turned his body toward me. I caught a glimpse of more of his tattoos as he moved. The body of a butterfly or something winged ran down the axis of his Adam's apple. Covering his right brow was another tattoo. This was a word written in wispy cursive, like smoke trailing off a cigarette on a cold night. I stretched out my hand, shook his, and just like that, the tattooed young man exited.

His departure seemed to signal that things were getting more personal. They were and they weren't. I talked more about the Gold Card and my hope that we could get Christian's knee pains under control. Norma talked about handouts, and how she'd avoided Ben Taub and the safety-net system because she felt like her family made enough. "I don't think that anymore," she said.

Only later did I learn that the stocky man on the bed was the youngest of Norma's sons, my new patient's brother, and that the tattoo on his face had still been fresh. It said "Christian." He'd had it done during his big brother's quest in Mexico.

Imprecise care is expensive care. It is wasteful care. The delay in Christian's diagnosis hadn't been caused by a lack of resources or a scarcity of doctors and procedures. It was caused by the opposite: the amount of excess and waste in the system overloaded the doctors caring for him.

In a 2012 special communication written for the *Journal of the American Medical Association*, Donald Berwick, the former head of the US Centers for Medicare & Medicaid Services, pleaded with the American public, particularly those complicit in Medicine Inc., to stop wasting money. "No matter how polarized politics in the United States have become, nearly everyone agrees that health care costs are unsustainable," Berwick and his coauthor, philosopher Andrew Hackbarth, wrote. With the debate over how the Affordable Care Act might or might not impact the raging cost of healthcare, the authors recommended focusing on what Americans lose by overspending. "Here is a better idea: cut waste."

Of the six areas of waste in American healthcare identified by the authors, Christian certainly endured five, and possibly all six. Most prominent, Christian had fallen victim to a failure of care coordination, whereby his care fell through the cracks because his doctors failed to coordinate with one another. When he received stem cells, Christian was subject to another form of waste, overtreatment, which the authors define as "the waste that comes from subjecting patients to care that, according to sound science and the patients' own preferences, cannot possibly help them—care rooted in outmoded habits, and ignoring science." Administrative complexity—the largest source of waste in America according to Berwick and Hackbarth—occurred when insurance prevented Christian from receiving the tests he required, as well as when Christian was denied health insurance on the basis, he believed, of a preexisting condition. He had also been subject to pricing failures. In fact, the vast majority of Americans not covered by Medicare or a group insurance plan are subject to this form of waste. We simply pay excessive amounts, more than what would be expected in a normal market, because of a lack of price transparency.

The sixth source of waste the authors identify—fraud and abuse, or scams and filing faulty claims—may well have occurred on Christian's quest for care, though we can never know.

What we lose with such waste is staggering. Berwick estimates that 20 percent of all healthcare expenditures amounts to waste. That's $200 billion every year, down the drain. That same $200 billion would provide every uninsured person in America with annual health coverage.

Medicine Inc. doesn't prioritize affordable healthcare for everyone. Medicine Inc. prioritizes profit. And profit occurs best in a system that generates excess healthcare for some rather than sufficient healthcare for everyone. Profit is best generated when healthcare is imprecise and impersonal, resulting in waste. Twenty cents of every dollar we spend on our own healthcare goes down the drain. We accept this because we cannot see an alternative to private health insurance. Our imaginations are constrained by the reality of what has been, rather than perceiving what could be. And millions of people like Christian who are un- or underinsured pay the price.

The same challenge of minimizing waste operates each day inside our own bodies. Diabetes is an illness of excess, whereby the body suffers the effects of excessive blood sugar. A wide variety of problems can cause this excess, including genetics, but the bulk of cases are caused by consuming excessive sugars and carbohydrates and high-calorie meals, and not exercising enough. Similarly, in healthcare, we consume too many high-cost procedures and diagnostic tests, and we don't utilize preventive care enough—a problem, as we've seen, that is especially acute for those without insurance. Putting the brakes on our healthcare spending excess, as well as what sugars we consume, can make our healthcare systems and bodies healthier.

It's impossible to stop wasting money within healthcare on command or immediately. But Berwick and Hackbarth warn that situating any reductions of waste within a "business as usual" model, whereby the financial incentives of Medicine Inc. continue, will do nothing. The authors stop short of thinking beyond the Affordable Care Act. They're careful not to use the word "rationing" or "government" in any solution. To stop wasting, however, we must be bold.

*   *   *

Sometimes the whirring of the machine keeps Christian awake at night. As he settles into bed and the machine atop his desk begins its work, thoughts take over. Is this really my life? Will I ever have sex again? How does this happen to a twenty-six-year-old?

Other nights, the mechanical sounds of filtering soothe him. He can relax into his own body and breathe easily, because there's no coughing, no vomiting, and the knee pains are subdued. The tiny clicks lull him to sleep. None of this is normal, but for Christian, at least it's a new normal. He can live like this.

The machine sits on top of his desk in the corner of his room. Without the supplies stacked beside it—cleaning solutions, gauze, face masks, alcohol swabs—somebody could easily confuse it for a laser printer. Make no mistake, though: this box is a medical marvel, one of those rare apparatuses that saves both lives *and* dollars. It is Christian's new kidney. At night while he sleeps, the machine pumps eleven liters, or nearly three gallons, of a special fluid called dialysate through a plastic tube that connects to another tube surgically implanted in Christian's belly.

By six a.m., the dialysis machine has drawn back the same volume of fluid it's pushed in; what's taken out is dumped into a toilet in the adjoining bathroom via a different tube. Inside Christian's belly, in a space called the peritoneum, is where the magic happens: the fluid going in sucks out the excess potassium and phosphorus and toxins in his bloodstream through osmosis, the natural passage of electrolytes through a membrane. In this case, it's the lining of Christian's abdomen that serves as the sieve. This coordination—getting precise materials into precise spaces safely and conveniently—is what it takes to keep Christian alive.

Christian knows it's pretty extraordinary. And he's just the right person for a machine requiring such precision and oversight. "As you can see, my son is pretty anal," says Norma, cackling, as Christian wipes one of the tubes with an alcohol swab.

This type of dialysis isn't for everyone. Comfort with routine and process—and the temperament of a master brewer—are prerequisites. Every night before connecting himself to the machine, Christian spends thirty minutes inspecting the tubes, warming the dialysate, measuring his weight and blood pressure. He wears a surgical mask during portions to prevent the lines from carrying infection—for instance, from an errant fungus from his breath. Christian takes this all very seriously, which is why he has boxes of alcohol swabs at the ready. Norma jests that he may be taking it *too* seriously, but Christian's used to it.

"I'm pretty prepared for coronavirus," he jokes back. It was early March 2020. One headline in the *New York Times* read: "'When Can We Go to School?' Nearly 300 Million Children Are Missing Class." The world was beginning to change. Christian focused on what he could control in front of him, removing the excess waste in his body from his kidney failure.

Peritoneal dialysis costs around $53,000 every year. When coming into Christian's house—at the moment, he lives with his grandparents—it's not hard to see where this money goes. Thirty-two boxes are stacked against the dining room wall. This represents a month's supply of the dialysate that enters Christian's belly at night. Another wall in his room is lined with more boxes of supplies to be used if the electricity fails.

Keeping things clean and workable is expensive. But home dialysis like this is also an investment. The treatment that most people with end-stage renal disease (ESRD) use is hemodialysis, the filtering of blood directly through a machine. Usually this happens three times weekly in a clinic, which is why dialysis like that costs almost 50 percent more than the home version.

In July 2019, the Trump administration, eyeing a way to shave costs from the health budget, announced that it would attempt to increase the number of people using Christian's version of at-home dialysis. In announcing the plan, Joe Grogan, head of the White House's Domestic Policy Council, noted just how deep the bill for kidney care runs in America: "Taxpayers spend more on kidney disease—over $110 billion—than we do on the National Institutes of Health, the Department of Homeland Security, and NASA combined," he said.

After Christian and I met, he received hemodialysis at Ben Taub, and then he started on a schedule at a nearby clinic, three times every week. Meanwhile, his kidney doctor organized a long-term plan of home dialysis. It took two months for Christian to receive sufficient training and to have the plastic connector surgically inserted into his belly. With everything in place, the hemodialysis catheter was removed and he could begin dialyzing himself at home.

At another hospital, Christian might never have had the option to start on home dialysis. Only around 25 percent of patients with ESRD in 1996 felt they had received adequate information about the different dialysis options, according to one study. A full 33 percent didn't even know that this type of dialysis existed. (Outside the United States—for instance, in Hong Kong—as much as 85 percent of ESRD patients receive dialysis at home.) The internet era seems to have pushed awareness, as a more recent 2011 study found that 58.6 percent of patients understood that peritoneal dialysis is an option. Still, the number should be higher. It's not hard to imagine how and why this miscommunication happens. A doctor might start talking with Christian, using medical terms like "glomerular filtration rate." They might tell Christian that the majority of people use hemodialysis at a clinic. One thing the nephrologist would probably avoid mentioning is that they get paid more if the dialysis happens at a clinic, and that this arrangement makes it easier for them to "optimize" their bill to Medicare. This is how easy it is to generate waste in American healthcare. One conversation with a doctor subject to financial incentives can direct patients toward imprecise care that is excessive and costly.

The kidney doctor at Ben Taub knew that self-dialysis like this would empower Christian, and, moreover, that he was capable of doing it. One type of dialysis didn't present a clear financial incentive over another. Christian wins, the system wins, and, if he cares more about his patient than he does about maximizing profit, the doctor wins, too.

At Harris Health, patients with kidney disease can receive home dialysis even if they don't qualify for Medicare, the way Christian did. The safety-net system's county-funded home dialysis program, one of the first of its kind, provides Christian's type of dialysis to any Gold Card holders who can perform the intricate tasks it requires.

One of my patients, an undocumented man who now self-dialyzes, remembers how, during the old days when he visited the ER twice a week, he nearly killed himself. His blood pressure was routinely 200/120. For many months, he could eat only applesauce and even the slightest movement made him dizzy. Now, years later, the self-dialysis allows him to run his own business as a computer programmer. He considers this opportunity a true miracle.

"I have created jobs," this patient told me while slumping comfortably into his desk chair. "Even for American citizens."

As a citizen covered by the federal government health insurance, Christian has set his sights beyond the machine. The ultimate treatment for ESRD is a kidney transplant. Medicare—the insurance for the elderly that Congress made available to Americans with end-stage renal disease—not only covers these surgeries but encourages them, since program officials have found that kidney transplants are even more cost-effective than home dialysis. Christian has sent emails to his inner circle of family and friends imploring them to think about donating a kidney, and so far, only two have visited the hospital for the requisite blood check.

It's a big ask, and Christian and Norma know it, but they can take hope from the science. A study in the *New England Journal of Medicine* showed that kidney donors survived for just as long as people who didn't donate kidneys (i.e., the general population). In fact, donors showed better physical and mental health than non-donors even after twenty years without a kidney. Which is kind of amazing: one of the most altruistic decisions a person can make—giving a part of oneself, literally, to another—not only saves money and helps the recipient but also helps the giver.

Until that donor steps forward, Christian and Norma wait patiently while counting their blessings. With Medicare coverage, Christian no longer needs the Gold Card. Medicare allows Christian to visit private dialysis centers outside of the safety-net system. If he were to receive a kidney transplant, it would have to occur outside of Harris Health, which does not offer this type of transplant currently. Doctors at Ben Taub have opened preliminary discussions on adding transplants, but this remains a hope for the future. In order to provide care for many, Ben Taub still has to make tough decisions about some expensive surgeries, organ transplants among them.

For now, Christian and Norma can visit a genetics clinic without feeling the shame of flinching at exorbitant prices. A geneticist has recommended a novel treatment for the Fabry, and Christian thinks he might try it. He's consulted with a Fabry group on Reddit, which has him thinking twice. It's possible Christian will never use the safety net again, but at least it was there, during his young adulthood, to put him on the right path toward solving the mystery of his pains.

Public + Private

Stephen didn't want to spend an extra minute at Ben Taub beyond what was absolutely necessary. After a night tossing and turning and trying to tune out the noise, he awoke before daybreak. He knew it was closer to morning than it was to two a.m. by the soreness of his jaw. Much of the pain medicine had worn off, but not all. No worries; he'd be able to ring his new nurse for the day. He glanced at the window in his room, which faced north and framed the glow from the city. There always seemed to be a race in the hospital at this hour. While those coming off the graveyard shift quickly tied up loose ends, workers scuttled to their stations, preparing to receive the new day's baton.

The race inside Stephen's room was something different altogether. Would the sun sneak in through the window and be the first to greet patients, or would somebody active during the wee hours—the kitchen personnel delivering breakfast trays, surgeons—flip on a switch and release fluorescence from above? It was unscientific to think it mattered which of these two old foes, the natural and the artificial, triumphed.

Musings like these made Stephen feel antsy. You can take the man out of the restaurant but can't take the restaurant out of the man. For six months now, Stephen had been a professional patient. He'd visited dozens of clinics and spent nearly a full month inside the hospital. Ben

Taub no longer scared him. If anything, he felt comfortable here. The old GM from the burger joint began to come out. To ensure he received the most efficient care, he had to stay active, he had to communicate. He couldn't just lie around and let healthcare happen. Just like in the restaurant, there were many working parts, and he had to make sure the staff was on track. After all, he was paying for this.

He pressed a button on the guardrail beside his dominant hand, and with that, a gear rumbled. Stephen's head chugged higher and higher until it was nearly upright, giving the bed the appearance of a padded throne. From here, Stephen assumed command of the day. The perch allowed him to verify what went into his body ("How many bags of antibiotics do I have today?"), to keep an eye on the consultants coming and going ("Are you a throat doctor?"), and to chat ("I don't know what political affiliation you are, but . . ."). The TV remote—as boxy and outdated as those found in nail salons on pedicure chairs—helped him during this downtime. Instead of offering variations of back rubs, the remote let Stephen flip between a patient information channel and Fox News—not his favorite, but given the circumstances, it would have to do.

Stephen's nurse contacted me before I'd even met him. "Patient wants to know why he's getting the pain medicine," she said. "He wants to talk with you."

It was early Monday, and I had yet to make it onto the wards. Instead, I sat in my cubicle, mapping out the day and week. Eleven other patients appeared on a list, all of whom I was newly responsible for. Notes appeared beside each name, gleaned from the electronic chart and from a checkout conducted with the departing doctor the previous evening. Some of what I wrote was legible, at least to other internal medicine doctors, but much of it was my own code. I glanced at the list. An open checkbox beside "D/C?"—or "Discharge?"—appeared next to Stephen's name. After reading through his vital signs and lab tests from the morning, I thought Stephen might be able to return home today, except now, he had a question.

"I'll take a look," I said. "Thanks for letting me know."

With that, my attention turned to the more urgent codes on my list, some circled and underlined. The oxygen level of one of my new COVID patients had dropped overnight. Another patient had spiked a fever to 102. Neither I nor the doctor preceding me could figure out why one patient was so confused. Stephen would have to wait. I took a final slug of coffee, picked up my face shield and list, and headed toward the wards.

By the time I made it to Stephen's room, lunch had started to make its way throughout the hospital. I peeked quickly at my list as if it was a cheat sheet, rubbed sanitizer into my hands, and entered.

"Mr. Hart?" I said.

He couldn't move his mouth much, but that didn't stop him from speaking. As I took my usual hovering position on his right, he straightened himself in bed. "Are you the new internal?" he said.

In their notes, surgeons had described Stephen as "well groomed." Doctors document prim appearances not to pander to their patients, necessarily, so much as to note that the opposite isn't the case. Someone characterized as "disheveled," for instance, may not be as meticulous about taking medications on schedule. Stephen did more than make himself presentable. He'd parted his hair at the side to create two salt-colored swoops, one dominant, the other diminutive, which he held in place with pomade. The ends of his mustache were thicker than the body and nearly lengthy enough to be waxed, so that, from the side, he looked like a card dealer from the set of *Deadwood*.

The grooming hid Stephen's scars well. Below his left jaw, in the area where responders check for a carotid pulse, stretched a pale flap of skin the size of a credit card. Two months before, this patch had been harvested from Stephen's left breast in the second part of a radical neck dissection. The amount of radiation absorbed by the Chernobyl firefighters—harnessed and beamed microscopically over the course of thirty-five sessions—had stymied but not stopped the cancer growing in

Stephen's tonsil. Nor had the 160 milligrams of accompanying chemo-therapy (an amount equivalent to the amount of caffeine in a Rockstar energy drink, except that it poisons DNA). The surgeons spent eight hours picking every bit of tumor away, tumor that the treatments had blasted without killing, leaving the inner architecture of the left side of Stephen's neck to appear matted, like gum in hair. Careful not to nick the jugular vein or the facial arteries or the essential cranial nerves, like the vagus or XI—which lets us shrug—the surgeons cut and cut and cut until the evil gum was gone. The remaining hole measured four by six inches. They covered it with the most accessible skin Stephen could spare.

With time, the patch had contracted. It was too soon yet for the area to look natural, and who knew if it ever would, but as I walked into Stephen's room, it wasn't the first thing I noticed.

But it did distract me after we started talking, so much so that I lost the flow of the conversation. As much as I tried to get it back, I was off, and so I pulled out the first thing I could think of.

"Are you eating okay?" I asked.

"I haven't eaten anything solid since this came in," he groaned, point-ing to the tube in his stomach.

Since its insertion four and a half months before, Stephen had lost fifty pounds. He'd endured five chemotherapy infusions, twenty-three office visits, thirty-eight radiation treatments, three tooth extractions (with forceps), six CAT scans, a PET scan, three biopsies, and one ten-hour dissection of his neck. And now, three days into his fourth hospital stay, this for an infection of the parotid gland, he wanted to leave, pronto.

I was holding him up.

"If I don't need to be here, just let me move along," he said. "I'm paying for this."

To call Stephen's accent "Texan" or even "East Texan" would be a bit of a misnomer. For sure, he extended vowel sounds into short melodies and lavished his sentences with diphthongs. His jaw might have been swollen but it didn't hurt "muuch," for instance. He could fill a sentence with as many curses as genteel praises, and often did when he felt listened to. All of this spoke to his rural roots. But his sentences were clipped and direct and compressed those vowels with the consonants of city life. His vocal tone, possibly an effect of the chemo and radiation on his throat, wavered between a baritone and a sonorous squeal. The mention of money brought a specific note out of him, one that perked up my ears.

"Do you have the Gold Card?" I asked.

"I'm self-pay," he murmured. Between past earnings and assets, he now had too much money to qualify for the Gold Card or Medicaid.

This was when I learned that he used to manage restaurants, individual branches of a homegrown burger franchise. Did I know the place?

My friends and I broke a neon sign playing spread eagle at a birthday party there—the best place for kids' parties. I'd confided to my dad what happened on the way home and he just laughed. "Yeah, definitely," I said.

His job had been all about customer care. The way he saw it, they paid him good money just to talk with people, whether that meant guests or staff. After he turned a profit at his first branch, corporate had moved him to a struggling bigger branch, and presto, he'd turned that place around too.

"I was that good," he murmured. "Wuuz."

Headlines about President Trump's defeat in the election—the votes had now been tallied—flashed across the screen. Both of us fought the urge to give the TV our attention.

I took a gamble and expressed some opinions. I didn't want him to distrust me or the hospital. "I've never been through what you're going through," I said, "and I know the cost is huge. But if I was in your position, I'd feel good that, at least, I wasn't being fleeced." Ben Taub was one of the best-priced hospitals in the United States, I explained.

These weren't just words. In 2019, the RAND Corporation, a nonprofit think tank, published a study detailing the billing practices of hospitals across the country. The study showed that, on average, hospitals billed private insurance nearly two and a half times more than they billed

Medicare for the exact same care. Two patients in neighboring rooms receiving the same antibiotics, seeing the same number of specialists every day, receiving the same number of CAT scans, received entirely different bills. It was like a restaurant charging one customer $7.50 for a burger, only to charge the very next guest $18.75. In Medicine Inc., markets set hospital prices. Only the state of Maryland has succeeded in regulating hospital prices at some governmental level. The government will regulate prices it pays for patients with Medicare but doesn't regulate prices paid by patients with private health insurance.

Medicare sets the benchmark for healthcare costs in America in large part because it doesn't negotiate with hospitals and doctors, but rather sets a price taking into account patients, providers, and taxpayers. Its prices hew most closely to the actual cost of services. Hospitals and doctors charge private insurance more because that is the way the system is set up. Because the insured are not protected by the regulations under Medicare, in all likelihood another hospital would have treated Stephen as it would have a private insurance patient and billed him at least 241 percent of what Medicare billed for the treatment he received.

He could feel confident we weren't overcharging him here. The RAND Corporation study listed Harris Health as the second-cheapest hospital in America according to these criteria, as it charged private insurance only 2 percent more than what it billed Medicare (a $7.65 burger). Since Harris Health is a public system and uses taxpayer funding, it doesn't need to turn a profit: it can charge patients for the actual cost of their healthcare.

It's also true that at Ben Taub, we performed fewer unnecessary tests and procedures than any hospital in Houston. Again, it's a claim backed up by data. In March 2019, the US Centers for Medicare & Medicaid Services released data collected from all the hospitals around the country on a website called Hospital Compare. At a local not-for-profit hospital no more than a ten-minute walk from Ben Taub, more than 50 percent of patients with lower-back pain received an MRI before trying treatments like physical therapy recommended by experts. This means that doctors at this hospital *ignored practice recommendations* and went straight to the MRI more than half the time. The national average was 43.2 percent. Ben Taub's number of back-pain patients who received MRIs was "N/A," meaning that "the number of cases/patients is too few to report."

The Hospital Compare data also showed that patients at Ben Taub received far fewer unnecessary heart tests before low-risk surgeries. Only 1.9 percent of patients received stress tests before surgeries like those for cataracts. The national average at the time was more than double that at 4.6 percent. The rate at the local not-for-profit hospital was 6 percent—or three times the rate at Ben Taub.

I told Stephen he could be confident of two things: first, that he was paying fair prices, and second, that he was only paying for the services that he needed to recover.

A few years after I started working as faculty at Ben Taub, Dr. Ken Mattox, Ben Taub's longtime chief of staff, invited me for a discussion in his office. I was writing an article on how Harris Health provided healthcare to people who couldn't afford health insurance and who didn't qualify for entitlement insurance like Medicaid. I had contacted his office, in part, to discuss how much the local government influenced healthcare decisions. Mattox responded immediately and invited me to speak with him. I knew that Mattox was a proud conservative—"I've been offered cabinet-level positions under Democrat and Republican presidents," I'd heard the trauma surgeon announce more than once—and that he wasn't one to mince words. I gathered my voice recorder and notepad and rushed to our appointment.

A colleague once described Mattox as a "showman," which seemed to capture the chief's penchant for delivering controversial statements with a grin. In the keynote addresses he gave to medical societies, Mattox, a trauma surgeon with more than two hundred publications to his name, discouraged the use of tourniquets. Better to place sphygmomanometers, or blood pressure cuffs, in the trash can rather than on the arm of a bleeding patient, he insisted, to protect patients from the IV fluids administered by scared doctors.* Mattox held a special scorn for ambulances, especially their flashing red lights—studied quite in-depth in the trauma literature—which, he believed, did more harm than good to bleeding patients. His strong opinions ran counter to many of the principles of medicine. And Mattox liked that just fine.

His secretary escorted me into the office, and Mattox waved for me to sit down at the front of his desk.

"Conference call," he boomed in his baritone before releasing the Mute button on his speakerphone. It was March 2014, and an outbreak of Ebola in western Africa threatened the United States. Patients with the virus had already started to appear in emergency rooms throughout the country, including in Dallas. Mattox had volunteered Ben Taub to lead the effort to design a national screening protocol to help emergency rooms identify the illness.

"Who owns the patient?" he said.

I was relieved to hear that even with government officials, Mattox spoke his mind.

As Mattox boomed on, I tried to limit my eavesdropping by scanning through his office from my seat. Alongside such titles as *Great Ideas in the History of Surgery* and *A Treatise on the Scurvy*, he kept a copy of *The Hospital* on his bookshelf. Above my head hung a framed old photograph of Jefferson Davis Hospital, complete with architectural plans and blueprints, the way a pop star might hang up their first platinum record.

---

* Mattox believes that IV fluids dilute the clotting factors necessary to help a hemorrhaging patient from bleeding out. He has published different studies looking at the benefit of IV fluids in this circumstance to support this theory.

Mattox had trained at old JD exactly when Jan de Hartog volunteered there. When *The Hospital* was published in 1965, Mattox didn't celebrate it. In fact, many trainees from that era eschewed it, sensing that de Hartog had cheapened their hard work at Jefferson Davis Hospital. In fact, when Jan was invited back to Houston in 1990 to mark the twenty-fifth anniversary of *The Hospital*'s publication, rumors spread throughout the Texas Medical Center that a group of doctors would protest the lecture, with Mattox leading the charge. Right before de Hartog took the podium, Ben Taub's perennial chief of staff took his seat in the auditorium, and for a moment, cordiality seemed to have emerged victorious.

In the ensuing Q & A, however, Mattox called for the microphone. He stood up, patted his starched white lab coat, and addressed de Hartog publicly.

"Mr. de Hartog, when you were here, I was a trainee, and I could not speak my mind," he said.

The lecture hall grew as silent as an operating room between cases. Mattox had a reputation for eviscerating residents and staff during weekly morbidity and mortality (M & M) conferences. No topic was off-limits during these hours when surgeons discussed how and why things had gone wrong for their patients. Mattox had even thrown fifth-year residents out of conference for attending in scrubs. As some in the audience wondered if Mattox might be going all M & M on the old ship captain turned dramatist, others noticed a tell appearing on his face, that showman's grin.

"Your book inspired me to stay at Ben Taub," Mattox continued. "I felt my calling was here."

It seemed fitting that *The Hospital* sat among titles that had helped Mattox tie off arterial bleeders and dissect damaged intestines. Ben Taub and its sister hospital, LBJ, kept Houston's workers at their construction jobs, building the city. Would Ben Taub be the civic institution it was without the book?

Once he finished with the Ebola conference call, I asked him about the photograph of the old Jefferson Davis Hospital.

It had been his teaching hospital, he explained quite simply.

We got to business. Mattox went through some napkin math with me. He divided Harris Health's $1.3 billion budget by the 311,000 unique patients in the system. It amounted to $4,180 per patient, compared to $8,900 per capita spent nationally.

"If we augment our revenue," he said—by utilizing a two-cent sales tax, for example—"we could take care of Houston's entire population."

The suggestion was a bit shocking, not for its ambition—Mattox trained beneath legendary surgeon Michael DeBakey, who performed the first successful coronary bypass in 1964—but for its principle. That government can provide healthcare, not just for a few, but for all, departed from the political ideology Mattox typically espoused. Mattox's showman side could well have been coming out, colored by his deep love of Ben Taub and his representation of the institution he led, but there seemed to be more.

What private hospitals charged was "highway robbery," he said. Not only that, Ben Taub helped Houston's nonprofit and corporate hospitals. Without the safety-net hospital, more uninsured patients would certainly visit these. I remembered what King Hillier had told me about the relationship between private and public healthcare in Houston: "If we go, they go." The safety-net system off-loaded nonpaying patients from private hospitals.

Both Mattox and I took care of patients in this safety-net system, so we had experienced (and been a part of) the limitations. But many of Houston's sickest and most vulnerable patients received excellent healthcare for pennies on the dollar. Many people loved the healthcare they received. Neither the hospital nor the system was motivated by profit. Many doctors, like the two of us, loved working here.

"I told President Barack Obama this is the purest form of medicine," he said, referencing the commander in chief's visit in the months preceding passage of the Affordable Care Act.

I couldn't help but agree. Medicine felt pure here. That's one of the big reasons I had wanted to work here, why I cried when I wasn't hired initially, why I revered this building. I could practice medicine the way I wanted. The local government subsidized that liberty.

He answered all my questions and, when I was done, jumped on another conference call. In addition to the Ebola outbreak, Houston was also dealing with a surge of child migrants from El Salvador, Honduras, and Guatemala. Many were housed in area shelters, and some required medical care. Harris Health was clearly the right medical venue for the job, but a process had to be organized. Problems like these decorated the chief of staff's calendar on a daily basis: how does one stretch the system to accommodate the newly sick and derelict, those left without jobs—and, therefore, health insurance—due to the latest hurricane? Or freeze? Or because oil prices have dipped?

Mattox seemed pleased that he had been able to show President Obama a system created in Houston, from local government. To Mattox, healthcare, like politics, should be all local.

"People in Bangor, Maine, have different healthcare needs than us Texans," he said.

As I gathered my recorder and notebook to leave, I overheard the start of the next Ebola phone call. I could hear the pride in his voice as he boomed some more, this time offering up the expertise he'd earned in public hospitals to private hospitals throughout the state.

Ben Taub was his baby. He wore the pride of a father in his grin and in the starch of his lab coat. The pride came out when he was showing off Ben Taub and its underlying idea, that pure medicine transcends politics. That this idea made Republicans and especially Democrats squirm a bit gave him a special delight. It was local government at its finest.

"I don't mind paying," Stephen said, his voice at a higher pitch now. "I'm not looking for free, I'm looking for reasonable."

We were starting to talk for real now, and so I asked if I could sit down.

"Please do," Stephen said.

With its minimalist furniture cut into right angles and decked with vinyl—including a boxy sleeper sofa—his room had the feel of a budget European hotel, one that seemed to say, This place is hygienic! I sat in the armchair to Stephen's left. The TV divulged that the Pfizer COVID vaccine was showing great promise and that President Trump was doubling down on contesting the election results. I asked Stephen how much all this—the surgery, the chemo, the radiation, the hospitalization—cost him. A few weeks later, he would show me the amount on his phone via an app developed by the hospital. But Stephen also knew the number by heart: it was $32,378.*

"I don't think it includes this visit," he said.

"That's nothing," I said.

Of course, it wasn't *nothing*; $32,378 was a boatload of money, to me, at least. It wasn't the kind of cash people had lying around. I'd seen ludicrous medical bills over the years. And Stephen's bill didn't seem too bad at all, considering all the healthcare he had received. And while the amount seemed a lot, I reminded myself that financial counselors verified that Stephen held valuable assets, including a house. Those earning beneath 150 percent of the federal poverty level and without assets received a Gold Card, with nearly full financial assistance. In Stephen's case, it would be difficult, but he could afford to pay it.

"Oh, I agree," he said. "You can't buy a new truck for forty thousand dollars."

His father had received radiation treatments for prostate cancer and a bill to his insurance totaling more than $700,000. It was impossible to know the true cost of that care, but going statistically by what hospitals and doctors billed private insurance, the real cost of his father's care was likely closer to $241,000.

---

* Stephen's original health insurance ended up paying a total of $1,200 toward his care. This figure had already been subtracted from his total.

Even if it seemed fair, Stephen was well aware what the low sticker price didn't buy him. The ideal healthcare system would provide low healthcare costs while minimizing wait times. Other features important to many patients, like added privacy and added thoroughness beyond what standards suggest, might also be accessible. Ben Taub had prioritized standard healthcare according to the scientific guidelines. But certainly, at other hospitals, Stephen might have experienced healthcare with more bells and whistles as well as real conveniences.

"I don't have a personal surgeon that comes by to check on me every day," he said, noting that doctors rotated on a weekly basis, sometimes even more frequently. The day before, a different internal had seen him; now it was me. Stephen could live with that, especially at this price. What he wasn't so sure about was the quality of care he received.

"I don't know that the surgeon did a great job or not," he said, brushing the patch on his neck with the pads of his fingers. "I've never seen one. I have nothing to compare this to."

Stephen had posed a highly complex question, one I happened to be obsessed with: Was Ben Taub any good?

Someone could easily point to the Hospital Compare rating of one star and conclude that Ben Taub was exactly what they expected: a really bad hospital. I questioned the basis of these ratings, and I wasn't the only one. In 2019, leaders from the Association of American Medical Colleges, the American Hospital Association, and America's Essential Hospitals—which represents US safety-net hospitals—wrote a letter to then-administrator of the Centers for Medicare & Medicaid Services Seema Verma requesting a suspension of the overall star rating. "We remain extremely concerned that [the] star ratings approach does not provide an accurate picture of hospital quality performance," they wrote. Star ratings were driven more by methodology than actual performance, the group argued. The ratings seemed to be unfairly biased toward smaller and for-profit hospitals.

There was also the problem of how to account for a patient's "social risk factors," meaning, the life factors that affected the care a hospital could provide. Safety-net hospital patients were more likely to take buses to the hospital, and some buses ran late, perhaps past the time a pharmacy closed: Should a hospital receive a lower rating because of the life obstacles its patients faced? Was it Ben Taub's fault that it was only one of two major trauma centers for a city of more than five million? The ratings suggested as much. "Without adjustment, star ratings will put hospitals caring for poor communities at an unfair disadvantage, and mislead the customer," the group concluded.

I told Stephen what I told my friends, that the quality at Ben Taub and the safety-net clinics depended on a lot of things.

Stephen eyed me suspiciously. "If it was you, would you come here?"

"For most illnesses, for sure," I said. "For some, probably not."

The wait time for gallstone and kidney stone surgeries was pretty long, I explained. Some of my patients lived months with tubes coming out of lower backs draining urine into a bag they wore around their legs. A screening colonoscopy could take six months to schedule.

I asked Stephen what he thought. What had been his experience with the system?

There is a young lady that stands by the door and takes people's temperatures as they walk in for their clinic appointments, Stephen said. Taking a page out of his restaurant managing days, he decided to let her know what he thought about her work with actions, not words. At his last clinic appointment, after she pointed the temperature gun at his forehead and cleared him to enter, he'd given her a $25 gift card and thanked her for always brightening up his day, even when he was at his lowest.

Everyone, in fact, had been exceedingly nice to him throughout his illness, from the ER to the business office to the clinics to the doctors, even me. The kindness made him nostalgic for the restaurant. It was hard to judge the quality of his treatment, but he knew that everyone here had treated him as a person. This had surprised him, since Ben Taub was public. "I would recommend this hospital at any cost," he said.

While he didn't buy scratch-offs anymore, it had been harder for Stephen to shake his betting nature. He still scoffed at the idea of spending real money on health insurance. Illness was definitely no longer an abstraction to him, but he still suspected insurance companies only sought to rip him off. Giving up his hard-earned cash to an insurance company he didn't trust simply wasn't in the cards.

Things had turned out well for him, though. He was happy with the hospital, happy with his care, and when he did the math, the cash price of $37,385 amounted to less than he would have paid in premiums counting back from his start at the burger chain in 2001. He realized that with good coverage and a connection to the healthcare system, his cancer might have been caught earlier, thereby lessening the amount of tissue resected and giving him more peace of mind. But overall, he felt like he'd played the game well, except now he believed he knew how to win.

Without a job, he would have to navigate unemployment and disability benefits. He planned to apply for Medicaid, which didn't require money out of his pocket (he's still not a fan of government insurance). All of this had been unimaginable to him previously. But seeing his cancer treated sequentially and effectively at Ben Taub had given Stephen confidence.

At some point, my phone began to chirp again, and a little after that, my pager.

"You need to go," Stephen said a bit ruefully.

"Hold on," I said as I ducked into the hallway. There, I dialed the numbers I'd missed, and for a few minutes, found myself back in the race, noting blood sugars, making sure discharges were in by eleven a.m., receiving new patients from the ER. When I returned, Stephen's attention was on the TV.

"I don't know what political affiliation you are . . . ," he crooned.

For the previous weeks, I'd talked politics only with people inside my bubble, and had done so obsessively. I didn't talk with my dad, and he didn't reach out to me. My daughter asked if she could see him again, since we'd spent so much time together during the COVID summer. "Maybe soon," I said.

Stephen aired out his concerns about the election—the fraud, how this might be a coup—and I listened. He said that Fox News was too mainstream and not conservative enough for him, and I nodded. I didn't lie when he asked me specific questions, but I also didn't fuel the discussion, either. Stephen was a people person, and so was I. He was our customer, and I had the opportunity to make his day or to ruin it.

When my phone chirped again, there was one thing left to do, and that was to put my hand on Stephen's face. His parotid gland was inflamed, the texture of the skin taut and warm and tough.

"I think you need another night of IV antibiotics," I said.

"You're the doc," Stephen said, touching the same area I'd touched.

I stopped by Stephen's room early the next morning. The wrinkles had returned to his cheek, and the gland felt more rubbery, less stiff. "You're good to go home," I said, except I couldn't help but reiterate something to him. This hospital existed in large part because of government, I said. This was public healthcare run by the local government. Property taxes picked up from the community subsidized what happened at Ben Taub.

Ben Taub hadn't looked much like a public hospital to Stephen, or, at least, what he thought a public hospital might look like. It was also changing. A large portion of the emergency room had completed its renovation. Now sixteen individual rooms with glass doors surrounded two central computer stations for nurses and doctors. The first time I saw this new pod, I stood stunned, as if I'd entered a new stadium.

"This is beautiful," I said to the nearest person wearing scrubs, a woman I'd never met.

"It really is," she said.

The McDonald's in the cafeteria was long gone after the flooding brought by Hurricane Harvey. Now there were plans for a cafeteria that served "international food" and a Subway. Certain parts of Ben Taub were starting to appear private. But the hospital was still publicly funded. I had no interest in igniting an argument, but I wanted my patient to know.

Stephen accepted this and thanked me. He thanked all his nurses before leaving.

The oncologists had used an acronym I hadn't seen much when describing the stage of Stephen's cancer. When he visited their clinic a week later, it appeared again in their note: "NED."

This time, I looked it up on Google, "NED Head and Neck Cancer," and was directed to a slew of websites. I clicked on the first one.

"No Evidence of Disease," it said.

— 14 —

Disaster Syndrome

Patients and doctors, nurses and social workers—most people who've entered an emergency room or a doctor's office know something is wrong with healthcare in America today. Instead of correcting the problem, however, we've all decided to accept the issues as permanent. We debate each other about the nuances of private insurance, like protections for preexisting conditions, but these discussions are nothing more than circumventions. We show no will to reinvent American healthcare: we think it would be impossible, that we're stuck with the status quo. We're making the best of it, we tell ourselves if we're lucky enough not to be sick. But the costs remain unaffordable; many millions of people cannot access healthcare when they need it. We Americans are suffering collectively from disaster syndrome.

We aren't the first to suffer from this ailment. A quick look at one of the great natural disasters of the last century—eerily reminiscent of some of the catastrophes we endure today—shows us how easily disaster syndrome sets in.

It had been a week since the waters of the North Sea breached Holland's dykes. *De Watersnoodramp*, the great flood of 1953, had spilled salt water on a tenth of the country's farmland. Seventy thousand people had evacuated their homes. Eighteen hundred would die. While US

Army helicopters rescued Dutchmen from their rooftops, a young Jan de Hartog navigated a hospital ship toward one of the Netherlands' most isolated towns. In a decade, Jan would write *The Hospital* after working as an orderly at Ben Taub's predecessor, Jefferson Davis Hospital, but for now, his attention fell squarely on skippering the ship and bringing supplies to his afflicted compatriots. For seven days and nights, the medical care for the town and its surrounding villages had fallen to one lone doctor and his wife.

The devastation was shocking. The village was in shambles. Planks of wood from what had been people's houses sat in heaps. Entire buildings had been swept from their foundations and abandoned a short distance downstream, their signature V-shaped roofs jutting up out of the earth like hands reaching from the grave.

When Jan arrived, he expected the doctor to run toward his ship weeping tears of joy. The ship captain had brought water, cans of food, dry clothes, and warm blankets. He'd brought nurses and medical personnel and soldiers ready to help organize the chaos and relieve first responders. Jan steered the ship through the village like a gondolier, navigating the avenues slowly with open eyes, except he wasn't looking for tourists. He called into abandoned homes, hoping to reach anyone in need, "Hallo?"

Rather than being greeted by enthusiasm and relief, he found the opposite:

> They lacked everything, even the most primitive nursing aids; but when we arrived they seemed almost resentful, as if the well-equipped hospital ship, suddenly emerging in the middle of their world of destruction and death, interrupted a battle when it was almost won. "We made the best of it," I heard the doctor say to ours, with ill-concealed resentment. "As a matter of fact, we did rather well."

What's wrong with these people? Jan thought. How can someone in these conditions eschew help?

Jan recalls this moment in *The Hospital* during his first volunteer shift at Jefferson Davis Hospital. With a long line of patients waiting for care in the hallways, he sees how bureaucracy weighs down the doctors and nurses and saps them of their motivation. The chief nurse tells Jan that they need more staff, but that the hospital makes the most of what they have. The conversation triggers memories of the great flood and the village doctor's reluctance to accept help. It also shows Jan how easily good people's judgment can be clouded when working through difficult conditions:

> In the chaotic aftermath of an unimaginable catastrophe, he and his wife had rallied with magnificent courage; but they had been able to do so only after relinquishing all usual standards for the practice of medicine . . . The disaster syndrome can be diagnosed when normal reactions of protest or outrage in the face of intolerable conditions are absent and the overriding reaction is not to correct those conditions but to accept them as permanent and to circumvent them.

Whenever an article on healthcare's brokenness flashes across our screen and we shake our heads in resignation, assured this problem can't be fixed, we're manifesting disaster syndrome. Disaster syndrome explains our unwillingness to change the healthcare conditions for ourselves and the greater society. It is awareness followed by inaction. It's all of us copping out.

What went wrong? Can we reverse this collective disaster syndrome?

No one group suffers more from disaster syndrome than doctors. Doctors are on the front line and deal with the inequities of the system every day. Many doctors would like to bring change, but, in a system that rewards profit over concern for people at virtually every level, inertia sets in. Others decide to leave the profession; the challenges feel too big to confront. When doctors weather these conflicts for too long, they can develop burnout, one of disaster syndrome's leading symptoms.

I saw signs of this in my dad growing up. Over time, the suits he wore every day to his clinic gave way to scrubs. Sometimes his pager went off two or three times before he answered it. He stopped exchanging the corkboards with baby photos in his office. Compare the man holding a child to the camera—mustachioed, a helmet of black hair, and a smile that, in the nineties, still appeared fresh —with the one moving stacks of paper around on his desk and sighing before entering an exam room, and it becomes clear: my dad was burned out.

Was he just getting older? Had we, his kids, worn him out? Just because he was burned out doesn't necessarily mean he suffered from disaster syndrome. Different illnesses can manifest similar symptoms. Some of his behaviors, however, indicated he was suffering from a burnout specific to American doctors. Manila folders had started to consume his office as he fell behind on paperwork. If his job came up in conversation, he immediately launched into a screed against insurance companies and Medicaid. The man who'd once claimed he'd work until the moment of death started to talk about retirement.

His level of disillusionment was not unique. In a survey of twenty thousand doctors worldwide, more than half of American doctors reported bureaucratic tasks as the top burnout factor. Only Portuguese doctors complained so much about bureaucracy. The survey showed similar levels of doctor burnout in all countries, including in France, Germany, and Spain, but for different reasons. American doctors craved more control and autonomy than their counterparts. Notably, UK doctors reported the lowest burnout and depression rate in this survey. These doctors, who, by and large, worked for the National Health Service, complained of government regulations more than doctors from other countries, but they didn't identify these regulations as factors for causing burnout as much as US doctors did bureaucracy.

Burnout is a problem because it affects patients and the cost of healthcare. It also worsens disaster syndrome. Nearly half of all doctors in America plan to decrease their work hours or leave the field altogether prior to retirement. They do so for a variety of reasons. For some, the ability to walk away earlier than at retirement age is a privilege afforded by the largesse of American healthcare. Others find less stressful opportunities. Some, unfortunately, die young. Researchers predict that with an aging and larger population, the United States will experience a shortage of 54,000–139,000 doctors by 2033. Burnout only accounts for a fraction of this shortfall, but when you consider the length of the training that doctors require, and how that training is often subsidized by state governments, losing even one doctor like this feels like a waste of resources.

The dearth of doctors is expected to go beyond primary care doctors and include the specialists who perform hip fracture surgeries, colon cancer screenings, and care essential to an aging population. Increased demand for healthcare and a decreased supply of doctors could mean higher prices, longer waits for clinic appointments and procedures, and worsening disparities.

Doctors' ditching their duties in the midst of dire need is its own disaster. Opening more medical schools and allowing more foreign medical graduates to work in the United States only places a Band-Aid on a larger problem: most doctors simply don't like practicing the American style of medicine anymore.

In a 2018 opinion piece published by Stat, a Harvard plastic surgeon and a military psychiatrist argued that the problem went beyond tired and downcast workers. "We believe that burnout is itself a symptom of something larger: our broken health care system," they wrote. "The increasingly complex web of providers' highly conflicted allegiances—to patients, to self, and to employers—and its attendant moral injury may be driving the healthcare ecosystem to a tipping point."

Dr. Zubin Damania, a hospitalist in Las Vegas who appears on You-Tube under the pseudonym ZDoggMD, posted a six-minute diatribe affirming this idea. "Burnout is a kind of victim shaming," he says in the clip, which has earned more than fifty thousand views. "It's saying, you're not resourceful enough, you're not resilient enough, you're not strong enough to adapt to a system, so maybe you should meditate? Maybe you should use some lavender essential oil? It's all bullshit."

Damania's TEDMED talk in 2013 titled "Are Zombie Doctors Taking Over America?" earned the attention of then–Zappos CEO Tony Hsieh. The businessman's deep pockets helped Damania start Turntable Health, a primary care clinic that aimed to provide personable healthcare to Las Vegas's less fortunate without a fee-for-service system. Instead of charging for each visit or for each procedure, Turntable used a subscription model and charged each patient a flat fee of $80 per month. If you remove the profit motive from medicine, Damania hypothesized, doctors will feel fulfilled and patients will stay safe. A model like this helped doctors stay in the profession more than wellness retreats, he surmised: "What's gonna happen to a good person in a bad system? They're gonna adapt, they're gonna adapt, they're gonna adapt, and then they're gonna fucking break. And that's what they call burnout."

Even though Turntable Health was able to please its doctors and achieve good outcomes for patients, the financial hurdles proved too high. Patients' insurance companies balked at the flat fee. The clinic's administrators attempted to coerce Damania into offering a fee-for-service option, as well as co-pays, which cut against Turntable's focus. With insurance companies refusing to pay their clients' flat fees, in January 2017, the medical start-up closed its doors. Damania now practices at UNLV medical school.

Burnout at Ben Taub is different. Here, the system adapts to doctors as much as doctors adapt to the system. For instance, each hospitalist can only see as many as fifteen patients in one day. Patient caps like these give doctors time to make safe and thoughtful decisions and to feel unhurried at the bedside. I know in advance when I may be responsible for a new patient thanks to an admissions schedule. Understanding the limits and timetable of my responsibilities allows me each morning to look at my list of patients and plan. I typically reserve afternoons for conversations while using the mornings for efficiency: getting patients home. Financial incentives, like bonuses for extra productivity, exist at Ben Taub, but they're calculated at the end of an entire work year, and they're not sufficient to affect how I manage my daily routine. At Ben Taub, I feel like I can balance medicine as a job and as a vocation. The system's flexibility has helped me keep my patients as the top priority whenever I'm working. And moral injury isn't so much a problem at Ben Taub, because the values of the safety-net system and the doctors are more likely to align.

So why, then, do doctors at Ben Taub like me and my colleagues still feel like we have to empty the tank every day?

Maybe it's because we see many more stage-four cancers than we do stage ones. Maybe it's because, since we deal with people who haven't had preventive care or early cancer screenings, we meet our patients not at their first sign of sickness but nearer to their last. Maybe it's because we usher people to humane deaths more often than we save lives. Or maybe it's because, in caring for our patients, we put our heads down and fail to notice what's going on with our own friends.

The coronavirus drifted into Houston like a gentle rain—floating over the city, collecting here and there. The first cases appeared in early March 2020. Hospitals didn't see a spike in admissions until early April. While infections mounted, Houston's medical capacity remained strong during those first months. There was no lack of beds for patients citywide, neither on the wards nor in the ICU.

Ben Taub remained busy, though if anything, with fewer people on the roads and most people locked down at home, our workload decreased. My colleagues and I held out hope that the storm would pass us by. We knew what hospital staff in hot spots endured. A Spanish ER doctor posted a video on Facebook describing how it felt to select who received the hospital's last ventilator and who died. An old friend working as a hospitalist at Evergreen hospital in Seattle, America's ground zero for the pandemic, described to me the cognitive dissonance of what the news portrayed and what she saw on the COVID wards: "I am continually amazed by the psychology of this disease and how it does its damage by making no one believe it is real until it is upon them."

We paid attention to the numbers every day. Still, we knew the truth even before it was reflected in bar graphs sent to us by our own virologists or on the *New York Times* website. COVID was starting to overtake our isolation beds. It was filling our wards.

Our days fell naturally into two parts: moments of caution, when we'd gown and enter our patient's room without touching them, and the liberated times, where we'd sit six feet apart and vent to one another about medicine and society and feel fortunate we weren't locked down in our homes. We shared theories that appeared in the *Lancet* and on our Facebooks. We debated whether using hydroxychloroquine actually made sense. We couldn't help but note the silver linings: the free coffees given to us by masked baristas, the empty freeways, the vacant garage with parking spots as close to the hospital as we'd ever been.

When the ICU began to fill, we expanded capacity. We moved the infected-but-not-so-sick onto cordoned-off wards to save time and staff and PPE and to give ourselves the feeling that this thing could be contained. Our fears got to us. We separated from our families. Before entering our own homes, we stripped to near nothing and carried our scrubs to the washing machine with used chopsticks. We lamented those who refused to wear masks. We wondered aloud what the hell our governor was thinking. How could he be so cavalier?

Though we never quite got there in Houston, we drafted ventilator algorithms designed to guide us through the most difficult and abstract questions: Who receives priority? Who doesn't? New faces showed up on the wards, nurses traveling from Utah, Arkansas, the Dakotas, and immediately, we felt relieved. More staff: this was real help.

The disaster syndrome at Ben Taub didn't look like the one Jan de Hartog encountered during the great flood. Our disaster syndrome was more insidious, its manifestations far-ranging. Some doctors became so disillusioned that they pretended they were impermeable to the virus and scampered in and out of patients' rooms without eye protection. Others treated each day as an airborne Armageddon, removing their ski goggles and gas masks only in their homes. And still others changed in ways that were difficult to detect.

You see a person you've admired for years walking down the hallway, for instance. "How's it going?" you ask, the way you always do. Instead of the usual, "Good, how're you?" the person looks hurt, even insulted, by your words. There is no eye contact, no exchange of pleasantries, just a shrug and "Eh, you know."

This happens again and again, to the point where, with everything going on—the COVID numbers starting to ramp up, more and more patients filling the ICUs, our resources starting to wane—you lose empathy for the person. When you see the person again, you take the stairs, to avoid the encounter. You think to yourself, Snap out of it! You want the problem to solve itself.

As COVID began to surge in early June 2020, something seemed amiss with the leader of our section, one of my best friends at Ben Taub. Those of us who knew him well talked about it in secret, in the hallways, always out of earshot of his office: "What's wrong with Dave?"

He preferred we use his name rather than any of his titles. When not in his presence, I proudly referred to him as my boss, but he was much more than that. He was a public health expert, an educator, and a scientist. He was an internationally recognized expert on how to treat the most common illness, high blood pressure. No matter how busy hospital administration duties kept him, he always found time for his patients. He loved them, and they loved him. He embodied what was right about Ben Taub.

It was Dave who'd decided not to hire me coming out of residency. Dave had also followed my progress at the People's Clinic and saw I was serious about the safety-net system: he brought me back to Ben Taub. Every couple of weeks or so, we would sit in his office and discuss Ben Taub's place in the world. That patients received more doctorly care at Ben Taub than at the fancy hospitals nearby made us feel like we knew one of the world's little secrets. Or could we have been drinking our own Kool-Aid? Dave never accepted an easy answer, and so our talks became part of a lifelong conversation about the topic of Ben Taub and how to make medicine in America better.

Once he told me he'd met my dad at a dinner for doctors. They had been assigned to the same table and, after going through the usual pleasantries, discovered their common link.

"Did you all get along?" I asked. How little I knew. They were both fathers to me in their way, but more than anything, they were both doctors who loved what they did, so of course they got along.

"We had a great time," Dave said. "Smart man. Funny."

When I asked him about that night, my dad described Dave in almost exactly the same way.

Apart from being a doctor, Dave spent the bulk of his day in one meeting or another—Operations Committee, Patient Wellness, Meds-to-Bed Program, you name it—administering to all the fine print that might inhibit us frontline doctors from doing our jobs. "I'm a bureaucrat," he liked to tell me, his eyes peeking above his glasses. Promotion in medicine brings many of these opportunities. An associate professor ten years in, for instance, might trade 10 percent of his time with patients for the opportunity to streamline the hospital's billing practices, or improve the discharge process, or teach a course on the physical exam. The incentive is clear: fewer patients, same money. Dave was a full professor. He could have devoted his time solely to the bureaucracy he may have enjoyed, but he kept seeing patients too. The two together turned out to be too much.

In early June 2020, as COVID surged through Houston and as disaster syndrome gripped our hospital, I entered the office to find one of my colleagues crying.

"What's wrong?" I asked.

She asked me to shut the door and then she gave me the news. Dave had killed himself.

For the next week, as I attempted to piece things together, images of Dave roving through Ben Taub's hallways flashed through my head. He had loved this hospital. He had found meaningful work here. Even though I had noticed that Dave was depressed, I never thought it was possible that he could break. Dave had bent so much, not just for himself, but for all of us.

From my cubicle at the hospital, I logged in to the funeral broadcast over Zoom. For the second time in my career, I tried to fight back tears at Ben Taub and the tears won.

Despite meeting with friends and colleagues and talking about what had happened, I couldn't stop thinking about Dave's death. I knew that something as complex as suicide depended on a variety of factors, and that work was just one of them. Still, it seemed inevitable: I began to think about suicide myself.

I didn't have a plan. It was more of an urge. Driving home, approaching a fast fork in the highway, I'd find my grip tightening on the steering wheel. I could swerve right into those barrels, I told myself.

We were all sick of the N95 masks pulling at our ears and pressing our faces. We were sick of the gowns. It exhausted us to no end to hear "Code Blue" announced again and again overhead. Our patients were alone—a strict visitation policy was enforced to curtail contagion—and had to make very difficult medical decisions via FaceTime. There was a palpable lack of human bodies in the hospital hallways. Added to this were the pressures outside. Tens of thousands of Houstonians had gathered in downtown to march in remembrance of the slain George Floyd, a native of the Third Ward, just a few weeks before. I was one of them. I couldn't help but think of Jefferson Davis Hospital while hearing George's family plead for justice. I was sad and angry.

Things weren't better at home. Even the smallest problems—such as the garbage not fitting perfectly into the can—irritated me. I snapped at my wife and kids. I asked my sisters to stop talking with me so that I wouldn't text them insults. I began punching myself in the thigh again, an old compulsion I thought I had dropped early in college. I felt alone. I didn't like being myself.

My health insurance listed therapists within my network. I emailed and called a few but couldn't quite establish a rapport with them. I found one therapist who specialized in working with creative types, and over the next few months, after many sessions aimed at identifying triggers for my anger, I rediscovered the rational part of myself. I controlled my emotions better. I went back to being me.

After I filed an out-of-network claim with my health insurance company, a representative contacted the therapist. Much of the information I had submitted "couldn't be read," he explained, even though I had submitted it using the company's online form. Once again, my therapist provided me with all the information requested, which I mailed to the insurance company, along with a letter.

"I'd like to share information with you regarding the claim and the circumstances of the last 8 months that are central to this claim," I wrote. I explained how, during the pandemic, I had served as the doctor to dozens of patients with COVID throughout the hospital, from the ER to the ICU, how my wife and I had contracted COVID ourselves, how my friend had committed suicide, and how I had searched through their network and had been unable to find a therapist who fit.

"I hope this explanation helps your decision-making process," I wrote. The claim was denied.

Without our leader, and with COVID surging, we returned to work.

We breathed. We regrouped. We turned our attention to our home lives, our families, our bills. Practicalities began to take us by surprise. The strict visitor policy started to make our patients' decisions harder. Renovations of the Ben Taub ER, planned years ago, limited our bed space and made us circumnavigate the ward to get from point B to point A. When the next surge came, we felt better prepared because science had given us weapons. Steroids—which we dispensed to patients multiple times a day every day—helped, a lot. So did blood thinners. So did explaining to the patient that she had to switch positions and rest awhile on her chest. It was now the fall of 2020. A vaccine, we read, was on the horizon.

We saw mortality plummet. We grew confident. We told patients right off the bat that we anticipated they would get better. We were weary but resolute. We began playing a ten-second segment of "Simply the Best" on the loudspeakers each time a COVID patient left the hospital recovered. But soon the repetition grew irksome. We discharged so many that the song stopped sounding like the triumphant Tina Turner and more like another interruption—the overhead call for a mop to the waiting area—made to distract us.

Politics divided us. So, at times, did race. If we found out that one of us supported the wrong candidate, we avoided that person and whispered about them to those with views nearer to our own. We endured the election, the challenges, the certification, the breach of our Capitol, another larger and deadlier wave of the pandemic. And once we received the vaccine, once we felt safe, once we felt relieved to live in a place that was looking forward, not behind, opening up, not locking down, that was when our real surge came, the one we didn't see coming. It was in

April 2021, more than a year after the birth of the pandemic, almost a year after Dave left us, that we truly felt overwhelmed.

So sweeping was this new influx of patients that Ben Taub administrators called a Code Purple.

Code Purple, what's that? we asked one another.

Immediately when setting foot onto the wards, we saw what this meant. Sets of partitions made of white nylon, like you'd find in a field hospital, lined the wall space between rooms. The privacy was such that we saw no faces, only IV tubing and yellow socks. We had started to board patients in the hallways.

Was this what JD looked like, way back when?

"My patients are sick," my colleagues kept telling me. It wasn't just me who felt we were busier than we'd ever been: we all did. We diverted patients away from our ER more than at any other time: our ER was now closed to ambulances more hours than it was open. And yet, our virologists sent us bar graphs showing how low the coronavirus hospitalization numbers had fallen. Even the *New York Times* had downgraded the infection risk within Harris County. We were in the middle of our most challenging surge of the pandemic, but very few of the patients flooding the hospital had COVID.

I thought about Roxana during this time. When she first came to Ben Taub, her medical care hadn't been particularly challenging. The infections, the amputations, even the ensuing physical therapy, these all required work and expertise, but none of it required extraordinary efforts. The largest challenge in caring for Roxana had been to plug her into the system. Once she received a Gold Card, individual efforts became collective ones: we could begin to rely on teamwork.

If, in a typical week before the pandemic, I was responsible for twelve patients, only one or two people would require us to plug them into the system. The rest already had Gold Cards. During this new surge, however, the number of patients new to Ben Taub and Harris Health seemed to double, if not triple.

Six hundred fifty thousand Texans lost their employer-sponsored health insurance during the pandemic. Correspondingly, enrollment with Obamacare increased by 15 percent in Texas, more than any other state in the nation. The number of uninsured people younger than sixty-five swelled to 29 percent. Texas Medicaid took on 12 percent more cases. An already sinking Medicine Inc. began to capsize. In the aftermath of the disaster, the safety-net system grew overloaded. Some standards—like space for patients—had fallen. My beloved Ben Taub didn't look so robust. Patients didn't move so swiftly through the system receiving the care they needed. Everything felt weighed down. We needed help.

One of my patients during this surge had been receiving cancer treatments at a nonprofit hospital when he lost his job. His health insurance disappeared along with his paycheck. For a few months, the hospital continued to give him treatments under a cash payment plan, but this was short-lived. Right before his third round of chemotherapy, the hospital informed him it was no longer offering this plan. After a few weeks of vomiting and enduring belly pain, he went to Ben Taub.

The newly un- and underinsured flooded into the safety-net system. COVID had also made caring for patients with Gold Cards a challenge. Elective surgeries for cancers and infections had been canceled. Even our own patients were coming into the hospital sicker.

We received pleas from administrators on GroupMe, the texting app, nearly every day: "Try to expedite discharges as much as possible! We have lots of patients boarding in the ED waiting on beds!" We attempted to off-load the pressure. We asked patients waiting in the ER if they wouldn't mind our transferring them elsewhere. Many said no, and so they waited for hours, sometimes days, for a room—or a set of partitions—on the wards.

"We're making the best of it." We said variations of this phrase to one another during each COVID surge and the surge of newly uninsured patients that followed. ICU nurses said it to one another. "We're making the best of it." We felt like we had been helping society. Now we were dealing with society's shortcomings, its inability to provide adequate coverage. Without help, without a restructuring of how healthcare is provided to those unable to afford it, how long could we hold on?

— 15 —

Tiers

Neo-Persia, 550 AD, three hundred kilometers due north of modern-day Kuwait, four hundred kilometers due south of the Silk Road city of Hamadan.

A sick person would have traveled for weeks to find the kind of attention for which American medicine later became known. There were no urgent cares, no same-day clinics. There were instead temples made of stone with dens where incense burned, day and night, to rid the air of putrefaction. A shaman would pray over the ill, and only those with souls considered unworthy handled wounds. If this provided relief, great. If not, it was on to the next village, the next temple.

Some made it their life's journey to find the proper care. Their ailments didn't have the names we know today. Medical language back then was more descriptive, which was why people said they had a cholera— an "angry diarrhea"—rather than gastroenteritis or gluten intolerance. Illnesses produced external patterns, or stigmata, visible to a doctor's discerning eye. Skin bubbling over with pus and scabs was a sign of the day's pandemic, what today we know as the plague.

They traveled through cities built by Romans, with aqueducts and sewers and public baths. The quality of the temples in the cities was no better, and if a patient wasn't careful, she might pick up a secondary illness from all the urban filth. Mosquitoes swarmed over the heads of children playing ball. Scab-ridden animals defecated in the middle of alleyways and streets. By the banks of the river it wasn't uncommon to see a decomposing human body. To us, this amounts to lunacy, but at the time, with so many other hazards—malaria, childbirth, TB, any trauma that went deeper than the subcutaneous fat—coming face-to-face with human death wasn't any more shocking than finding our favorite waterfall or walking trail today strewn with old beer cans and used plastic forks.

There were people who purported to have all the answers. I don't mean priests, though this special band was uniformly male. They traveled from city to city and to the very extremes of the empire to hold open forums on a topic of the people's choosing. Healthcare—or how to mend an ailing body—was often discussed. These men won over crowds with words, not actions; that was their trick. They were called sophists. Today a person might sit in the comfort of their home or office and grow an audience with the use of video and a connection to the internet, but at the time, working as a sophist generally meant one had to travel. Sometimes, these journeys were fraught with peril. The most desperate of the sick would pay these men many times over to receive nothing more than their words. Others were once bitten, twice shy.

Rumors have always carried outsize weight with the ill, then as much as now. Norma, for instance, sent her son Christian to Mexico to receive stem cells—or something like stem cells—based on little more than whisperings. She was a reasonable woman with a job, a taxpayer who had raised two sons on her own, living hand-to-mouth. Solving Christian's suffering served as much of an economic purpose for her as it did a motherly one, all of which is to say that, for the sick, rumors must be heard out, they must be weighed. Which was why the rumor spreading in Southern Europe and Asia Minor and the Middle East in 550 AD was so hard to dismiss. The pandemic had already ravaged Constantinople, the seat of the Byzantine Empire. Carthage, Jerusalem, and what is now

Marseille had all suffered through the scourge. The rumor in the midst of such sickness was startling: there is hope.

Perhaps it's a tribute to the progress we've made in healthcare that we, in modern times, can't even fathom how somebody looking for a cure might have phrased this rumor. They can't have said, "There's this incredible hospital!" because, in 550 AD, there were no hospitals, only treatment areas cobbled together in poorhouses and temples. I imagine instead they might have called it by its name: Jundi-Shapur, which translates to "Beautiful Garden."

Jundi-Shapur was, foremost, a great medical university with faculty and student doctors from all over Eurasia. Greek physicians flocked there, as well as Jewish ones, first responders from Roman cities, Zoroastrians, and doctors from India. They convened in an atmosphere of tolerance to share ideas on medicine and to train the next generation of caretakers. Hard-core supporters of Galen mingled with practitioners of Ayurveda. The Talmud was cited for its wisdom alongside the teachings of Zarathus-tra. Sometimes, these experts of different cloaks even rounded on patients together, the whole team of teachers and learners focusing singularly on one thing: sickness. The hospital—known as a *bimaristan* after the ensu-ing Islamic conquest—was intimately connected to the medical school. It was where the concepts from books and lectures could be observed in human bodies. Jundi-Shapur was, above all else, a teaching hospital.

For anyone on a journey in search of relief, the sense of discovery at finding the doctors of Jundi-Shapur must have been exhilarating. Some patients had traveled hundreds of miles, with limbs that looked rotten. Some had visited shaman upon shaman. Some showed signs of plague. What they found at Jundi-Shapur was an irresistible idea: putting science together with people was the best way to control the pandemic's costs.

Today, some of America's most prestigious healthcare institutions implement the Jundi-Shapur model, where elder doctors teach medicine to students and residents at the bedside while providing care to patients. The academic model is in Ben Taub's DNA. I learned medicine at Ben

Taub as a student and then as a resident. I've stayed to teach learners how to care for patients in the hospital. Ben Taub was the destination at the end of my own healthcare journey, as it was for so many uninsured patients like Roxana and Christian and Ebonie.

But the rumors about Jundi-Shapur went beyond what this strange grouping of doctors could do. The rumor driving people across half a continent was even more revolutionary: any person, female or male, from any race, of any class, could go there to receive care. This new type of building opened its doors to everyone. There were no tiers. People didn't even have to pay.

This is the dream: Science applied impartially to illness. Disease analyzed and cured without the interference of money or a higher authority. Equality. When I read about Jundi-Shapur, I envision a Nightingale ward with beautifully tiled floors kept immaculately clean. There are partitions between beds—somehow in this pre-industrial world, the beds still shift up and down, back and forth, at the push of a button—and boxes of alcohol swabs at the central nurse's station. The doctors are dressed like background players in *Star Wars*, representing the sage wisdom of different peoples. There is no beeping of IV pumps, no interruptions, just patients receiving treatment.

When I imagine this moment in history a little more deeply, I can see the pandemonium of peoples. I hear different languages—Farsi, Greek, dialects of Latin with recognizable hints of Spanish—bouncing against the walls. I smell the sweat of sepsis and the blood of dysentery. I see offerings—goods from the Silk Road, animals, weaponry, foods cooked with faraway spices—given to doctors to help cajole them toward a loved one's bedside. I feel the tension of the grand authority, the caliph, walking through the hallways. The patient rooms look more like cells, maybe even dungeons. I see unhappy patients with incurable conditions, doctors having bad days. It also gives me hope for the future. If the first plague made Jundi-Shapur possible, who knows what the most recent plague will bring?

I really have no idea how it felt to work at Jundi-Shapur, but the idea behind it—treating everyone equally in a single-tiered system based on science—is one that has lingered in our collective imaginations. Countries like Canada have organized healthcare to achieve this goal, while in the United States, the use of private health insurance as a requirement for entry into healthcare has resulted in a multitude of tiers and wide inequality. The question is, if the United States wants to achieve more equality in healthcare, can it jump from the many tiers created by Medicine Inc. toward a more equitable single-tier system like Medicare for All?

The Affordable Care Act, or Obamacare, attempted to make healthcare more equally accessible by building on the existing employer-sponsored private health insurance model. States that expanded their Medicaid programs brought more equal access to American citizens earning below 133 percent of the federal poverty level. But the legislation hasn't made healthcare more affordable for those who don't qualify for Medicaid or for subsidies for Obamacare, or for those who require more healthcare than what basic Obamacare plans provide. Healthcare remains linked to the question of worthiness. The question of who deserves healthcare and who doesn't remains fundamental to how Americans access doctors and hospitals.

In late 2000, 25 percent of the patients admitted to Ben Taub from the emergency room had the following characteristics: nonfunctional kidneys, visited ERs for the same symptoms twice every week, Latino, deathly ill, and undocumented. Walking through the holding area in the ER was like entering chaos. Two rows of stretchers faced each other, with patients separated by only half a thigh's girth, and there was a busy thoroughfare of doctors in between. There was yelling, nudity, the smell of bile from people's retchings. Among the alcoholics and orange-jumpered jailbirds and abandoned elderly—patients one might expect to see at a safety-net hospital—was a group of young Hispanics: these were undocumented patients with end-stage renal disease. Trainee doctors held these patients' chest X-rays to the fluorescent lighting to reveal lungs whited out by fluid where there should have been air. Crinkled EKGs—a ton of them piled on the patient, inside the chart, speared through the IV pole—showed aberrant heart rhythms, some of which, as smooth as a sine wave, portended death. Who were these patients with green skin who, in the middle of summer, wrapped themselves in cardigans and florid quilts? Who were these people emergency room staffers recognized and greeted with "Back again?" What kind of care did these people deserve?

It depended on who you asked.

One camp believed these patients were only entitled to receive emergency care at Ben Taub. This camp believed that while the federal law EMTALA still applied, any further care given to these patients—including clinic visits and preventive care—constituted misuse of public dollars, since those dollars were going to help people who had entered the country illegally. This camp was comprised not only of doctors but also politicians. Then–Texas attorney general and now–US senator John Cornyn became a leading voice for this group in 2001 when, writing in the *Houston Chronicle*, he opined that any nonemergent care provided to undocumented immigrants violated federal law.

Ben Taub had long provided one standard of healthcare to all its patients. But the number of undocumented patients, and the question of how much providing them with a standard level of care might cost, had led to the creation of a lower tier and a lower standard. Those patients who qualified for Medicare or the Gold Card received a certain standard of healthcare, while the undocumented received a lower one.

Over time, something became evident. Dialyzing patients on an emergency basis may have solved short-term problems, but when patients returned to the emergency room looking much sicker, some doctors began to feel like they were chasing their own tails. Soon enough, they felt more than just frustrated.

A protocol emerged for how to deal with these patients when lab results or symptoms were severe enough to warrant emergent dialysis: admit them into the intensive care unit or medicine ward, place a temporary catheter into one of the major accessible veins—either in the neck, below the clavicle, or in the groin—dialyze three days, then discharge. Doctors utilized this protocol regardless of whether it was the patient's first visit or fifth.

In practice, the consequences of this protocol were awful. One of the problems that started to crop up in these patients was a higher number of amputations. When major veins are damaged by needles over and again, clots form, and eventually, the clots block blood flow. This begets infection, sometimes even gangrene. But even with a limb amputated, these patients still needed dialysis, and so doctors would turn their attention to the next available major vein connected to the adjoining limb. And, eventually, this vein, too, would clot, leading to another amputation, and on and on, until all the major veins of a person's body were clotted, at which point, dialysis couldn't be performed. Some patients were discharged when that happened. Those patients never returned.

A growing number of doctors and leaders began to fear the worst: that they were part of a system that caused patient suffering, rather than alleviating it. Overseeing amputation after amputation on their patients, some questioned whether they were fulfilling the Hippocratic oath they had taken. They asked themselves, Am I the bad guy here?

What made it harder was knowing that the US government had already solved this problem for most of its citizens with ESRD. In 1972, the End Stage Renal Disease Program authorized the payment of chronic treatments for ESRD (including transplantation) under Medicare, extending this benefit to ten thousand Americans—a large portion, but not everyone—living with the illness. The story behind how this enormous entitlement, accounting today for nearly $50 billion of Medicare's budget, passed through Congress is not much more than a one-liner on Wikipedia, but it required a dramatic flourish to capture the attention of the decision-makers. During a House Ways and Means Committee meeting in 1971, as Democratic and Republican representatives heard testimony from people with failing kidneys, doctors wheeled a dialysis machine into the meeting, hooked it up to a patient, and performed the filtration on a living human being right before the members of Congress.

A senior aide to a representative expressed his shock: "What the fuck is going on here?"

The scene stuck in the mind of Americans and future members of Congress, and many pieces of legislation have honed this entitlement—the US government paying for the treatment of a specific disease—including, most recently, the American Taxpayer Relief Act of 2012. The process of how chronic dialysis is initiated, continued, and paid for remains, today, deeply connected to Medicare, even for the 10 percent of Americans with ESRD not covered by Medicare but by private health insurance.

Today, American citizens with ESRD receive Medicare benefits if they've paid enough into the system, via deductions from paychecks, or if they've been disabled long enough. Americans with ESRD who don't qualify for Medicare often find their scheduled dialysis paid for by Medicaid, which is partially funded and administered by a patient's home state. Other avenues available to US citizens who don't have enough work credits for Medicare and who earn too much income to qualify for Medicaid are Social Security Disability Insurance (SSDI) and Supplemental Security Income (SSI), both of which confer coverage based on the disabilities incurred by ESRD. Obtaining the funding for this type of treatment can take as long as five months, during which time patients receive emergent dialysis, with the crucial distinction that eventually, if they survive, they will receive scheduled dialysis, paid for in part by federal funds.

As has been the case with all federal healthcare legislation, undocumented immigrants—including the ESRD patients at Ben Taub—were explicitly forbidden from receiving federal funding through Medicare. There was no Ways and Means Committee before which to perform a dialysis session to change hearts and minds. In a system built on public money, but without any of that public money available to treat undocumented patients suffering from this illness, doctors would have to think outside the box to help their patients.

The most compelling argument for changing the system, they decided, didn't rely on ethics alone but also on economics. The safety-net system's administrators had a hard time understanding the emotional tug of the substandard care. But they responded to budgets. Doctors felt that the moral costs were likely also financially exorbitant, and so they set out to study this.

Two doctor-researchers at Ben Taub, Drs. Sheikh-Hamad and Shandera, began to compare patients who received dialysis on schedule versus those who relied on the emergency room. How many times in the past year had each group of patients visited the ER? How often had the patients been admitted to the hospital or ICU? What was the cost of treating the undocumented differently from the standard?

In a 2007 issue of *Texas Medicine*, the duo published the results of this study in a paper demonstrating that the emergent dialysis protocol cost more than $280,000 per patient per year, a third of which was spent on hospital and emergency room costs. Chronic-care patients, on the other hand—those on thrice-weekly scheduled dialysis—only cost $77,000 a year. Emergent dialysis patients visited the ER, on average, twenty-six times in eight months, while patients receiving dialysis on a schedule visited it only once in eighteen months. Emergent dialysis patients spent more days in the hospital (one hundred thirty-five days versus five), required many more blood transfusions (twenty-five versus two), and were four times more likely to be admitted to the ICU than patients on scheduled dialysis. Clearly, there was no economic justification for emergent dialysis. This second tier of care proved exorbitant.

The science had spoken and administrators listened. Thanks to this study, in 2008, Harris Health decided to open the Riverside Dialysis Center, a health center where people with a Gold Card could receive scheduled dialysis just like those with Medicare. The center helped off-load patients from the Ben Taub wards and its ER. By 2014, Riverside accommodated one hundred seventy-five patients with end-stage renal disease. That is one hundred seventy-five people helped to thrive, not to mention millions of local taxpayer dollars saved.

Right now, Riverside is the most active dialysis center in the city, running four shifts (versus the typical three) Monday through Saturday. Patients assigned to the night shift finish their dialysis session at one a.m., which is late, but far more tolerable than the hours and days they spent in the ER. Demand for one of these spots keeps growing as more people develop diabetes and high blood pressure and as these chronic illnesses wear down kidneys. At one point, the number of Gold Card holders on the wait list—whose only option was to receive dialysis in the ER—grew so high that Harris Health began outsourcing patients to other area dialysis centers, which likely meant that the safety-net system paid a higher amount per patient, depending on how it nego-tiated with these centers. In an informal, unscientific way, I've asked some of these patients visiting alternate sites about their experiences. They've all said that they hope to visit Riverside, the facility connected to Ben Taub.

But the living patients who save the system the most dollars are the ones who don't even visit Riverside. Their dialysis occurs in a place where there are no extra hands to help. These are the patients like Christian, who carry out their dialysis treatments in their own homes. It requires more than just showing up for an appointment; it depends on the person themselves to make good and consistent decisions. It might demand more from a patient, but it gives more too: freedom, empowerment, and savings.

As we saw with Christian, Harris Health now offers peritoneal dialysis. Considering how preferable this type of dialysis is for people like Christian, and how few Americans know about the alternatives, the safety net has in this case surpassed the national standard. It's a point worth repeating: the undocumented with end-stage renal disease can now receive better care in the Houston safety-net system than the routine care given to citizens with Medicare at nonprofit and for-profit hospitals simply because they know they have more options.

This is just one example of how offering coverage to everyone can improve the quality of healthcare. The inclination might be, then, to conclude that the United States should move to a single-tier healthcare system. Medicare for All proposes such a system: one standard of care, one method of healthcare, one insurer—the US government—for everyone. I'm not sure the majority of Americans would accept such a system, especially because of what they would relinquish. Private health insurance allows a person to experience healthcare in private. It also allows people to make more choices in their healthcare and to receive certain types of healthcare—particularly specialty care—faster. We shouldn't take these benefits lightly. Any time I walk into a room shared by four patients and hear the heaves of somebody vomiting, or even the smell of excrement, I can feel how preferable it is to have a private room. The question is whether the privacy is worth what we're paying for it. We're not only paying a premium financially, we are also sacrificing fairness, equality, and, in many cases, quality of care.

A two-tier system that allows people to purchase additional health insurance to ensure privacy or faster healthcare solves this problem. Such a system would require a national standard of healthcare for everyone, regardless of citizenship. Americans would have to decide what falls under that standard—would it go beyond Harris Health's standard, for instance, and offer liver transplants?—as well as whether it would be administered at the national, state, or local level (or a combination).

This type of system wouldn't be based on worthiness: it would aim to provide healthcare to everyone. It wouldn't be perfect, just like, no doubt, Jundi-Shapur wasn't perfect, but a national safety net would help us place people at the center of medicine.

*   *   *

For nearly every Memorial Day weekend during my childhood, my parents loaded me and my two sisters into the car and drove to our beach house in Galveston. As much as he liked his work, my father revered his time away from the hospital and his patients. The familiar shrieks we heard from his pager—at restaurants, during movies, sometimes at three a.m.—quieted during these holidays, if only for a few days. Instead, we heard the grinding of blenders, the clamor of conversation, and of course, somewhere in the background, the waves of the gulf.

But one Fourth of July, I awoke to find him and my mother gone. My relatives told me they'd left for the day and would be back later in the evening. They returned that same night, dressed not in beach gear but formally, as if for a banquet.

Much later, I learned they had driven to a funeral. One of my father's patients had died the third day after giving birth. Though the cause of death was nothing my father could have prevented, he felt the tragedy of the situation—a dead mother. He and my mother drove three hours to the funeral to pay their respects, but the woman's family wasn't prepared to receive the doctor. How could something like this happen? Could it have been his fault? It took only a few moments before my father realized his presence only worsened the family's grief. He and my mother climbed back into the car and returned to the beach.

The death—the first and last of his practice—impacted my father. Many years later, after I finished my internal medicine residency and began working at Ben Taub as a teacher and hospitalist, I told him that I constantly dealt with death. Many of my patients had incurable cancer or organ failure. I filled out so many death certificates and held so many end-of-life conversations. I loved my work too, but at times it exhausted me.

He smiled at me knowingly. It was one of the reasons he had chosen to become an ob-gyn in the first place. My dad referred high-risk patients like Ebonie to maternal-fetal medicine doctors. "Ricky," he said, "my patients are healthy."

For the most part, he was right: women entering pregnancy are generally healthy. But when medicine focuses on generalities, groups of patients, particularly the marginalized and dispossessed, fall through the cracks. Tiers of care develop. These are exacerbated by the cost of healthcare: those with insurance receive one standard, those without receive another. Disparities in how certain groups of women receive their healthcare—particularly African Americans and those with low incomes, like Ebonie—have dispelled the notion, once considered gospel, that childbearing women are healthy.

In May 2018, eighteen months after the news of the maternal mortality spike in Texas went viral, two facts emerged. The first was that the death rate of mothers within six weeks of childbirth was much lower than initially reported. The spike observed in maternal deaths had been largely due to an accounting error caused by doctors filling out death certificates incorrectly. The addition of a question on death certificates in 2006, and the migration to filing these certificates electronically in 2012, had led to confusion and inaccuracies in reporting. The question asked doctors to slot female decedents into one of five categories: not pregnant within the past year; pregnant at the time of death; not pregnant, but pregnant within forty-two days of death; not pregnant, but pregnant forty-three days to one year before death; or unknown if pregnant within the past year. It's not hard to see how this question may have generated inaccuracies. In the end, a review of data showed the maternal mortality rate was lower than previously reported. Texas wasn't like Mongolia. It was more like France.

But the spike in maternal deaths also illuminated how we've become inured to a different standard of care for minorities. A 2016 study in the journal *Obstetrics & Gynecology* showed that Black soon-to-be mothers like Ebonie were at far greater risk than white, Hispanic, and Asian mothers, not only in Texas, but in the entire United States. The disparity was so pronounced that the authors argued that a state's racial composition played more of a role in the maternal mortality rate (MMR) than the quality of its medical care. Washington, DC, for instance, has the nation's highest MMR at 38.8 maternal deaths per 100,000 live births. A graph in this study shows how the rate for African American women has remained consistently high for decades. White mothers in the District, however, have the nation's lowest rate. Not a single white mother died in DC within forty-two days of childbirth from 2005 to 2014.

It wasn't that Black mothers were only now starting to die at higher rates. They had been dying at much higher rates than white, Hispanic, and Asian mothers *all along*. A lack of health coverage in Texas put Ebonie's life in even greater peril.

"Excellent care is apparently available but is not reaching all the people," the authors concluded.

Doctors and healthcare workers need to consider how much their biases exacerbate these tiers.

All doctors are taught to stereotype. Without stereotyping, a middle-aged smoker clutching his chest and gasping for air wouldn't trigger the words "heart attack" in the minds of emergency room workers. But new evidence suggests that stereotyping can start before a doctor lays eyes on a patient. It can start when a woman tells the scheduler that she has Medicaid or when she sits down for a blood pressure check. Stereotyping during these moments can lead to different treatments offered, or worse, a lower standard of care.

Over the years, I noticed a difference in how I asked certain women about their drug history. With most women, I asked, "Any drugs?" while with others—specifically, elderly Hispanic ladies who reminded me of my grandmother—I said it almost as a joke: "No drugs, right?" Certainly this was a result of an implicit bias on my part, an unconscious attitude. I couldn't really control this attitude because of my heritage, but if I was being true to my job as a doctor, I would have known that the way I phrased this question could change the way a patient responded. "No drugs, right?" might push the rare Hispanic grandmother who actually used drugs to say no to please me.

The attitudes a doctor or a nurse brings into the examination room can affect how a patient responds to questions, how they listen, and whether they take the medications you prescribe. It's one of the reasons the Council on Patient Safety in Women's Health Care developed a set of standard practices to reduce peripartum racial and ethnic disparities. The point of this safety bundle isn't to eliminate implicit bias but to reduce variations in care by calling doctors' attention to these attitudes.

In one of its policy statements, the American College of Obstetricians and Gynecologists acknowledged the effect of racial bias on its patients: "There is a growing body of literature that validates the public health impact of racial bias, implicit and explicit, on the lives and health of people of color." In addition to recommending that each physician become aware of their own biases, ACOG encouraged research projects that focused on women of color and that also linked biases with outcomes. "We recognize that structural and institutional racism contribute to and exacerbate these biases, which further marginalize women of color in the health care system," the statement concluded.

A short while after taking over as Ben Taub's chief of obstetrics, Carey Eppes began administering an implicit-bias questionnaire to OBs-in-practice at Ben Taub. The impact of this questionnaire remains to be seen, but Carey finds value in calling attention to the topic, even if the scientific results don't pan out. She believes that calling attention to doctors' attitudes in this way will help reduce variations in care.

Ebonie, however, wasn't heading toward a hospital that utilized safety mechanisms like weighing blood and bias training. Ben Taub was not going to be an option for her.

A voice from the front of the ambulance explained the situation to Ebonie: Ben Taub was full. Any ambulance that radioed in was being diverted to another hospital, in this case, a not-for-profit hospital nearby. Ebonie couldn't go to the hospital where she had planned to deliver her child.

"In the five years I have been here, we have never been on diversion," Carey Eppes told me. Ben Taub's ER often diverted patients—roughly for four hours every day—but, as a matter of policy, the labor and delivery ward never did. Needless to say, Carey was not very happy that her patient unnecessarily ended up at a different hospital, though she wasn't surprised either. Just as her patients had to contend with late buses, she knew that ambulance drivers often didn't listen to them.

Patients say it's not uncommon to end up at a different hospital from the one they've requested. Some of them feel that the ambulance drivers make their decisions based on whether the patient is insured or not, or even the type of insurance they have. Financial counselors at Ben Taub had helped Ebonie apply for Texas Medicaid during her prior admission. By the time she started to bleed again, her coverage had kicked in: Ebonie was no longer uninsured. She was evaluated at the not-for-profit hospital, where her new doctors determined that her water had broken. They decided that the best course of action was to keep her hospitalized until it was safe to deliver the child, which wasn't due for two months.

There's no way to know whether the doctors and administrators at the hospital would have kept Ebonie admitted for so long if she lacked insurance, or whether they did the math to figure out if such a long stay might be offset by what little Texas Medicaid paid. I'd like to think it was a purely medical decision. It seemed to be the right one, too. A neonatologist told Ebonie that a baby born at that point, less than twenty-four weeks into the pregnancy, would have only a 34 percent chance of surviving and a 90 percent chance of being born with a severe developmental problem. While the new hospital used a protocol to deal with bleeding, nurses did not weigh pads to quantify blood loss. Instead they eyeballed it. Ebonie's C-section was scheduled for the start of her thirty-fourth week of pregnancy, in September 2017. Unaware that she had the option to request a transfer to Ben Taub, she settled in.

Some of the differences between the safety-net hospital and this nonprofit one came to light as the weeks passed. Ebonie enjoyed more privacy at this hospital, for instance, as she was assigned her own room. Nurses wrote daily goals on the whiteboard by her bed: "Stay pregnant! No seizures!" To chase away boredom, the hospital outfitted Ebonie's room with DVDs to watch and books to read. But Ebonie's mind was whirling so much she hardly noticed.

Once a week, her family came to visit her. Ebonie's sister and brother (who also lived in Houston) could only bring Blessn every so often due to their work schedules—one worked at Walmart, the other drove for Uber—and the expense of parking. Still, Ebonie spoke with Blessn every night on the phone. Sometimes Blessn cried and pleaded for her mother to return home. "No," Ebonie told her. "Mommy got to wait until the doctors take the baby out of her stomach."

When Blessn's father called from California, Ebonie explained that, even with a C-section, her risk of significant bleeding after the delivery was still high with the placenta blocking the birth canal. "Are you serious?" he said. "Is this a life-and-death situation?"

"I'm dead serious."

Some days, the solitude and the sporadic bleeding overwhelmed her, and Ebonie began to think about what might happen if things went wrong. She prayed constantly. But nothing seemed to comfort her. Her fear grew so intense that she began to question whether she should have made a different choice.

"A baby is precious, but I don't want to die," she recalled thinking. "What will my family do if I die?"

Three weeks after doctors admitted Ebonie into her new hospital's labor and delivery ward, she began to feel cramps in her lower belly. She called the nurse and told her she thought she was having contractions.

"Are you in labor?" the nurse asked. She lifted up the bedsheet and, very quickly, covered Ebonie back up. "You're in labor," she said. "We need to call the doctor."

Ebonie was twenty-five weeks and six days into her pregnancy. Her C-section wasn't scheduled for another two months, but now it looked as though the calendar was eluding her control.

The nurse went to let the doctors know. When she returned, she checked Ebonie again.

She could hardly believe what she was seeing: the baby's head was emerging. Ebonie felt a burst of pressure in her rectum.

"I need to push," she said.

"Don't push!" cautioned the nurse.

"Bitch, my baby is pushing his own self out!" Ebonie later recalled saying.

What the hospital had tried to prevent was happening: Ebonie was having her baby in one of the most dangerous manners possible, through a birth canal blocked by the placenta.

"Don't push! Don't push!" yelled the nurse.

With so much pressure, Ebonie couldn't help it. Within minutes, the labor was over, and her newborn boy was immediately taken to the neonatal ICU, since he couldn't breathe on his own. Ebonie had only glanced at him before he was whisked away.

As Ebonie lay there, she started to bleed again. For forty-five minutes, doctors attempted to deliver the placenta by pushing up and down on her belly, to no avail. Ebonie, who was already drowsy from the pain of childbirth, began to cry. The bleeding wouldn't stop.

The documentation in her chart is unclear about what occurred after her child was delivered. She started to bleed again. Doctors rushed her to emergency surgery to remove the placenta. "Breathe some of this air," she remembers the anesthesiologist telling her, before everything went black.

Ebonie's blood level, the doctors discovered, was very low. The surgeons transfused her with two bags of blood as they worked, and even as they did so, she continued to bleed. They removed the placenta and sent it to the pathology lab for analysis. Eventually, the bleeding finally stopped.

Ebonie awoke from the anesthesia with a sore throat and pain in her belly. Doctors transferred her to a recovery room, where another blood test revealed that the two bags weren't enough. She received another two bags of blood, for a total of more than two liters postdelivery.

This was, by any measure, a traumatic delivery and surgery. Yet forty-eight hours later, Ebonie was discharged. The documentation, again, is unclear, but it appears that once doctors felt sure that she was no longer bleeding, they decided it was safe to send her home.

Though Ebonie's doctors weren't sure how she managed to deliver her child with the placenta blocking the birth canal, her attending obstetrician speculated that, over the preceding weeks, the placenta had migrated into a position that allowed a premature child, who was very small, to squeeze out. During her three weeks in the hospital, no ultrasound was performed to confirm the position of the placenta. Analysis of the placenta in the pathology lab offered no clues. Her doctors seemed to have sent her home with many questions hanging in the air.

Discrepancies like these can happen with any patient, regardless of their level of insurance or wealth or even their race. Nothing in my reading of Ebonie's chart suggests that she received lesser care at the nonprofit hospital. Tracking Ebonie's bleeding in a precise way would have been preferable, but ultimately this didn't make her delivery a near miss. The nonprofit hospital provided a standard level of care. It could've been more personalized and precise, but it wasn't incorrect.

A few weeks later, I met with Ebonie in a children's play area outside the neonatal ICU. That was where her newborn son, King, was staying. Since he was born so prematurely, the neonatologists told her that they intended to keep him in the hospital until his original due date, for a total of three months, so that his young organs could develop. Ebonie had brought Blessn to visit her baby brother. While we talked, Blessn relished pushing herself up and down on a little seesaw.

I asked Ebonie how she was doing.

"Blessn," she said, making sure her daughter didn't hurt herself on the jungle gym.

Ebonie was still rocked by her traumatic delivery. She was no longer in physical danger, but she continued to fear for her life.

"Even when I went home, I was still scared," she said.

When I asked Ebonie if she was still having seizures, she smiled. "No," she said. One of the positive outcomes of her recent hospitalization was a thorough study of her seizures, which led the neurologists to conclude that they were the result of the emotional stress of having been the victim of abuse, an illness known as conversion disorder. Mothering seemed to have ameliorated the condition, at least for the moment. It was certainly a better remedy than the seizure medicines she had been taking.

I thought about how near of a miss she'd had. I thought about the moments she had spent in the hospital, alone, bored, scared, and waiting. I thought about the tattoo on her neck and the boundless love she had for her child. I also thought about how dangerous it was for people like me to believe the problems she faced were beyond us. To call Ebonie "healthy" after a birth as traumatic as hers disregarded the obstacles she still faced. Poverty meant an unreliable supply of food and work and education for her children. Even her own healthcare wasn't guaranteed. Medicaid helped, but what if she arrived late at an appointment for reasons beyond her control? Life was that unstable. Thankfully, this time, she had survived.

"I'm very happy that you're okay," I told her as we stood up to leave.

Ebonie nodded in the manner of someone who is multitasking. With all the things going through her mind—King's lungs, Blessn's school, finding her own place eventually so she wouldn't have to impose on her sister—how could she worry about reciprocating a small courtesy? How could she worry about her own health, even? As we walked toward the door, she quickly turned around.

"Come on, Blessn," she said. "We got two buses to catch."

PART FOUR

Faith

As Hurricane Harvey made its way through the city, I received a text from a number I didn't immediately recognize. The city was inundated. Houstonians rich and poor were losing their homes. Those who escaped unscathed helped those most in need.

Roxana withstood the rains in her apartment. From there, as the waters began to recede, she texted me.

"Hola. Doctor," she wrote. "Espero en Dios que estem Todos bien usted y familia." *I hope to God that you and your family are well.*

It had been less than a month since her legs had been amputated. She still felt pain on her shins—"phantom" limb pain is common in amputees—but Roxana was getting used to the stumps and was beginning to prepare for the surgery to remove the dead parts of her arms. As the rains poured down, she thought to check in on me and my family.

"We're fine, thanks," I responded, using Spanish grammar I double-checked with my wife. "Are you all okay?"

"Yes," she wrote, I imagined with that same stylus crammed into her fingers. "May God watch over us . . ."

A few days before Roxana's scheduled surgery, I received a phone call from a number I didn't recognize. When I answered, a woman with a San Antonio accent was on the line.

"You're a doctor, right?" she said.

"Yes, definitely I'm a doctor," I said awkwardly.

She said her name was Nelda, and it didn't take her long to explain the purpose of her call. Her husband was a podiatrist who also made prostheses at a hospital on Houston's southwest side as part of the family business, which had gotten harder and harder as of late.

"A lot of snakes in this profession," she said.

Nelda had heard about "Roxanne" and was inspired by her story. She wanted to help. Before the arm amputations, they really had to get cracking on the legs, she explained. She was in contact with a Christian group that would be able to cover the costs of the actual prostheses, but there were so many other costs to account for, including labor. We all had to get moving quickly if this was going to happen.

I didn't understand, I told her. Roxana had a Gold Card. She was seeing the prosthesis people from the safety-net hospital. Was this some sort of miscommunication?

"Roxanne didn't tell you?"

What I hadn't heard from Roxana was this: the prostheses contractor for the hospital district had quoted her a price. She would have to pay $30,000 for each prosthetic limb. Cash.

Much later, I found out why. Even though Roxana had decided to forgo cancer treatment while the dead arms and legs lingered on her body, the cancer remained inside, and the diagnosis persisted in her chart. Prostheses are expensive, and in a safety-net system, expensive items have to be doled out judiciously, out of fairness. This was one of Ben Taub's limitations. Not all amputees received prostheses. They were evaluated by specialists who decided whether the benefit of the apparatus matched the cost. So it was with prostheses. The Gold Card didn't cover prostheses for patients with metastatic cancer. If Roxana wanted the prostheses now, she'd have to pay out of pocket.

It's not difficult to see the utilitarian argument behind this, particularly in a safety-net system. It makes sense—every penny, especially if it comes from a taxpayer, ought to be spent wisely. And very expensive prostheses for someone with an incurable illness sits low on the list of community necessities. I get that. But it was hard to confront that personally, especially with someone like Roxana, who had struggled so mightily.

Still, there was hope. Nelda had made it her mission to find the money and equipment through charity. She'd contacted some of the organizations she had worked with over the years, most of them Christian based. But some wouldn't work with the undocumented. Nelda looked past this, though she admitted how difficult Roxana's visa status made it to find her the right charity.

"People are scared to help an illegal because they think it's illegal to help an illegal," she explained. Roxana's story had moved Nelda. She considered it part of her Christian faith to help another in need.

Roxana received amputations of both hands without any complications. It had been ten months since her friend Mariam brought her to the emergency room for a lingering pain in her stomach. She had no hands and feet now, but at least the charcoal-black parts had been removed. The sisters still cared for her around the clock, but she had hope that with prostheses she'd walk again.

She met with Nelda a few weeks after the amputation, and then I met Nelda at her office in southwest Houston. She welcomed me warmly, with a hug, her big Texan hair never moving an inch. Over a cup of instant coffee, we talked about the patient we shared.

"I thought Roxanne was incredible," Nelda said.

They had spoken multiple times on the phone over the past month, Roxana with her accent, Nelda with hers. The topic of conversation had naturally shifted from tragedy to religion, the two of them trading stories of their faith in God's plan.

But seeing Roxana had left her with an indelible image of a woman in desperate need.

After recounting this, Nelda took a sip of her coffee and leaned in toward me. She had just found something out that day, something that she felt compelled to ask me about, something that had stuck with her. Now that I was in front of her, she decided to ask.

"Did you know she's a Muslim?" she said.

It had taken me a few months to put the pieces together. When we'd first met, Roxana mentioned some "sisters" who tended to her wounds. I never considered it more than a term of endearment, until I visited her in the days following the leg amputations and met some of these "sisters" at her bedside. They wore hijabs. Things started to click. Then one day, after I explained to Roxana and her visitors why all the doctors were so concerned about infection, one of the sisters raised her hand and asked me if I believed in God.

"I went to Catholic school all my life," I said.

It was an answer I'd cultivated throughout my years at Ben Taub, one I delivered confidently, the way a community theater actor might. Usually, it put the topic of faith to bed.

The sister wasn't satisfied. She wore big bifocals with their tips buried beneath her hijab and arms pinched close to her temples. This created a hinge effect, so that whenever the sister smiled or furrowed her brow, the bifocals moved up and down her face.

I told her I believed human beings had limits, even here at this bedside. I wasn't lying, but I wasn't speaking from my soul either. The truth was that I believed in something, I just didn't know what to call it. I didn't want to assign a proper name to my belief like "God" or "Jesus Christ" or "nirvana," because I'd met faithful people in different parts of the world—Hindus in Bangalore, Protestants in Wittenberg, Catholics in Port-au-Prince, Muslims in Hyderabad—who lived similarly to one another, according to a code that I knew as "Do unto others as you would have done unto you." If I didn't believe in one specific name for it, I believed in the behavior, the idea. I believed in meaning and mystery, how, as much as we humans might have tried, we would never find answers to some of these larger-than-life questions (which I also believed was kind of great). I believed in people.

But I didn't say that. Instead, I opted to sound courteous. "I know I'm not God," I said.

She gave a quick glance at Roxana and then turned back toward me. The bifocals slunk down her nose. Rather than push them in, she peered at me over the lenses.

"I want to tell you about my faith," she said.

Few places on earth evoke the conflict between the physical world and what exists beyond quite like the hospital bedside. Americans die in the hospital today as often as they do in their own homes, and so hospital beds have become touchstones, where patients and loved ones test and pour out their faith. Ben Taub can't be much different from other American hospitals in this regard, except that the lamentations happen in Farsi, or Vietnamese, or an Ethiopian dialect, or K'iche'.

I've seen many doctors deal with religion at the bedside in different ways. Some ignore it, maintaining a strict adherence to science. These doctors often use a passive, statistical voice in conversations: nothing is ever definitive, it is "likely" or "unlikely." Some doctors can revel in it. They use terms like "miracle" and "blessed" and connect their ability to prescribe medications safely to the purpose of serving their God.

Many of Roxana's sisters spoke with me about their beliefs over the coming months. I joined a WhatsApp group titled "Roxana's Journey," which kept those invested in Roxana's progress, including Nelda, updated. One of the sisters organized a GoFundMe campaign to raise money for the prostheses. It raised $13,320 in one month, which was enough for Nelda to start. After the usual fees and deductions, Roxana should have had $12,267.72, but she only received $8,000. I sent an inquiry to GoFundMe. The missing money, it turned out, had been withdrawn by another of Roxana's sisters. Roxana had given it to her.

"She hears and she aches for others," the organizer of the campaign told me over the phone. She was frustrated that another sister had gone so far as to ask Roxana, in her vulnerable state, for money like that. But Roxana wanted to help.

"Faith has a lot to do with this," the organizer said. "Roxana has to hold on to faith."

As Nelda ordered the prostheses and the sisters organized the finances, the world began to spin around Roxana. It happened suddenly. She awoke one morning and quickly had to shut her eyes again to avoid vomiting. It was like she was on a merry-go-round, one that moved faster and faster and never stopped. She visited a same-day clinic, where a doctor optimistically prescribed her meclizine, hoping this might all just be a little motion sickness. Four days later, Roxana returned to the Ben Taub ER, where a CAT scan of the head uncovered the culprit, a grape-size mass in the part of the brain called the cerebellum. The tumor blocked the flow of fluid around her brain and spine.

A whole year had passed since Roxana's first surgery, which had removed the cancer around her heart and liver at the cost of her limbs. Those limbs had finally been removed from her body, but now the cancer had spread to her brain. As the neurosurgeons detailed their recommendations—burr holes into the skull, perform a sharp dissection of the mass with their scalpels, and after the surgery, deliver radiation to the brain—Roxana couldn't help but feel that this path God had made for her was too much.

Twenty years earlier, Roxana had sat alone in a café after another day working beneath the store's bright lights. As her body took rest and absorbed nutrients, different worries ping-ponged throughout her mind: her mother, her daughter, the money she sent back home, work. It was while she was in this cloud that a woman approached the table, extending toward her what appeared to be a pamphlet, which Roxana took into her hand.

"God created the Universe," it stated.

Roxana read on.

"The order of the Universe is proof of God's intelligence. The Quran is God's revelation to people. We can all have a relationship with God."

The pamphlet proceeded according to a logic that Roxana recognized had been buried inside of her. She'd never been one for gambling, for instance, or buying lottery tickets. She believed in meaning. All the store's glamour that surrounded her, not to mention the extremely rich—celebrities, dignitaries, heads of state—who dropped thirty thousand dollars on fashion items like it was nothing: there had to be more than this.

Right then and there, in the café, she acknowledged something: she had always been in search of this faith.

Roxana converted to Islam that moment. The parlance of her old faith—for instance, "*iglesia*"—stayed with her, as did her devotion to her family and her sense of elegance. She learned rituals that became a part of her, like the worship she offered five times every day even after she lost her limbs. Prayer sustained her through a change in jobs and through the toughest moments of her life, including when the cancer caused the blood vessels in her brain to throb. Even at her lowest—rolling on the floor after having fallen from the bed, crying out for anybody who might hear, pushing buttons with her nubs, allowing her bladder to release urine into her sweatpants—faith sustained her.

Faith will always be a part of practicing medicine. Science explains the phenomena that allow us to treat patients effectively, but it can't explain everything. What happens the moment a Code Blue ends will always be a mystery. Doctors will always have to believe in one possibility or another for which data can't be collected.

While I've never experienced a conversion like Roxana's, I've felt how faith has impacted my work as a doctor. I've seen how a person can will themselves to hold on to life for extra minutes or days. I've also seen, as in the case of Mr. Alvaro, the man I told, "It's okay if you die," that sometimes bodies allow people to choose when to release themselves. Faith has also affected me personally. Each morning when I walk into work, I pass a brass plaque in the parking garage. It's nothing special. The words emblazoned on it give nothing more than information: the architect, the politicians in office the year the building opened, the inspectors. To me, the plaque signifies that our society holds compassion and cooperation as core values.

It's only minutes after passing the plaque that I feel my daily dose of faith. It hits me as I walk through the lobby, past the security guards and up the stairs, across the walkway, through the double doors, at the corner of the hallway that leads to my office. My faith comes from the people I've greeted in the short walk from the parking garage, from their professionalism. Here we are at a hospital for people who can't afford healthcare, I tell myself, where you might see prisoners and drug addicts and the homeless, and the people I greet each morning with a "How are you?" show up here *every day*. They could work somewhere else—there are healthcare jobs to go around in this city—but they choose to work here. They all look so different, too. They're from south India and the Philippines and Honduras and the Fifth Ward. They wear lab coats and purple scrubs and bolo ties. This place works because of them.

They aren't anything like the people Jan de Hartog described in *The Hospital*. They aren't cynical or downtrodden. Some are at Ben Taub only to train. Others, like me, have decided to stay. They're why I'm optimistic about healthcare in America, despite all the problems we encounter every day. They believe in the medicine happening at Ben Taub. Some of the staff, in time, will decide to move on to more lucrative salaries in the surrounding nonprofit hospitals, which is okay. But for now, they work like they're part of something bigger than a paycheck. They feel for their patients. They have their bad days, but the kindness and empathy emanate. That's what healthcare is at its best, what I see at Ben Taub: science coming together with people. It's why I continue to believe in medicine. My faith comes full circle when I imagine myself through each of their eyes and I realize I'm one of them.

I'd be lying if I said this moment of faith happens every day, but it happens often, probably once a week. And in medicine's most difficult moments, when it's clear that a problem isn't fixable, I take solace in the fact that it's not just me working for a patient: it's a community, a people.

Just as all people are responsible for their larger community, so too are communities responsible for people. If someone is suffering, and there is the capacity within the community to help, in a way that doesn't harm anyone else, then we not only owe it to that person; we also owe it to ourselves to help. I'm not really sure how to try to do my job without that belief.

*　　*　　*

The numbers meant it was always going to be close. Emma heard us describe what they meant each day, how her son Geronimo's liver was failing, how this organ's failure placed increasing pressure on his other organs, how these other organs were starting to fail, too. She heard the numbers each day from the medical student on our team, and then the residents, and then from me—the bilirubin, his coagulation factors, the sodium and creatinine, all of these continued to worsen. No doctor or nurse wanted to voice what was becoming unavoidable: Geronimo, at the young age of thirty-six, was dying. Only a liver transplant could save him, but to receive one, even here, the numbers were too close: Geronimo's disability check exceeded the lowest threshold to qualify for Medicaid, and Medicaid was his only hope; without it, Geronimo would die. The numbers said so.

I wrote an email to Geronimo's congressman detailing the crisis. The tone was even, slightly deferential, sticking carefully to the facts, like what you might find in a catastrophic weather forecast. A few hours after I sent it, I knew it wasn't enough. There simply wasn't enough time. With every path at the safety-net hospital exhausted, the medical team decided to call Geronimo's representative to see if our patient might qualify for Medicaid and eventually receive a liver transplant.

John Culberson had represented Texas's Seventh Congressional District for fifteen years. He had voted against Obamacare and opposed the Medicaid expansion. The team knew that convincing Representative Culberson was a long shot, but the breakdown of Geronimo's liver was pushing the rest of his body to its limit. Fluid continued to compress his lungs, causing his oxygen saturation level to drop whenever he turned in his bed. No matter how much Emma rubbed his feet, they kept puffing with edema. If Geronimo didn't receive a new liver soon, he would die.

Culberson's staff took down their constituent's information. The resident on my team explained how Geronimo had been approved for Medicaid, but that this coverage had been taken away on account of his $912 disability check exceeding the limit. Purchasing health insurance outright wasn't feasible. The open-enrollment period for Obamacare had passed, and private insurers told Emma that her son's illness did not meet their criteria for a "qualifying life event," which is middleman-speak for a major change in life, like divorce, losing a job, or the birth of a child, that allows one to change health insurance plans. Dying didn't qualify. We asked Culberson's staff. What if Geronimo halted his disability checks? Could Texas Medicaid then consider his application ASAP?

Two staffers from Culberson's office began asking officials around the state who might be able to fund a transplant evaluation. Two days later, Dr. Emilie Becker, the medical director on call for the Texas Medicaid program, phoned me directly to say that several administrators at her office were working on the case, too. They needed one more piece of documentation, though—Geronimo's latest bank statement. Could we expedite things by faxing it over?

Emma left her son's bedside to search for the document. The very next morning, I found her in the recliner that had become a second home.

"Aquí está," she said, handing me the bank statement. *Here it is.*

I reviewed the paper. Three entries appeared in Geronimo's transaction history: a deposit of nine hundred and eighteen dollars from the Social Security Administration, a cash withdrawal the next day in the amount of nine hundred dollars, and another deposit of nine hundred and eighteen dollars twenty-nine days later.

The team stood by the fax machine on the nursing unit as the document filtered through. Nobody else on the team was older than twenty-six. I was the team's attending and leader. I had worked more than ten years at Ben Taub as a student and a resident and now, for the last five years, as an internist with a medical license. As much as I tried to put on a strong face, the team could see my faith was shaken.

"I'm worried about the numbers," I said. The total on the Social Security check exceeded Medicaid's limit by a measly $179, but that was enough for any administrator to deny Geronimo coverage. "I'm worried none of this will make a difference."

One of the social workers was so confident of this that she wrote as much in a note, appending it to Geronimo's chart: "He will be denied this benefit."

Later the same afternoon, however, I received a call from the Medicaid office. Geronimo had been approved.

As we hurried to transfer him to a transplant center, a staffer at Culberson's office called for an update. I thanked her for her help.

"Of course," she said. "This was someone's life at stake."

Although she and her colleagues had not dealt with a situation like this before, staffers for two other US representatives in the Houston area recalled instances in which a direct appeal to Congress had helped a critically ill patient obtain coverage. I spoke with financial counselors at several liver-transplant centers around Texas, who estimated that, in a given three-month period, between one and nine patients are disqualified from Medicaid because their disability payments are too high. Nobody could say what becomes of these patients—whether they somehow purchase insurance or move to states with less stringent Medicaid rules, or whether they simply die from lack of a transplant.

"I'm sure that happens," Representative Gene Green, of Texas's Twenty-Ninth Congressional District, which serves eastern Houston, told me.

I called Dr. Becker to thank her, too.

"You're so welcome," she said. I could hear in her voice that she really was happy for Geronimo and hoped everything would work out. Toward the end of our conversation, I asked her how, in the end, Geronimo had qualified.

Dr. Becker didn't have an answer. "It seems like you got the right people involved," she said.

Geronimo and his mother were overjoyed by the news.

"I trusted in God," Emma said. As she thanked the team, I noted that this was the first of many steps that had to occur before Geronimo received a new liver. It was a vital one, but the real medical work— posting him on the list, matching him with a donor, harvesting the organ, and all the technical challenges of connecting it to a body shutting down—still lay ahead.

"We have faith," Emma said.

Surgeons call it a Lazarus procedure for a reason. The idea is simple, but how a real liver transplant occurs is nothing short of a marvel. The first attempt at a human-to-human liver transplant occurred in 1963 in Colorado, and for the half century that's followed, the process has been refined both medically and socially. What used to be an experimental Hail Mary performed by a few surgeons now involves teams of highly specialized people—social workers, pilots, immunologists, ethicists, government workers—dedicated to making the best use of a precious resource: a healthy liver no longer used by its original body. Each time a liver is implanted into a new host, it's the medical equivalent of a rocket breaking through the atmosphere. The surgeon releases the clamps on the arteries and veins, blood begins to flow through an unfamiliar but fully functional organ, and we have orbit. The results are spectacular. The yellow blemishing the whites of a person's eyes immediately starts to wash away. Bleeding orifices clot. Gallons of excess fluid in the belly become liters and then milliliters until all that appears on ultrasound is viscera. Dying people stand up from their hospital beds and walk.

Witnessing this is like seeing a human being bounce gleefully on the surface of the moon. You can't keep the words from spewing from your mouth: "I can't believe we can do this."

Success is the product of analysis and execution, but more than anything, it's a result of human beings masterfully organizing time and space. A liver needs to make its way from a dead body into an ailing one. A surgeon trains for no less than eleven years to gain the technical expertise to harvest a liver from a dying body and to connect it to a dying person's circulatory system. But technical prowess only gets you through the door: making sure the liver survives after implantation involves teams of experts.

A liver can't just go into any ailing body. It must go into the *right* ailing body. What constitutes the right body depends on biology and ethics. The liver must be viable and fit size-wise into the body. Its cells have to be similar enough to the recipient's to avoid rejection. And so more experts are needed, including critical care doctors to keep the brain-dead donor's circulation going until the time of harvest, and immunologists, not to mention lab technicians, to ensure the cells of two different bodies match sufficiently. Without this, the satellite explodes in the stratosphere: a liver implanted into an unsuitable body literally dissolves right then and there as a result of liquefactive necrosis. It's a tragedy, a punch in the gut. Everyone involved is left staring, thinking, What went wrong?

The right body also means the sickest body, and here is where ethics demands even deeper organizing. A new liver is the most precious resource on the planet for a person dying of liver failure, and at any one time in the United States, there are at least seventeen thousand people—and likely many more—in need of one. Consequently, the US Department of Health and Human Services (HHS) has decided to prioritize the sickest people, or those closest to death. HHS lets the United Network for Organ Sharing (UNOS), a private group, organize lists of people most in need of a liver in eleven different regions around the United States. Numbers play a seminal role in determining who is sickest. Each potential liver transplant patient gives blood, and from this blood, sodium, clotting, bilirubin, and kidney function levels are gleaned and plugged into a complex formula. The product is a number: the Model for End-Stage Liver Disease (MELD) score. The higher the score, the sicker the patient.

The MELD score is supposed to be the most important factor determining someone's position on the list. Every transplant center has a committee made up of nurses, psychiatrists, social workers, and surgeons that evaluates each potential patient, to make sure nothing's lost in the numbers. Will this person take their anti-rejection medicines? Does this person have enough support at home to heal well? Can the person handle the stress of the process, or are they at high risk to start drinking again? Once the committee gives its thumbs-up, the patient is entered into a network run by UNOS that matches the highest score with a biologically suitable liver in the region. When there's a match, two important alerts go out: one to the harvesting doctor, who must now fly to the hospital where the liver is being kept alive, and another to the surgeon of the waiting patient. The harvest team flies back with the liver in a preservative vat and hands it off to the surgeon (yes, it has happened that a liver has slipped out of someone's hands during the handoff). When all goes smoothly, it's beautiful, and more so than seeing one of us in space. There's a sense that justice has prevailed. We can look at one another in moments of success and say we cured one of the sickest people on earth.

Eight thousand liver transplants happen every year in the United States, adding more than $5 billion to our national healthcare costs. To say that liver transplants aren't cheap is an understatement. Yet it's hard to imagine this procedure surviving without so much money. There's no way around affording all these experts and all this organizing without paying for it. Money definitely greases the wheels and makes this many high-quality liver transplants possible, but it also complicates the procedure. There are loopholes in the transplant network. MELD scores are inflated.* People game the system. Famous people can receive preference. Look no further than Steve Jobs, who received a liver in Tennessee two years before he died in 2011 (his new liver died with him). Jobs realized that his best chance at receiving a liver was to have doctors list him in multiple regions. It's no surprise that more livers were available in this part of the country. One of the effects of the opioid crisis was to make many, many more livers available. These were healthy livers, too, generally young and pristine, since fentanyl and heroin and Dilaudid aren't toxic to this part of the body. One transplant surgeon told me that whenever his patient is matched with a liver harvested from someone who's died of opioid overdose, he's ecstatic. He wasn't too pleased that someone like Steve Jobs could fly in and receive one of these livers ahead of the people living in his state.

These inconsistencies aside, the system is based on a more fundamental disparity, which is the price of entry into this market. Anyone, including the undocumented and poor, can donate a liver, but to receive a liver transplant, you must either be wealthy or have a generous health insurance. Bronze Obamacare policies, the lowest-level plans, for instance, generally don't cover transplants. Before the MELD points system was introduced for transplants in 2002, more minorities died waiting for a liver than white people. The new system, which provided urban regions the ability to procure organs harvested in more rural regions, has eliminated that gap, meaning those posted on the list now receive a fair shot race-wise, but the initial barriers for those who can't afford good insurance still exist. At an average cost of $878,000 (which includes follow-up care and medications for six months after the procedure), Lazarus surgeries are simply too expensive for any safety-net system, including ours.

---

* Lab results are lab results: these numbers can't be inflated. But committees can award "exception points" that are supposed to give priority to a patient whose level of illness isn't reflected by their MELD score. Some transplant surgeons have accused others of massaging the numbers by adding exception points when not indicated.

I don't know how to reconcile this fact with what I know about Ben Taub. The hospital where I work gives doctors and nurses the best opportunity to provide people with excellent healthcare even when they don't have the money for it. Coverage and an expensive procedure were exactly what Geronimo needed to live. While arranging for Geronimo to leave Ben Taub, I felt some pangs I recognized as disaster syndrome. If he stayed here, I thought, I know he'd continue to receive our best efforts. But our best wasn't enough for Geronimo—not with what the safety net had to provide for Houston's uninsured and those who couldn't afford healthcare—and so he had to leave.

Three days after we contacted Representative Culberson, Geronimo was transferred to a not-for-profit hospital in the Texas Medical Center. The transplant team quickly evaluated him, drew blood, and began checking all the boxes necessary for him to receive a new liver. Emma accompanied her son to the hospital and found a new seat beside him.

The first sign of trouble came when Geronimo's blood pressure dropped shortly after his transfer. He was intubated and placed on a ventilator. His doctors began dialysis, to take the strain off his kidneys, and set up a constant stream of IV medications to stabilize his blood pressure. Very quickly, the documentation of Geronimo's treatment, prepared for billing purposes, took on an ominous tone: "This patient has a high probability of sudden, clinically significant deterioration, which requires the highest level of physician preparedness to intervene urgently."

Once Geronimo was stabilized, the transplant team decided to place him on the transplant list. I visited him shortly afterward. It had been years since I had found myself lost inside a hospital, not counting the birth of my daughter, when dad delirium led me to a loading dock instead of the cafeteria. When I finally made it into the ICU and then into Geronimo's room, he was unrecognizable beneath the tubes and machinery. I placed my hand on his foot, which was considerably less swollen.

Emma stood up from her chair. I hugged her.

"Cómo estás, señora?" I asked. *How are you?*

It wasn't a very smart question. She looked fatigued and fragile. Even though she continued to pray, she told me the way he looked now worried her. I told her to hold on. The liver specialist said he had a high probability of receiving a liver based on his very high MELD score.

That same day, however, the nurses noticed that something wasn't right. When they inserted a needle into Geronimo's arm to draw blood, a procedure that, even in a heavily sedated patient, would cause a flinch, he didn't move. Even more concerning, when the doctors moved Geronimo's breathing tube around to test whether it would still provoke a natural coughing response, he only lay there—no cough, no fidgeting, nothing.

A CAT scan confirmed the worst: as a result of his liver failure, which increased his propensity to bleed spontaneously, Geronimo had bled into his brain. Surgery was not an option, since the bleeding was too widespread. The doctors waited five days to see whether Geronimo would regain basic brain function, performing the same reflex checks over and over. Once it became clear that he would never recover, Geronimo was taken off the transplant list. On May 10, a month to the day after he came to the ER at Ben Taub, Emma asked the medical team to remove her son from life support. It's very likely that if Geronimo hadn't lost Medicaid—if the state hadn't taken it away because of the extra $179 from his disability check—he would have been living with a transplanted liver on that day.

Geronimo's wake was held two days later, at Santana Funeral Directors, a squat red brick building on the service road for one of Houston's busiest freeways. I arrived late in the afternoon, after finishing my rounds at the hospital. Emma greeted me at the entrance and walked me to her son's casket. "Look at him," she said, pointing out how the yellow in Geronimo's skin had darkened into a dusky brown. "We didn't have to use much makeup."

I expressed my condolences as best I could. "Por lo menos, no esta sufriendo," I said: *At least he's not suffering*. I told her she had inspired my colleagues with her devotion to him. Emma bent her head and looked a little longer at her son. She asked me if I might say some words to the few who had gathered there that afternoon.

To the ten or twelve people sitting in clusters, I said what I believed: what happened to Geronimo was a tragedy—"Fue una tragedia." I noted how kind Geronimo and his mother were at all times despite the harshness of his illness. And then I apologized. Not for any harm I or the other doctors had caused. I just said I was sorry.

More than a few were dressed in ranch wear, as if upon hearing the news, they had put down the reins of whatever animal or machine they handled and found a way to make it into town. I was the only person wearing a sports coat. I said I knew Geronimo so little, but that it was always a privilege to serve as a person's doctor, something I continue to believe like it's dogma, medicine's only dogma.

I haven't reflected much on what I said that afternoon. I have wondered, however, what drove me to apologize. It's possible the apology was just my rote way of trying to make sad people feel better, but I also think that my desire to apologize meant something. It meant that I felt sorry I had gotten Emma and her son's hopes up. It also meant, "I'm sorry I didn't yell 'Help!' loud enough." It meant, "I'm sorry I feel this right now and won't be so alarmed the next time it happens." It meant, "I'm sorry we're in the richest and most innovative country in the world, and we couldn't find a way to help your thirty-six-year-old son over a hundred and seventy-nine bucks." And finally, it also meant, "I'm sorry I will continue to do my job tomorrow as if this never happened."

I say this aware of my own hypocrisy. I've allowed other tragic deaths to pass without as much attention.

Were I a preacher, I'd have said more. I'd have talked about where the responsibility for this death falls: on all of us. We accept these tragedies because we don't demand anything different. I'd have said that each premium we pay passively reinforces the idea that some people deserve healthcare and others do not. I'd have said that Medicine Inc. isn't working, not for medicine or patients, and that in the name of profit it's usurped this beautiful combination of art and science that doctors and nurses practice. We suffer from disaster syndrome, I would have said, because we can't imagine anything better than what we have. I would have noted how joyless it can be to see a doctor today, the waiting, the middlemen, the upselling, the bills aimed at us from every direction. And then I would've shared my vision: more *affordable* healthcare for all, the type that Geronimo could access even as a gas station attendant. Maybe he uses a system like the one at Harris Health, except this one's not so overloaded. Maybe he or his employer pays for insurance to access grades of care not covered by this standard. Choosing one or the other doesn't spell the difference between life and death—that's the big point, I tell everyone. I would've ended with a note about faith: The people in this country value life and decency. They want to do the right thing. We have already improved since the days of Jefferson Davis, I'd have said, we just have to have the courage to change. We have good people working in this field, we just need to organize them properly.

I didn't say any of those things. It just wasn't my role that day. I thanked everyone in attendance for giving me the opportunity to talk, took one last look at the casket, and headed toward the back.

Geronimo's wasn't the last funeral for a Ben Taub patient I attended.

Each time, I've wondered if my being there was appropriate. They'll understand if you don't make it, I tell myself, it doesn't really matter. And each time, after standing through formalities and spontaneous demonstrations of love, through rituals and anecdotes, a family member asks me if I might say some words.

I don't think I'm asked just for personal reasons. I don't think I'm asked only to represent science, either. I think it's a little of both. I think these people who've gathered to mourn want to believe that the very basics happened:

Your loved one was *worthy* of our attention and our care.

Your loved one was *exactly* the type of person doctors go into the field to treat.

Money didn't stop us from trying what we could to help.

He was at a public hospital, yes, but he got the same care he would've received at a private hospital.

Before I started seeing patients as a medical student at Ben Taub, I assumed these statements to be inherently true of medicine in America. I continue to work where I work because I can stand before a small gathering of bereaved and saddened people, say this to them, and know I'm not lying.

Emma caught me before I made it out of the funeral parlor. She wanted me to pass along a message to the team—not just the doctors, but also the social workers, the administrators, the nurses, and a congressional staffer who had visited with her and her son. It was something Geronimo had told her toward the end, when it looked as though he might indeed receive a transplant. "I feel so important," he had said. "Everyone treats me like I'm rich."

Addendum

It is August in Houston, the peak of summer, and Roxana is running a bit late for an appointment. I wait for her on the fifth floor of an old Fifth Ward hospital retrofitted by Harris Health into a rehabilitation center. It's a part of the safety net I've never seen myself, though I've referred many patients here. The fluorescent lamps, grade-school-style mats, and smell of old steel give the gym a CrossFit vibe. As I make my way deeper into the rehab center, signs of more technical calisthenics start to appear. Posters of tai chi sequences don the partition walls; Hula-Hoops, bunched according to their diameter, lie atop workbenches. A few patients are speed-walking on the treadmills connected to pulse monitors and oximeters. I scan the area for clues to point me toward the amputee section, but it's clear I'm a fish out of water here, and so a therapist escorts me to an office chair beside a padded mechanical platform. I tell her I'm here to visit with my old patient Roxana.

"She'll be here soon, I'm sure," she says.

Outside, it's sweltering. The peaks of the great Texas Medical Center hospitals are visible here, a three-mile distance along Brays Bayou. A year earlier, Hurricane Harvey engorged those waters with fifty-one inches of rain over five days. The medical schools and hospitals of the Texas Medical Center, prepared for such an event, enacted their disaster

329

plans, which included sealing doors as thick as those on submarines. The flooding still managed to reach Ben Taub's basement, however. Patient care continued on the floors above unabated. All in all, Harvey crippled very little of Ben Taub or the safety-net system's infrastructure. I wish I could say the same about its patients.

Many who had lost homes still lived in temporary housing. One of my patients, a single mother who couldn't walk to the bathroom or trail after her three young children without feeling breathless, had been forced to move in with a family from her church. The city had cleared thirteen million cubic yards of physical debris, but the healthcare debris—the unchecked liver disease and uncontrolled diabetes and advanced heart failure—would remain strewn for months.

The waters never entered Roxana's west-side apartment, but she experienced flooding of a different sort. The cancer found in Roxana's brain led to two brain surgeries and a cycle of radiation. Oncologists discovered more cancer in her hip, her lung, and the inferior vena cava, the great vein where it had been found originally twenty months before. Time was a factor in the amount of healthcare doctors offered her over the years, as Roxana's cancer was slow growing. She was also able to demonstrate a robust activity level that meant she was less likely to suffer risks from the procedures. Her doctors felt each bit of healthcare provided her with some gain in the quality of her life.

As she approaches the amputee section, I can't help but think about her illness and how she is still alive. I notice her hair first. It's colored blond and looks styled, short in length but voluminous, like the *peinados* you see at fancy Salvadoran weddings. The mass of hair heads straight at me, toward my hip, cutting through the Hula-Hoop station and then the free weights. Soon I see that Roxana's eyebrows are arched high on her forehead. Her pearls are on. I've seen her smile many times before, but this, I notice, is Roxana at her happiest.

"Doctorcito," she says, raising the stub of her arm out toward me, "do you like my Mercedes?"

Roxana's new mode of transportation is a peacock-blue Permobil power wheelchair with elevation and tilt. Thanks to higher torque, deeper tire treads, and increased horsepower, it's more sophisticated than the one used by Stephen Hawking, only instead of a laptop, Roxana employs a joystick to thread through traffic. The machine is a gift from a previous owner donated to an organization known to Roxana's physical therapist. Now it is Roxana's pride.

"It's beautiful," I say, hugging her.

The Mercedes is a large part of why I've come today to visit. Today is Roxana's graduation day. For the past four months, she has attended rehabilitation here on the fifth floor to learn how to walk and survive on her own. While physical therapy sessions focused on strengthening Roxana's core to help mobilize her leg prostheses, occupational therapy helped her develop the skills to keep herself alive: cleaning, toileting, feeding, calling for help. Roxana has graduated from occupational therapy because she's managed to arrive at the therapy on her own.

She started the day by calling MetroLift, the city's transportation service for the disabled, and arranging a pickup time. Then she moved from her bed onto the Mercedes. From there, Roxana fed herself, used the bathroom herself, put on her own makeup (and pearls), and brushed her hair. When the time came for her appointments, she drove the Mercedes onto the bus. Roxana is no longer a burden. She has reached her goals for independence.

"What about the big party?" she asks. "Where are the balloons?"

The physical therapist laughs. "The county didn't give us money for that."

It didn't come easy. Only a month ago, she nearly gave up after walking with her new leg prostheses. What an enormous feat. Roxana wore black Nikes for it, above which extended two metal pipes, her shins. Over her prostheses, she wore black running shorts, and wrapped around her head was a desert scarf. With her elbows strapped onto a walker, Roxana took a series of deep breaths and then slid the apparatus forward a few inches. Once she had pushed it far enough, she swung one prosthetic leg forward, followed by the other, and voilà, a step. She repeated the motion for fifteen full feet.

While Roxana had exceeded her therapists' expectations, she encountered a stark reality: she would never be able to do this without two therapists by her side. This wasn't just my opinion. There were anatomical reasons for her struggles. The cerebellum orchestrates movements. It is the GPS part of the brain, signaling precise coordinates to our arms and legs. Whenever we walk in a straight line or juggle, we have the cerebellum to thank for pinpointing the right movements. Roxana had to contend not only with four amputated limbs but also with the metastatic cancer that had migrated to this part of her brain.

A simple invention has helped. It's a band of silicone—also peacock blue—Roxana straps on her dominant stump. She can thread a stylus through the holes on either end, or a pen, or the pointy end of a hairbrush. As a repairman fixes a loose seat belt strap on the Mercedes, Roxana uses the tool to draw. She turns in a colored-in printout of the Hagia Sofia to her occupational therapist at the end of the session. The repairman nods in approval.

"Que Dios lo bendiga," she says.

With graduation complete, it's on to an amputee support group on the other side of town. Roxana has a tight schedule and must leave immediately.

"What are you going to do about food?" asks her therapist.

She gazes inquisitively into the air. "I hadn't thought about that," says Roxana. "I hope they have food."

It's no matter, she can deal with the hunger. As her therapists move on to their next patients, I tell Roxana I'd like to walk her out.

"Hurry," she says, "we can't be late."

The elevator drops us at the front door, where the MetroLift bus driver waits.

"I'm sorry!" Roxana says.

The driver nods. I take the opportunity to tell her something I've been meaning to say for a while, except now, in this rush, I'm not exactly sure how to say it. As the Mercedes begins to inch forward, the words just spill out.

"Me inspiras," I say. *You inspire me.* I somehow get the words out in a mixture of English and Spanish: she is the most resilient person I've ever met.

"Ay mi doctorcito," she says, putting her stubs together.

It's another of those little secrets about Ben Taub, like the ones Dave and I used to share. This one I treasure. It makes me feel special. There are people like Roxana *everywhere.* They live, they exist despite ridiculous odds, and nobody knows the absolute strength of their character except the people working at Ben Taub. That's my joy. I entered medical school with the ambition to care for sports stars. But these stories, these people—this, to me, is medicine.

We hug again, and with a quick push of her joystick, the Mercedes lurches toward the bus, stopping at the ramp, where the driver greets Roxana. He's a large African American man in uniform. He bows down and says something to her I can't hear.

For a moment, I'm concerned that something's gone wrong—the bus is full, or she's made the wrong reservation—but then a hearty laugh fills the air. Roxana wags her stubs joyfully in the air.

"Thank you kindly, sir," she says as the Mercedes pulls up the ramp.

It is the final time I see Roxana in the flesh, a moment that lives on with me now as much as when it happened. The moment is frozen in time, like blood cells trapped on a microscope's slide. I can focus in on some of the details—like her hair, the treads on the Mercedes—but I can also pull back. There's a bigger picture here beyond the cancer and the disability. I see one person helping another in need, but I also see more. When I use the widest lens, I see it's the people of a city getting the best out of one of their own. It's every penny from our pockets well spent.

Acknowledgments

Thank you to Roxana, Stephen, Ebonie, Christian, Geronimo, and Aqueria, along with your families and loved ones. This book wouldn't exist without your bravery, patience, and trust.

One of my favorite parts of writing this book was discovering the history and importance of the institution where I work, the Harris Health System. Kitty Allen, George Masi, and King Hillier all understood my aim from the start and gave me the space to write the most accurate portrayal of a civic institution I could produce. I also want to thank all of the spectacular social workers, therapists, case managers, and nurses I work with, especially those in units 3A, 4A, 4B, 5E, 5G/F, 5A, 5B, 5C, 6A, 6B, 6D, and the ER.

Thank you also to my colleagues in the Department of General Internal Medicine and everyone I ran into in the hallways over the years who encouraged me to write about Ben Taub Hospital. Thank you to Arthur "Tim" Garson and Stephen Linder, for offering a free and expansive health policy course to the Texas Medical Center community.

Dave, you're no longer around, but you believed in this book from very early on and you gave me the space to write it. This book wouldn't exist without you. I miss you. Thank you also to Joey Fisher, for serving as a supportive leader during a difficult time.

Thank you to Robert Graham, for serving as my mentor. Thank you also to Drs. Rush Lynch and Daniel Musher, both of whom encouraged me to find a way to blend the practice of medicine with writing. John Gavin and Norma Tilden gave me this same advice in college. Thank you also to Robert Cremins, Willard Volding, and Jeffrey Shulman for being amazing and impactful teachers.

Burke Nixon is not only one of my best friends; he's also a gifted teacher. On top of that, he's one of the kindest people I know. I've been uniquely lucky to write alongside someone with these qualities. He gave an immeasurable amount of time and insight to this book. Thanks, Burke, for everything.

Time and space away from the hospital proved vital to this book. I'd like to thank Alejandro and Scott Winters, as well as my in-laws, Gerald and Celinda Schillaci, for their generosity. Thank you to the Texas Institute of Letters and the University of Texas Dobie Paisano Fellowship Program, for providing the beautiful Paisano Ranch for me and my family. Michael Adams helped make this time special for me and my family. Fellowships at MacDowell, Yaddo, Ucross, and the Logan Nonfiction Program introduced me to a community of writers—many of whom are now friends—and gave me the perfect environment to push this book where it had to go.

Anna Stein recognized the scope and the ambition of this project from our first conversation. Thanks for your vision and dedication and for being such a smart and insightful reader—you're the best, Anna. Thanks also to Paul Reyes, Anthony Lydgate, and Jeff Salamon, who shepherded the articles from which this book took shape.

Kathy Belden has fought for this book from the day I submitted the proposal. Writing a book for the first time oftentimes made me feel nervous, tired, and small, the way patients can feel. Kathy, you were the trusted doctor throughout it all. You spoke straight to me when I needed it, you were also humane and experienced and thoughtful. I never doubted. Thank you for believing in this book and in me.

Thank you also to Rebekah Jett and the whole Scribner team—Nan, Colin, Stu, Paul Samuelson, Zoey Cole, and everyone who made it clear from the get-go that this book had a home. Thanks also to Aja Pollock and Jason Chappell for the wonderful copyediting and to Maya Shoukri for checking this book's facts. Dan Raeburn and Mark Bowden read this book at critical points and offered essential advice. Vivian Ho and Mark Pauly took time away from their extremely busy and important academic lives to read portions of this book and help me understand some key healthcare ideas—thank you.

I've been lucky to have a whole legion of friends and family supporting me. Thanks to my sisters, Jenny and Jackie, who have kept me in line over the years and have always encouraged my desire to write. Thanks to Vu Tran for your guidance and radical listening. Coco, you've done more than your share to help this book get here: thanks, bro, for throwing your hat in the ring. Thank you to my parents for everything. Mom, you provided me with a model of empathy my whole life, and, Dad, you modeled resilience: I couldn't have finished this book without either of you. To my beloved family, Valentina, Théo, and Valeria, you've been my source of light throughout it all. Thank you for tolerating me during my busy and not-so-great moments and for showing me compassion when I needed it. Without you I'd be rudderless.

Author's Note

I received written authorization from the patients named in this book to share their medical details and stories. I interviewed each patient on multiple occasions, recorded notes, and reviewed medical charts to ensure an accurate portrayal. The ideas and opinions expressed in this book come from my own analysis and thinking while working on the wards; they do not represent the hospital I work at or the medical college that employs me.

Notes

Chapter 1 **Histories**

3 *Texas, the state with the nation's largest uninsured population*: "Health Insurance Coverage of Nonelderly 0-64, 2019," Kaiser Family Foundation, May 15, 2022, https://www.kff.org/other/state-indicator/nonelderly-0-64/?data View=1&currentTimeframe=0&sortModel=%7B%22colId%22:%22 Uninsured%22,%22sort%22:%22desc%22%7D.

5 *John Cornyn wrote a legal opinion*: John Cornyn, JC-0394 Opinion, Office of the Attorney General of Texas, July 10, 2001.

6 *America spends a larger percentage of its gross domestic product on healthcare*: "Current Health Expenditures (% of GDP) – United States," World Bank, January 30, 2022, https://data.worldbank.org/indicator/SH.XPD.CHEX .GD.ZS?locations=US.

6 *In 2015, Ben Taub Hospital and Harris Health spent*: "Financial Statements as of December 31, 2015," Harris Health System, December 31, 2015, www .harrishealth.org/SiteCollectionDocuments/financials/monthly/2015 /december-2015.pdf.

6 *Compare that to national health expenditure data*: Anne B. Martin, Micah Hartman, Benjamin Washington, and Aaron Catlin, "National Health Spending: Faster Growth in 2015 as Coverage Expands and Utilization Increases," *Health Affairs* 36, no. 1 (January 2017): 166–67.

6 *In 2015, Ben Taub demonstrated itself to be the* best hospital in the country: Francisco Cota, Scott Bassett, Razvan Dadu, Ana Davis, Jaromir Bobek,

and Nassir Lakkis, "A Multidisciplinary Team Approach for a Successful STEMI Program in a Public Hospital System with Limited Resources," *Journal of Heart and Stroke*, no. 2 (June 2017): 1034.

9 *"The smell of poverty":* Jan de Hartog, *The Hospital* (1964; repr., New York: HarperPerennial, 1991), 22–23.

15 *Chekhov traveled:* Anton Chekhov, *A Life in Letters*, ed. Rosamund Bartlett (London: Penguin Books, 2004).

Chapter 2 **The Dead Parts**

29 *Nearly half of all people in the United States receive their health insurance through their job:* "Health Insurance Coverage of the Total Population, 2019 (Distribution: Employer)," Kaiser Family Foundation, May 15, 2022, https://www.kff.org/other/state-indicator/total-population/?currentTimeframe=0&sortModel=%7B%22colId%22:%22Location%22,%22sort%22:%22asc%22%7D.

30 *According to federal law, those who are not citizens:* 111th Congress of the United States, Patient Protection and Affordable Care Act, HR 3590, Section 1312(f)(3), https://www.govinfo.gov/content/pkg/BILLS-111hr3590enr/pdf/BILLS-111hr3590enr.pdf.

30 *Social Security Administration denies two-thirds of disability claims:* "Medical Decisions at the Initial Adjudicative Level, by Year of Application and Program, 1992–2010," *Annual Statistical Report on the Social Security Disability Program, 2011*, Social Security Administration, https://www.ssa.gov/policy/docs/statcomps/di_asr/2011/sect04.html#table60.

30 *Texas is the least generous state:* "Texas Medicaid," Benefits.gov, https://www.benefits.gov/benefit/1640.

30 *earning more than $8,796 per year . . . disqualifies Texans:* "Understanding Supplemental Security Income SSI Benefits—2021 Edition," Social Security Administration, https://www.ssa.gov/ssi/text-benefits-ussi.htm (accessed February 3, 2022).

30 *And another forty million are underinsured:* Sara R. Collins, Munira Z. Gunja, and Gabriella N. Aboulafia, "US Health Insurance Coverage in 2020: A Looming Crisis in Affordability," Commonwealth Fund, August 19, 2020, https://www.commonwealthfund.org/publications/issue-briefs/2020/aug/looming-crisis-health-coverage-2020-biennial.

31 *66 percent of all bankruptcies . . . were due to medical bills*: David U. Himmelstein et al., "Medical Bankruptcy: Still Common Despite the Affordable Care Act," *American Journal of Public Health* 109, no. 3 (March 2019): 431–33.

35 *The rate of mothers' dying shortly after childbirth*: Marian F. MacDorman, Eugene Declercq, Howard Cabral, and Christine Morton, "US Maternal Mortality Trends," *Obstetrics & Gynecology* 128, no. 3 (September 2016): 447–55.

35 *Ebonie's home state of California was bucking that trend*: Elliott K. Main et al., "Addressing Maternal Mortality and Morbidity in California Through Public-Private Partnerships," *Health Affairs*, no. 37 (September 2018): 1484–93.

36 *In 1980, Arnold Relman*: Arnold S. Relman, "The New Medical-Industrial Complex," *New England Journal of Medicine* 303 (1980): 963–70.

Chapter 3 Doctors

46 *"One patient, one doctor"*: This and other AMA principles of healthcare in "Proceedings of the Cleveland Session: Minutes of the Eighty-Fifth Annual Session of the American Medical Association, Held at Cleveland, June 11–15, 1934," *Journal of the American Medical Association* 102, no. 26 (June 30, 1934): 2200–2201.

47 *the doctors' lobby launched ad campaigns that painted change as tantamount to socialism*: Paul Starr, *The Social Transformation of American Medicine* (1982; repr., Philadelphia: Basic Books, 2017), 215–32.

47 *As Paul Starr notes*: Starr, *Social Transformation of American Medicine*, 61–63, 84, 248.

51 *Despite the original intention of HMOs to bring costs down*: Starr, *Social Transformation of American Medicine*, 456.

Chapter 4 Coverage

61 *Credit for the idea goes to Justin Ford Kimball*: Helen Jerman, "How a Baptist Educator and Businessman's Simple Plan Gave Rise to the Health Insurance Industry," *Baptist News Global*, November 16, 2020, https://baptistnews .com/article/how-a-baptist-educator-and-businessmans-simple-plan-gave -rise-to-the-health-insurance-industry/#.Yjp87zfMLX1.

64 *In insurance theory, this is known as "moral hazard"*: Liran Einav and Amy Finkelstein, "Moral Hazard in Health Insurance: What We Know and How We Know It," *Journal of the European Economic Association* 16, no. 4 (August 2018): 957–82.

64n *This idea has been proven false*: Ibid., 963–70.

65 *The age of employer-sponsored health insurance was born*: Stephen Mihm, "Employer-Based Health Care Was a Wartime Accident," *Chicago Tribune*, February 24, 2017, https://www.chicagotribune.com/opinion/commentary /ct-obamacare-health-care-employers-20170224-story.html.

65 *Politicians going back to Theodore Roosevelt had proposed a social insurance*: Starr, *Social Transformation of American Medicine*, 243.

70 *Between 1960 and 1965, national health expenditures had increased from $142 to $198 per capita*: Elaine L. Chao, "100 Years of US Consumer Spending," US Bureau of Labor Statistics, May 2006, https://www.bls.gov/opub/100 -years-of-u-s-consumer-spending.pdf.

71 *Today, a direct descendant of Kimball's plan, Anthem, ranks number 20*: Fortune 500 rankings, *Fortune*, https://fortune.com/company/anthem /fortune500/.

Chapter 5 **Hospitals**

79 *emergency Medicaid funds*: "Section 4.3.1 Client Eligibility: Emergency Only," *Texas Medicaid Provider Procedures Manual*, vol. 1, October 2019, Texas Health and Human Services website, https://www.tmhp.com/sites /default/files/file-library/resources/provider-manuals/tmppm/pdf-chapters /2020/2020-09-september/1_04_Client_Eligibility.pdf.

79 *"Woman taken to Ben Taub"*: Fox 26 Houston staff, "Woman taken to Ben Taub after crashing stolen ambulance from Ben Taub," Fox 26 Houston, https://www.fox26houston.com/news/woman-taken-to-ben-taub -after-crashing-stolen-ambulance-from-ben-taub.

82 *The first American hospitals grew out of almshouses*: Starr, *Social Transformation of American Medicine*, 149–51.

82 *Most of these hospitals were founded in the early 1800s by religious institutions*: David Oshinsky, *Bellevue: Three Centuries of Medicine and Mayhem at America's Most Storied Hospital* (New York: Doubleday, 2016), 48–65.

84 *voluntary hospitals homed in on the problems that science could address rather than people's social problems*: Jeanne Kisacky, *Rise of the Modern Hospital: An Architectural History of Health and Healing, 1870–1940* (Pittsburgh: University of Pittsburgh Press, 2017), 293.

85 *One system grew wealthy while the other floundered*: Starr, *Social Transformation of American Medicine*, 154.

85 *With Hill-Burton money, the institutions of the Texas Medical Center*: Committee of Energy and Commerce, US House of Representatives, *Report on Hill-Burton Hospitals and Their Obligations* (Washington, DC: US Government Printing Office, 1984), 71.

86 *Houston Negro Hospital only received limited funds*: "Riverside General Hospital History," Riverside General Hospital, http://www.riversidegeneralhospital .org/getpage.php?name=Houston.

86 *the IRS allowed hospitals to report themselves as charities*: Ge Bai and David A. Hyman, "Tax Exemptions for Nonprofit Hospitals: It's Time Taxpayers Get Their Money's Worth," Stat, April 5, 2021, https://www .statnews.com/2021/04/05/tax-exemptions-nonprofit-hospitals-bad-deal -taxpayers/.

86 *"Houston, 1963, is a remnant of the Middle Ages"*: De Hartog, *Hospital*, 145–46.

87 *to plug the poor into the mainstream of American medicine*: Starr, *Social Transformation of American Medicine*, 370–74.

88 *Today, the tax breaks nonprofits receive every year*: Sara Rosenbaum et al., "The Value of the Nonprofit Hospital Tax Exemption Was $24.6 Billion in 2011," *Health Affairs* 34, no. 7 (July 2015): 1225–33, https://www.healthaffairs .org/doi/full/10.1377/hlthaff.2014.1424.

88 *almost a third do not*: Michael Ollove, "Some Nonprofit Hospitals Aren't Earning Their Tax Breaks, Critics Say," Stateline, Pew, February 7, 2020, https:// www.pewtrusts.org/en/research-and-analysis/blogs/stateline/2020/02/07 /some-nonprofit-hospitals-arent-earning-their-tax-breaks-critics-say.

88 *To achieve their mission, safety nets rely on multiple funding sources*: John Galbraith Simmons, "A History of Public Hospitals in the United States," *Safety Net* 20, no. 1 (Spring 2006): 7–10.

89 *"Houston's Zoo Air Conditioned, Charity Hospitals Are Not"*: De Hartog, *Hospital*, 342.

Chapter 6 **Wards**

93   *In 1984, an eighteen-year-old arrived at Parkland Memorial Hospital*: David A. Ansell and Robert L. Schiff, "Patient Dumping: Status, Implications, and Policy Recommendations," *Journal of the American Medical Association* 257, no. 11 (March 20, 1987): 1500–1502.

94   *dumping uninsured patients onto safety-net hospitals was a rampant practice*: Robert Schiff, David Ansell et al., "Transfers to a Public Hospital," *New England Journal of Medicine* 314 (1986): 552–57.

94   *Texas became the first state in the country to pass anti-dumping laws*: Arnold S. Relman, "Texas Eliminates Dumping," *New England Journal of Medicine* 314 (1986): 578–79.

95   *EMTALA*: "Emergency Medical Treatment & Labor Act (EMTALA)," Center for Medicare & Medicaid Services, https://www.cms.gov/Regulations -and-Guidance/Legislation/EMTALA.

95   *as waiting rooms in the ER became more crowded than hospital lobbies*: A. Haas, "Designing for Emergencies," *Healthcare Design*, August 31, 2002, https://healthcaredesignmagazine.com/architecture/designing-emergencies/.

99   *one Level 1 trauma center for every million people*: American College of Surgeons Committee on Trauma, "Trauma System Consultation: State of Texas," Texas Department of Health Services, https://www.dshs.texas.gov /injury/registry/ACS-Report.doc?terms=trauma+systems+special+report +analysis+of+need.

99   *yearly hospital ratings*: "Overall Hospital Quality Star Rating," Centers for Medicare & Medicaid Services, https://data.cms.gov/provider-data/topics /hospitals/overall-hospital-quality-star-rating.

101 *Over the last one hundred years, the architecture of emergency rooms and medical wards has changed*: Tom Gormley, "The History of Hospitals and Wards," *Healthcare Design*, March 11, 2010, https://healthcaredesignmagazine.com /architecture/history-hospitals-and-wards/.

101 *Hospitals accommodated the middle class with semiprivate rooms*: Starr, *Social Transformation of American Medicine*, 159.

102 *The open ward kept patients safe*: G. C. Cook, "Henry Currey FRIBA (1820–1900): Leading Victorian Hospital Architect, and Early Exponent of the 'Pavilion Principle,'" *Postgraduate Medical Journal* 78, no. 920 (2002): 352–59, https://pmj.bmj.com/content/78/920/352.info.

107n *if the same situation happened today, Ebonie would probably not be offered an abortion to save her life*: Eleanor Klibanoff, "Doctors Report Compromising Care out of Fear of Texas Abortion Law," *Texas Tribune*, June 23, 2022, https://www.texastribune.org/2022/06/23/texas-abortion-law-doctors-delay-care/.

111 *Researchers found that the mortality rate doubled*: Steve Brewer, "Delays in Trauma Care Called Life-Threatening," *Houston Chronicle*, July 18, 2002, https://www.chron.com/news/houston-texas/article/Delays-in-trauma-care-called-life-threatening-2075575.php.

Chapter 7 **Assumptions**

122 *In 2017,* Annals of Internal Medicine *published a review*: Steffie Woolhandler and David U. Himmelstein, "The Relationship of Health Insurance and Mortality: Is Lacking Health Insurance Deadly?" *Annals of Internal Medicine* 167, no. 6 (September 2017): 424–31.

122 *It was a randomized control study*: Katherine Baicker et al. for the Oregon Health Study Group, "The Oregon Experiment: Effects of Medicaid on Clinical Outcomes," *New England Journal of Medicine* 368 (2013): 1713–22, doi:10.1056/NEJMsa1212321.

123 *Diabetes is a very expensive illness*: American Diabetes Association, "Economic Costs of Diabetes in the US in 2017," *Diabetes Care* 41, no. 5 (May 2018): 917–28, https://doi.org/10.2337/dci18-0007.

123 *adds up to nearly $4,800 every year on average*: Amanda Nguyen and Katie Mui, "The Staggering True Cost of Diabetes," GoodRx Health, April 7, 2020, https://assets.ctfassets.net/4f3rgqwzdznj/6Q5qUjkrhppOzC9n M23vhW/867883e7208f529a8f24f1e7da67993e/Diabetes-Cost-White -Paper.pdf.

136 *We assume that healthcare isn't rationed in this country, but that isn't the case*: Peter Singer, "Why We Must Ration Health Care," *New York Times Magazine*, July 15, 2009, https://www.nytimes.com/2009/07/19/magazine /19healthcare-t.html.

139n *non-alcoholic steatohepatitis is recognized as the leading cause of cirrhosis*: Guadalupe Garcia Tsao, "Nonalcoholic Steatohepatitis—Opportunities and Challenges," *New England Journal of Medicine* 385 (2021): 1615–17, https:doi.org/10.1056/NEJMe2110989.

Chapter 8 **Beliefs**

143 *the Scientific Charity Movement*: Michael Katz, *In the Shadow of the Poorhouse: A Social History of Welfare in America* (1986; repr., New York: Basic Books, 1996), 60–78.

143 *The movement gathered data about the poor*: A. G. Warner, "Scientific Charity," *Popular Science Monthly* 35 (August 1889): 488–94.

144 *Statistical analysis, driven by social Darwinism*: Linda S. Stuhler, "Scientific Charity Movement and Charity Organization Societies," Virginia Commonwealth University Libraries Social Welfare History Project, https://socialwelfare.library.vcu.edu/programs/mental-health/scientific-charity-movement-charity-organization-societies/.

144 *Oliver Wendell Holmes . . . echoed the Scientific Charity Movement's ideas*: *Buck v. Bell*, Superintendent of State Colony for Epileptics and Feeble Minded, 274 US 200 (1927).

144 *The eight states that have approved legislation requiring that patients work in order to receive Medicaid*: Rachel Garfield et al., "Work Among Medicaid Adults: Implications of Economic Downturn and Work Requirements," Kaiser Family Foundation, February 11, 2021, https://www.kff.org/report-section/work-among-medicaid-adults-implications-of-economic-downturn-and-work-requirements-issue-brief/.

145 *the Trump administration noted that those Medicaid programs*: Centers for Medicare & Medicaid Services (CMS), "Dear State Medicaid Director Letter #18-002, Opportunities to Promote Work and Community Engagement Among Medicaid Beneficiaries (Jan. 11, 2018)," https://www.medicaid.gov/federal-policy-guidance/downloads/smd18002.pdf (accessed October 5, 2019).

148 *Everyone living in the county is eligible for the Gold Card*: "Patient Eligibility," Harris Health System, https://www.harrishealth.org/access-care/patient-eligibility.

149n *Harris Health reduced the income threshold for financial assistance from 200 percent of the federal poverty level*: Markian Hawryluk, "Harris Health Slashes Eligibility for Subsidized Care; Will Encourage Obamacare Enrollment," *Houston Chronicle*, September 24, 2015, https://www.houstonchronicle.com/news/health/article/Harris-Health-slashes-eligibility-for-subsidized-6527864.php.

164 *For instance, in 2018, researchers compared the quality of care at Veterans Affairs hospitals*: Rebecca Ahnang Price et al., "Comparing Quality of Care

in Veterans Affairs and Non–Veterans Affairs Settings," *Journal of General Internal Medicine* 33, no. 10 (October 2018): 1631–38.

164n *The Inflation Reduction Act of 2022*: Juliette Cubanski, Tricia Neuman, Meredith Freed, and Anthony Damico, "How Will the Prescription Drug Provisions in the Inflation Reduction Act Affect Medicare Beneficiaries," Kaiser Family Foundation, August 18, 2022, https://www.kff.org/medicare /issue-brief/how-will-the-prescription-drug-provisions-in-the-inflation -reduction-act-affect-medicare-beneficiaries/.

165 *One study performed by the Congressional Budget Office*: "Comparing the Costs of the Veterans' Health Care System with Private-Sector Costs," Congressional Budget Office, December 10, 2014, https://www.cbo.gov /publication/49763.

Chapter 9 **Misperceptions**

171 *A 2018 article in the* Journal of the American Medical Association: Jeremy Snyder, Leigh Turner, and Valorie A. Crooks, "Crowdfunding for Unproven Stem Cell–Based Interventions," *Journal of the American Medical Association* 319, no. 18 (2018): 1935–36, https://doi.org/10.1001/jama.2018.3057.

172 *"They cater to people whose needs reach beyond the powers of current medicine"*: Erin Allday, "Merchants of Hope," *San Francisco Chronicle*, August 2, 2018, https://projects.sfchronicle.com/2018/stem-cells/clinics/.

172 *According to a study in the* New England Journal of Medicine: Scott Ratzan, Eric C. Schneider, Hilary Hatch, and Joseph Cacchione, "Missing the Point—How Primary Care Can Overcome Covid-19 Vaccine 'Hesitancy,'" *New England Journal of Medicine* 384 (2021): e100, https://doi.org/10.1056 /NEJMp2106137.

Chapter 10 **Miscalculations**

193 *No SSI, no Medicaid*: "Supplemental Security Income (SSI) Disability & Medicaid coverage," HealthCare.gov, https://www.healthcare.gov/people -with-disabilities/ssi-and-medicaid/.

194 *but Aqueria's path to HAART medications came through claiming disability*: "List of Conditions for Compassionate Allowances, US Social Security Administration (SSA)," Center for HIV Law & Policy, October 2008, https://www.hivlaw

andpolicy.org/resources/list-conditions-compassionate-allowances-us-social
-security-administration-ssa.

199 *Ziad Obermeyer, a doctor and public health scientist*: Ziad Obermeyer, Brian
     Powers, Christine Vogeli, and Sendhil Mullainathan, "Dissecting Racial Bias
     in an Algorithm Used to Manage the Health of Populations," *Science* 366
     (2019): 447–53.

200 *"Algorithms can do terrible things"*: Kara Manke, "Widely Used Health Care
     Prediction Algorithm Biased Against Black People," University of California
     Berkeley Research, October 24, 2019, https://vcresearch.berkeley.edu/news
     /widely-used-health-care-prediction-algorithm-biased-against-black-people.

201 *She offers the example of Medicaid in Indiana*: Virginia Eubanks, *Automating
     Inequality: How High-Tech Tools Profile, Police, and Punish the Poor* (New
     York: Picador, 2019), 11–15.

209 *Geronimo lived in Texas District Seven*: "Texas's 7th Congressional District,"
     GovTrack.us, https://www.govtrack.us/congress/members/TX/7.

210 *Republican John Culberson*: Alec MacGillis, "Meet the House Republican
     Who Compared Himself to the Flight 93 Heroes," *New Republic*, September
     30, 2013, https://newrepublic.com/article/114924/meet-john-culberson
     -house-republican-who-said-lets-roll.

Chapter 11 **Algorithmania**

213 *As far back as the sixteenth century*: Noha Abokrysha, "Shajarat al-Tibb (a Tree
     of Medicine), the History of the Medical Algorithms," *Journal of Research
     on History of Medicine* 10, no. 2 (2021): 75–80.

213 *healthcare workers started to use algorithms in their protocols when treating
     emergencies*: A. L. Komaroff, "Algorithms and the 'Art' of Medicine," *Amer-
     ican Journal of Public Health* 72, no. 1 (January 1982): 10–12.

214 *This algorithm, published by the Institute for Clinical Systems Improvement*:
     "Health Care Guideline: Assessment and Management of Acute Pain,"
     Institute for Clinical Systems Improvement, March 2008, http://almacen
     -gpc.dynalias.org/webdav/publico/Tratamiento%20dolor%20agudo%20
     ICSI.pdf.

228 *This meant he had a 99 percent chance of a full recovery*: Molly McNett, "A
     Review of the Predictive Ability of Glasgow Coma Scale Scores in Head-
     Injured Patients," *Journal of Neuroscience Nursing* 39, no. 2 (2007): 68–75.

232 *listed by the* New York Times: Reed Abelson, "Many Hospitals Charge Double or Even Triple What Medicare Would Pay," *New York Times*, May 9, 2019, https://www.nytimes.com/2019/05/09/health/hospitals-prices-medicare.html.

Chapter 12 **Excess**

240 *In 2016, a group of researchers decided to survey the healthcare team members*: O. Mazurenko, "Who Is a Hospital's 'Customer'?," *Journal of Healthcare Management* 61, no. 5 (September/October 2016): 319–33.

243 *In a 2012 special communication*: Donald M. Berwick and Andrew D. Hackbarth, "Eliminating Waste in US Health Care," *Journal of the American Medical Association* 307, no. 14 (2012): 1513–16, https://doi.org/10.1001/jama.2012.362.

244 *That same $200 billion would provide every uninsured person*: Decision-Data Team, "How Much Universal Healthcare Would Cost in the US," DecisionData.org, March 27, 2020, https://decisiondata.org/news/how-much-single-payer-uhc-would-cost-usa/.

247 *In July 2019, the Trump administration*: Selena Simmons-Duffin and Carmel Wroth, "Trump Administration Announces Plans to Shake Up the Kidney Care Industry," NPR.org, July 10, 2019, https://www.npr.org/sections/health-shots/2019/07/10/740276389/trump-administration-announces-plans-to-shake-up-the-kidney-care-industry.

247 *Only around 25 percent of patients with ESRD in 1996*: Nancy G. Kutner, Rebecca Zhang, Yijian Huang, and Haimanot Wasse, "Patient Awareness and Initiation of Peritoneal Dialysis," *Archives of Internal Medicine* 171, no. 2 (2011): 119–24, https://doi.org/10.1001/archinternmed.2010.361.

249 *A study in the* New England Journal of Medicine *showed*: Hassan N. Ibrahim et al., "Long-Term Consequences of Kidney Donation," *New England Journal of Medicine* 360 (2009): 459–69.

Chapter 13 **Public + Private**

255 *In 2019, the RAND Corporation, a nonprofit think tank, published a study*: Chapin White and Christopher M. Whaley, "Prices Paid to Hospitals by Private Health Plans Are High Relative to Medicare and Vary Widely," RAND Corporation, 2019, https://doi.org/10.7249/RR3033.

256 *In March 2019, the US Centers for Medicare & Medicaid Services released data*: "Hospital Compare," Centers for Medicare & Medicaid Services, https://www.cms.gov/Medicare/Quality-Initiatives-Patient-Assessment -Instruments/HospitalQualityInits/HospitalCompare.

258 *Better to place sphygmomanometers . . . in the trash can rather than on the arm of a bleeding patient . . . to protect patients from the IV fluids administered by scared doctors:* William Bickell et al., "Immediate versus Delayed Fluid Resuscitation for Hypotensive Patients with Penetrating Torso Injuries," *New England Journal of Medicine* 331 (1994): 1105-1109.

Chapter 14 Disaster Syndrome

269 De Watersnoodramp, *the great flood of 1953*: De Hartog, *Hospital*, 35.

272 *In a survey of twenty thousand doctors worldwide*: Tim Locke, "Medscape Global Physicians' Burnout and Lifestyle Comparisons," Medscape Internal Medicine, February 24, 2019.

273 *the United States will experience a shortage*: Association of American Medical Colleges, *The Complexities of Physician Supply and Demand: Projections from 2018 to 2033*, June 2020, https://www.aamc.org/media/45976/download? attachment.

273 *In a 2018 opinion piece published by Stat*: Simon G. Talbot and Wendy Dean, "Physicians Aren't 'Burning Out.' They're Suffering from Moral Injury," Stat, July 26, 2018, https://www.statnews.com/2018/07/26/physicians-not -burning-out-they-are-suffering-moral-injury/.

274 *Dr. Zubin Damania . . . posted a six-minute diatribe*: ZDoggMD, "It's Not Burnout, It's Moral Injury: Dr. Zubin Damania on Physician 'Burnout,'" You-Tube, March 8, 2019, https://www.youtube.com/watch?v=L_1PNZdHq6Q.

283 *Six hundred fifty thousand Texans lost their employer-sponsored health insurance*: Sarah R. Champagne, "Texas Has the Highest Uninsured Rate in the US. and During the Pandemic, an Estimated 659,000 Texans Lost Their Health Care," *Texas Tribune*, July 14, 2020, https://www.texastribune .org/2020/07/14/texans-health-insurance-jobs-pandemic/.

Chapter 15 **Tiers**

286 *The pandemic had already ravaged Constantinople*: William Rosen, *Justinian's Flea: The First Great Plague and the End of the Roman Empire* (2007; repr., New York: Penguin Books, 2008).

287 *Jundi-Shapur was, foremost, a great medical university*: H. D. Modanlou, "Historical Evidence for the Origin of Teaching Hospital, Medical School and the Rise of Academic Medicine," *Journal of Perinatology* 31 (2011): 236–39.

287 *Today, some of America's most prestigious healthcare institutions implement the Jundi-Shapur model*: Andrew C. Miller, "Jundi-Shapur, Bimaristans, and the Rise of Academic Medical Centers," *Journal of the Royal Society of Medicine* 99 (2006): 615–17.

291 *In 1972, the End Stage Renal Disease Program*: Christopher R. Blagg, "The Early History of Dialysis for Chronic Renal Failure in the United States: A View from Seattle," *American Journal of Kidney Diseases* 49, no. 3 (March 2007): 482–96.

293 *Two doctor-researchers at Ben Taub, Drs. Sheikh-Hamad and Shandera, began to compare patients*: David Sheikh-Hamad et al., "Care for Immigrants with End-Stage Renal Disease in Houston: A Comparison of Two Practices," *Texas Medicine* 103, no. 4 (April 2007): 54–58, 53.

295 *A two-tier system*: Jonathan Gruber, "The Case for a Two-Tier Health System," *Pathways*, Winter 2009, 9–13, https://inequality.stanford.edu/sites/default/files/media/_media/pdf/pathways/winter_2009/Gruber.pdf.

297 *The spike observed in maternal deaths had been largely due to an accounting error*: Sonia Baeva et al., "Identifying Maternal Deaths in Texas Using an Enhanced Method, 2012," *Obstetrics & Gynecology* 131, no. 5 (May 2018): 762–69.

298 *A 2016 study in the journal* Obstetrics & Gynecology: Amirhossein Moaddab et al., "Health Care Disparity and State-Specific Pregnancy-Related Mortality in the United States, 2005–2014," *Obstetrics & Gynecology* 128, no. 4 (October 2016): 869–75.

PART FOUR **Faith**

313 *Americans die in the hospital today as often as they do in their own homes*: Robert H. Shmerling, "Where People Die," Harvard Health Blog,

October 31, 2018, https://www.health.harvard.edu/blog/where-people
-die-2018103115278.

320 *The first attempt at a human-to-human liver transplant*: Roberto Ferreira
Meirelles Júnior et al., "Liver Transplantation: History, Outcomes and Per-
spectives," *Einstein (São Paulo)* 13, no. 1 (January–March 2015): 149–52.

321 *there are at least seventeen thousand people*: Organ Procurement and Transplantation Network, "National Data," US Department of Health and
Human Services, https://optn.transplant.hrsa.gov/data/view-data-reports
/national-data/.

322 *Yet it's hard to imagine this procedure surviving without so much money*: Dany
Habka, David Mann, Ronald Landes, and Alejandro Soto-Gutierrez, "Future
Economics of Liver Transplantation: A 20-Year Cost Modeling Forecast and
the Prospect of Bioengineering Autologous Liver Grafts," *PLoS One* 10,
no. 7 (2015): e0131764.

323 *Before the MELD points system was introduced for transplants in 2002, more
minorities died*: Nyingi Kemmer, "Ethnic Disparities in Liver Transplantation," *Gastroenterology & Hepatology (NY)* 7, no. 5 (May 2011): 302–7.

323 *At an average cost of $878,000*: T. Scott Bentley and Nick J. Ortner, "2020
U.S. Organ and Tissue Transplants: Cost Estimates, Discussion, and Emerging Issues," Milliman Research Report, January 2020, https://www.milliman
.com/-/media/milliman/pdfs/articles/2020-us-organ-tissue-transplants
.ashx.

Index

Page numbers in *italics* refer to graphs.

abortion, 107–8, 210
Abuelita (author's grandmother), 217–25, 224–25, 226, 231
addictions, 104, 162–63, 194
administrative complexity, 243
Affordable Care Act (ACA), 7, 35, 38, 39, 97, 162, 174, 243, 245, 260
  exclusions from, 30
  limitations of, 289
  Medicaid expansion provision in, 207
  open-enrollment period in, 318
  opposition to, 210, 317
  provisions of, 5, 29, 154–55
  in Texas, 283
African Americans, 90, 94, 180, 297, 298–99
  healthcare rates of, 70, 200
  uninsured, 34–35
AIDS, *see* HIV/AIDS
AKA (above-the-knee amputation), 157
alcohol use, 82, 139
algorithmania:
  impersonal approach of, 222–23
  use of term, 211, 212–17
algorithms, 184, *212*
  advantages and disadvantages of, 214–17, 221–23
  in allocation of funds, 198–202

bias in, 200–202
cost factor in, 223
in COVID response, 276–77
in diagnosis and monitoring, 199–202
for esophageal cancer, 220–21
faulty presumptions of, 216–17, 225
healthcare's dependence on, 211–33
historical perspective on, 213–14
in predicting costs of treatment, 200–202
in search for certainty, 229
Allday, Erin, 172
Allison, Tropical Storm, 90
almshouses, 82, 84
alpha-galactosidase, 176
Alvaro, Mr. (patient), 10–14, 315
Alzheimer's disease, 119, 121
ambulatory surgical centers, 90
American Academy of Neurology, 68
American College of Obstetricians and Gynecologists (ACOG), 299
American Health Care Act, 154
American Hospital Association, 263
American Journal of Public Health, 31
American Medical Association, ten principles of, 46–47
American Taxpayer Relief Act (2012), 292

America's Essential Hospitals, 263
amputations, 28–29, 36, 111, 113, 151–53, 230, 291, 309, 311, 329–33
amputee support groups, 332
anesthesiologists, 99
Annals of Internal Medicine, 122
Anthem, 71
antibiotics, 137, 152, 167
antibiotic stewardship, 137
anti-dumping laws, 94–95
A-P (assessment and the plan), 135
Aqueria (HIV patient), 191–98
"Are Zombie Doctors Taking Over America?" (TEDMED talk), 274
arthrocentesis, 66–67
Asians, 298
Association of American Medical Colleges, 263
asylums, 144
Ativan, 80, 81
atrial fibrillation, 218, 220
autism, 171
auto-amputation, 28–29
Automating Inequality (Eubanks), 201–2
Ayurveda, 287
AZT, 193

back pain, 256–57
bacterial meningitis, 93–94
bankruptcies, medical costs in, 31–32
barium swallow, 219, 231
basic metabolic panel, 72
Baylor College of Medicine, 53
Baylor University, 61
Bellevue (Oshinsky), 87
Ben Taub Hospital, 79
  author's essays about, 231–32
  author's father as volunteer at, 53–54
  author's roles at, 8, 10–14, 117–22, 226, 232–33, 257
  balance of algorithms and arguments at, 231
  burnout countermeasures at, 274–75
  care as priority at, 132–33
  Carey's tenure at, 183–84
  cost control measures in, 256–57
  cost of care at, 166–67, 255
  COVID response of, 275–84
  disaster syndrome at, 277, 279
  discharge from, 187–88, 266–67, 283
  diverse staff base at, 316
  doctors' regard for, 260–61
  dumping at, 93–94
  educational mission of, 5–6
  emergency room procedures and treatment at, 100–114, 118–22, 161–63, 166–67, 266, 282, 314
  evolution of, 9–10, 89–91
  feeder clinics of, 205
  in Hurricane Harvey, 330
  ICU at, 205
  Jundi-Shapur model in, 287–88
  as last resort, 177
  as Level 1 trauma center, 99–100
  limitations of, 8–9, 124, 161, 263, 264, 310, 324
  maternity care at, 181–82
  medical milestones of, 3
  misconception about, 104–5
  mission and focus of, 98
  ongoing patient care at, 133–35
  organizational structure at, 240
  patient admission to, 109, 113–14
  patient base of, 3
  quality of care star rating of, 263
  rationing at, 137–38
  renovations and upgrades at, 266–67, 281
  services provided by, 2, 4–5, 26, 79–81
  staff-patient relationship in, 264–65
  step-down unit at, 207
  see also specific staff and patients
Bernard Mevs Hospital, 226–27, 230
Berwick, Donald, 243–44
bias:
  in predictive algorithms, 200–201
  stereotyping in, 298–99
Big Pharma, 36–37
bilirubin, 134
biopsies, 163, 165–66, 175, 237, 254
birthing hospitals, 186
BKA (below-the-knee amputation), 153
black markets, 136

Blessn (Ebonie's daughter), 180, 301, 304, 305
blood loss, 107–8, 185, 185–86, 205, 230, 301–5, 325
blood pressure, 179–80, 217, 298
blood thinners, 281
blood transfusions, 205, 293
Blue Cross Blue Shield, 71, 147, 175
bone cancer, 198, 230
bone marrow transplants, 138
bowel function, 134
brain cancer, 315, 330, 332
brain function, 325, 332
brain surgeries, 330
brain tumor, of McCain, 158–60
bureaucracy, doctors burdened by, 272, 278–79
Bureau of Labor Statistics, 123
burnout, 272–75
Butler, Win, 211
Byzantine Empire, 286

California, 180–81, 185
    healthcare in, 35, 172, 180–81, 185
Camp YOLO, 194–95
Canada, 71
    healthcare in, 129, 289
cancer, 78, 151, 195, 265, 267, 275, 283, 310, 315
    complication of surgery for, 167
    cost of treatment for, 166–67
    diagnosis of, 25–26
    metastatic, 221, 223, 310, 330, 332
    radiation treatment for, 253–54
    see also specific types of cancer
capitalism, 163
Capitol, US, breach of, 281
cardiopulmonary bypass machine, 27n
Career Days, 43–45
Carthage, 286
castration, 144
cataracts, 257
Catholics, 312
CAT scans, 61, 68, 127, 166, 227–28, 230, 254, 256, 314, 325
CD4 counts, 197–98
CDC, 185

Centers for Medicare & Medicaid Services, US (CMS), 99, 243, 256, 263
cerebellum, 314, 332
cerebral palsy, 171
cesarean section, 44, 109, 180, 301–2
charity, 86
    Christian, 310–11
    healthcare funded through, 15, 82
    health services provided by, 78–79
    hospitals taxed as, 86–88
charity clinics, volunteers at, 42
Checklist Manifesto, The (Gawande), 212–13
Chekhov, Anton, 14–17, 85
chemo-resistant leukemia, 171
chemotherapies, 7, 138, 159, 166, 167, 230, 254, 262, 283
    hospice care vs., 222
chest pains, 197, 213–17, 215, 219
child abuse, 194
childbirth, 95, 177–89, 286
    author's personal crisis with, 178–80
    costs of, 72
    coverage in, 59
    discharge from hospital after, 303
    labor in, 129
    mortality rates in, 35
    uninsured in, 146–47
    see also Ebonie; maternal care
children:
    illness in, 16
    in immigration, 261
cholera, 225, 285
chronic care, 91, 200
civil war, in El Salvador, 158
Civil War, US, 45
climate change, 210
Clinton, Bill and Hillary, 97
Cloak and Dagger (film), 120
COBRA, limitations of, 174
Code Blue, 315
colon cancer, 11
colonoscopies, 264
complete placenta previa, 107
concentration camp survivors, 9
concussion, 60–61, 68–69
Confessions (Augustine), 120

Congress, US, 85–86, 95
  in appeals for medical help, 317–19
  dialysis demonstration for, 292
  Medicaid cuts debated in, 154
Congressional Budget Office,
      VA hospital study of, 165
congressmen, healthcare intervention by,
      209–10
Constantinople, 286
conversion disorder, 304
Cook County Hospital (Chicago, Ill.), 94
co-payments, 136, 153
Cornyn, John, 5, 290
coronary bypass, 260
corporate medicine, 37, 50–51, 113, 260
Council on Patient Safety in Women's
      Health Care, 299
county hospitals, 84
coverage gaps, 59
COVID-19 pandemic, 1–2, 14, 15, 23,
      105, 136, 149, 163, 246, 266
  alternative treatments in, 172–73
  Ben Taub in, 275–84
  restaurant business affected by, 24
COVID-19 tests, 161
COVID-19 vaccines, 262, 281
  opposition to, 172–73
crack, 83
crack babies, 194
creatinine, 73
Crimean War, 102
Cruz, Ted, 210
Culberson, John, 210, 317, 324
customers, use of term, 240–41

Dallas (TV show), 209
Dallas Morning News, 62–63
Damania, Zubin, 274
Darwin, Charles, 143–44
Darwinism, 143–44, 199
Dave (chief of internal medicine at
      Ben Taub), 226, 231–32, 333
  in Ben Taub's COVID response, 277–82
  death of, 279–82
death:
  choosing release in, 315
  dignity in, 224–25

impact of insurance on rates of, 122–23
impact on doctors of, 296–97
medical procedure in, 13
preparations for, 12–13
of uninsured, 32
DeBakey, Michael, 260
decision trees, 212–14, 215, 222
deductibles, 29
de Hartog, Jan, 9–10, 86–87, 89–90, 277,
      316
  Mattox's opposition to, 259
  in Netherlands flood disaster, 270
dementia, 122, 124
Democratic Party, 257
  healthcare stance of, 159
depression, 279
Depression, Great, 46, 63
De Watersnoodramp (great flood of 1953),
      269–71
diabetes, 122, 175, 205, 213, 244–45,
      294, 330
  costs of, 123, 125, 132
  diagnosing and treating of, 124–27
  long-term effects of, 124–25, 139n,
      121
diagnoses, 126–29
  costs determined by, 184
  errors in, 220
  tools of, 199
diagnostic tests, rationing of, 138
dialysate, 245–46
dialysis, 182, 232, 242, 324
  costs of, 246–47, 293–94
  at home, 245–48
  ongoing, 290–91
  study of protocol for, 293–94
dialysis machines, 245–48, 292
diarrhea, 191
diet, in diabetes treatment, 127
Dilaudid, 77, 323
disability, 163, 167, 194, 195, 206–8
  presumptions about, 201
  rating scales for, 152–53
disability benefits, 265
disability checks, 317, 318–19
disability claims, denial of, 30
disabled, transportation for, 331–32

disaster syndrome, 269–84, 271, 324, 327
    at Ben Taub during COVID pandemic,
        277, 279
disproportionate share, 95
divorce, 226
DNA, 254
DNR orders, 12–13
doctor-patient relationships:
    complexity of, 183
    evolution of, 41–58
    listening in, 217
    see also specific doctors and patients
doctors:
    burnout in, 272–75
    disaster syndrome evidenced in, 271–75
    financial incentives for, 275
    increasing costs to, 52–53
    reimbursement for, 95
    science interpreted by, 173–74
    shortage of, 273–74
    in transition from care to business,
        41–55, 177, 275
domestic abuse, 203
Domestic Policy Council, 247
drug rehabilitation, 97
drugs, cost of, 112
drug trade, 203
drug use, 83
dry gangrene, 27–31, 83, 149–50, 152, 156
dumping, of uninsured and indigent
        patients, 93–95
dysphagia, 218–19

earthquake, in Haiti, 225–29
Ebola, in US, 258–59
Ebonie (uninsured patient), 33–36, 37,
        39, 107, 177–78, 185, 186–89, 288,
        297, 298, 300
    at Ben Taub, 100
    childbirth trauma of, 300–305
    Medicaid coverage for, 300
    pregnancy history of, 180–81
ECOG scale, 153
EKGs, 290
elderly, healthcare for, 39, 69–70
election, US, of 2020, 255, 266, 281
elective surgeries, 138, 154, 283

Elliott, Bill, 89–90
El Salvador, 219, 261
    healthcare in, 223–25
    medical training and practice in, 52
    specific accent of, 150
    violence in, 157–58
emergency care, mandated, 95
Emergency Medicaid, 91
Emergency Medical Treatment and Labor
        Act (EMTALA), 95–96, 98, 101, 131,
        290
emergency rooms, 33–34, 64, 78–80,
        181, 197
    atmosphere of, 289
    author's personal experience in, 72
    at Ben Taub, 100–101, 103–4, 118–22,
        161, 266, 282, 314
    capacity of, 110–11
    chronic patients at, 290–91
    costs of, 25, 31–32, 56, 72
    death in, 94
    insurance coverage for, 60–61
    limitations of, 174
    open wards in, 101–4
    overcrowding of, 95, 110–11, 283
    overuse of, 214, 216
    procedures for, 100–101
    protocol for chronic patients at, 291
    rating of, 99
    wait times at, 100
emergent dialysis, 293
Emma (Geronimo's mother), 133–34,
        203–6, 208, 317–20, 324–26, 328
empathy, 103–4, 316
EMTs, 189
end-of-life care, 77, 221–22
endoscopy, 205, 220–21
End Stage Renal Disease Program, 291–92
enduring, use of term, 32
England, healthcare in, 65, 129
epilepsy, 133–34, 180, 187, 203, 204, 207
Eppes, Carey, 178–79, 182–86, 187–88,
        189, 299–300
ER (TV show), 94
esophageal blood, 205
esophageal cancer, 219–25, 231
esophagogastroduodenoscopy (EGD), 219

ESRD (end-stage renal disease), 247–49, 290–95
Eubanks, Virginia, 201–2
Europe, healthcare in, 46, 51, 65
Evergreen hospital, 276
evolutionary theory, 143–44, 199
exception points, 323n
exercise, in diabetes treatment, 126–27
eyeballing, 181–82

Fabry disease, 175–76, 237, 239, 242, 249
Facebook, 170, 193, 196, 276
FaceTime, 279
faith:
    author's experience of, 312–17
    hope in, 320
Family Dollar, 192, 197
Fauci, Anthony, 199
fear:
    in patients, 10, 12
    after trauma, 304
federal law, 113, 188
federal poverty level, 149n, 198, 262, 289
fee-for-service billing, 47–48, 49, 51, 71, 184, 274
    group coverage vs., 65–66
fee negotiations, 50, 52
fee schedules, 44–46
fentanyl, 77, 323
"Fight Against Tuberculosis" campaign, 15
financial counselors, 106, 165, 187–88, 300
Floyd, George, 280
fluoroscopy, 219
follow-up visits, 82, 112, 180, 197, 215, 323
food stamps, 202
forced sterilization, 143–44
for-profit clinics, 172
for-profit hospitals, 3, 88, 95, 99, 132, 155, 240, 263, 295
    VA hospitals compared to, 164–65
Fox News, 252, 266
fraud, 244
fulminant liver failure, 140
funerals, 326–28
fungal infection, 198

Galen, 287
gallbladder surgery, 27, 29
gallstones, 154, 264
gambling, 162, 265, 315
gangrene, 27–31, 83, 109, 111, 149–50, 152, 156, 291
Garza, Christian (uninsured patient), 55–58, 66–68, 72–74, 169–77, 237–49, 286, 288, 294–95
gastroenteritis, 285
Gawande, Atul, 212
genetic defects, 176
genetics, 176, 244, 249
genetics clinics, 242
Geronimo (hepatitis C patient), 133–35, 138–41, 202–10, 317–20, 319, 324
    death and funeral of, 325–28
Glasgow Coma Scale, 228
glomerular filtration rate, 248
glucose levels, 125
gluten intolerance, 285
GoFundMe, 313
Gold Card (Harris County program), 147–54, 160, 204–6, 242, 248–49, 255, 262, 282, 283, 290, 294, 310
    basic premise of, 148
    financial caps on, 255
    levels of support offered by, 153
gout, 66
government, healthcare involvement of, 39, 69–70, 135, 145, 164–65, 198–202
Graham, Robert ("Cowboy Doctor"), 119–22, 125–33
Great Depression, 46, 63
Green, Gene, 319
green cards, 30, 48, 204, 206
Grogan, Joe, 247
group coverage:
    defined, 29
    establishment of, 62–63
    fee-for-service vs., 65–66
GroupMe, 283
Guatemala, 261
Gulfton neighborhood, 210
gun rights, 210
gunshot wounds, 104
Gurteen, Reverend, 144

HAART (highly active anti-retroviral
    treatment), 192–94, 197, 198
Hackbarth, Andrew, 243–44
Haiti, author's volunteer work in, 225–31
Hamadan, 285
handouts, 177
Harris County, 232, 242, 282
    Gold Card program of, *see* Gold Card
Harris County Medical Society, 90
Harris Health, 5–6, 8, 90–91, 188, 193,
    211, 241–42, 261, 282, 327, 329
    controlled costs of, 256–57
    dialysis program of, 294–95
    eligibility requirements for, 149
    financial counseling by, 165–67
    home dialysis program of, 248
    house call service of, 152
    indigent patients in, 4–5, 98–99, 148–50
    limitations of, 249
    outsourcing by, 154
    per-patient cost of, 260
    pharmacies of, 138
    rationing at, 137
    restrictions of, 138
    see also safety-net system
Harrison's Principles of Internal Medicine, 199
Hart, Stephen (professional patient),
    21–26, 29, 37, 39, 104–7, 161–63,
    251–57, 260–67
Harvey, Hurricane, 90, 266, 309, 329–30
Hawking, Stephen, 331
head and neck cancer, 266–67
Health and Human Services Department,
    US (HHS), 321
healthcare:
    algorithms in, 211–33
    alternative sources for, 169–74
    assumptions about, 117–41
    author's vision for, 327–28, 333
    beliefs about, 143–67
    as big business, *see* Medicine Inc.
    caregivers' stress in, 124
    community support in, 151–53, 157
    costs vs. care in, 29, 41–58, 63, 70–72,
        88, 97–98, 106, 112–14, 121–25,
        130–33, 136, 146–47, 176, 184, 201,
        232–33, 244, 248, 293

cost variations in, 63, 101, 256
employer-funded, 240
excess and waste in, 237–49
governmental vs. corporate control of,
    137
government involvement in, 39,
    69–70, 135, 145, 164–65, 198–202
historical perspective on, 45–48, 61–65,
    69–72, 81, 143–45, 285–89
hope in, 172
ideal of equality in, 288–89
for indigent persons, *see* indigent
    healthcare
individual states' responses to, 35
inequalities in, 9, 14, 39, 43, 69–70,
    75–76, 84–88, 136, 140, 180, 198–
    99, 200–202, 201, 225, 285–305,
    289, 297, 326
inflated costs of, 262
local oversight of, 261
misperceptions about, 169–89
navigators' role in, 174–75
obstacles in search for sources of,
    169–89
ongoing preventive measures in, 199
oversight of, 261
paradox of, 36–39
people as factor in, 183–86
political implications of, 38–39, 90,
    96–99, 113, 159, 209–10, 243, 261,
    290
practitioners bias in, 298–99
preventive, 124–25
price of certainty in, 229
priorities of, 130–33, *131*
private and public costs in, 260
as public good vs. business, 46
rationing in, 136–41
as a right, 95, 112
rising costs of, 43–44, 47–48, 55,
    69–70, 71
science in, 173
six identified sources of waste in,
    243–44
social factors in, 183–84
state-based differences in, 207–8
statistical analysis in, 182–86

healthcare (*cont.*)
  as tax deductible, 66
  tier system in, 285–305
  unwillingness to remedy, 269–84
  US costs of, 6
  US vs. global level of, 71
  volunteerism in, 52–53
  weighted costs in, 200–202
  worthiness factor in, 145
healthcare for all:
  Gold Card as access to, 148–54
  limited choice in, 148
  public and private funding for, 260
healthcare inflation, 48
health insurance:
  brokers of, 65
  claims in, 280–81
  different grades of, 24, 29
  doctors' opposition to, 65
  employer-employee funded, 59, 65–68, 69
  employer-sponsored, 29, 65, 283, 289, 327
  evolution of, 59–74
  health maintenance impacted by, 121–25
  historical perspective of, 61–63
  insufficient, 25
  lost during COVID pandemic, 283
  marketplace in, 154
  moral hazard in, 64–65
  options available with, 58
  rising cost of, 67
  scams in, 244
  search for, 141, 174–75
  self-purchased, 29
  see also various types of health insurance
health insurance, private, 41, 42, 51, 52, 101, 113, 165, 289, 292, 295
  billing in, 44–45
  decline in, 53
  failures of, 155
  inflated costs of, 256
  as root of healthcare problems, 37–39
health insurance companies:
  avoidance and resistance procedures of, 73
  coverage denied by, 67
  exploitation by, 265
  hospitals owned by, 70–71
health maintenance organizations (HMOs), 49–51
health trauma, 227–28
heart attacks, 6–7
  algorithm in diagnosis in, 214, 216–17
heart disease, 214
heart failure, 165, 330
heart tumors, 36
Hematology Outpatient Services clinic, 170
hemodialysis, 247
hemorrhaging, 181–82, 258
hepatic encephalopathy, 209
hepatitis C infection, 139, 205
heroin, 83, 323
high blood pressure, 175, 186, 199, 212, 248, 277, 294
Hill-Burton Act (1946), 85–86, 89
Hillier, King, 155, 260
Hindus, 312
Hispanics, 94, 133–35, 298
history and physical assessments, 81, 134–35
HIV/AIDS, 90, 97, 191–98
  medications for, 7, 192
HIV clinics, 90
Holmes, Oliver Wendell, 144
home dialysis, 245–48
home hospice care, 32, 76–79, 91, 155
Homeland Security Department, US, 247
homelessness, 108, 187
Honduras, 261
Hong Kong, 247
hope, 189, 287
  cure vs., 172
  dignity and, 224–25
hospice care, 155, 160, 221–22, 225
hospital, use of term, 81
Hospital, The (de Hartog), 9–10, 89, 258–59, 270, 316
hospital billing study, 255–56
Hospital Compare, 256–57, 263
hospital costs, exploitation in, 256
hospital districts, tax base for, 90–91

hospitality, 226
hospitals:
    CMS rating of, 99
    financially vulnerable, 32
    historical perspectives on, 81–85, 102, 287
    incorporation of, 70–71
    inequalities in care at, 84–88
    organism analogy for, 110–11
    patient selectivity in, 83
    privacy issues in, 100–101
    star ratings of, 263–64
    taxed as charities, 86–88
    in transition from care to business, 75–92
    see also specific institutions and types
house calls, 48
House Ways and Means Committee, 292–93
Houston, Tex.:
    COVID pandemic in, 275–76
    proliferation of hospitals in, 85–86
    undocumented immigrants in, 203
    wealthy districts in, 209–10
Houston Chronicle, 86, 89, 290
Houston Methodist, 3
Houston Negro Hospital, 86
Hsieh, Tony, 274
Humana, 51
Hurricane Harvey, 90, 266, 309, 329–30
hydroxychloroquine, 172, 276

IBM, Indiana's lawsuit with, 202
ICUs, 205, 277, 284, 324
    in COVID pandemic, 276
    neonatal, 302, 304
identity politics, 113
immigration, immigrants:
    in author's family background, 42
    children in, 261
    healthcare for, 1, 5
    undocumented, see undocumented immigrants
implicit-bias questionnaire, 299
Indiana, rigged Medicaid coverage in, 201–2
indigent healthcare, 87, 98, 108, 323
    definition of, 148–49
    dumping in, 93–95

in Harris Health system, 4–5, 98–99, 148–50
inequality in, 69–70, 84–88, 200–201
Scientific Charity Movement study of, 143–45
infrastructure bills, 85
Institute for Clinical Systems Improvement, 214
insulin, use of, 126–27
intensive care program, 200
Internet, medical information on, 247
intracerebral hemorrhage, 227
IRS, 86
Islam, 312–15
Islamic conquest, 287
isolation, 279
ivermectin, 172–73
IV fluids, 258

jaundice, 133
Jefferson Davis Hospital, 86, 89–90, 240, 258–60, 270, 280, 282, 327
    de Hartog at, 271
    deplorable conditions at, 86–87
    as predecessor to Ben Taub, 9–10
Jersey Village, 209
Jerusalem, 286
Jesuit education, 97
Job Corps, 204
Jobs, Steve, 323
Johnson, Lyndon, 69, 87
Journal of General Internal Medicine, 164
Journal of Healthcare Management, 240
Journal of the American Medical Association, 94, 243
Jundi-Shapur (Beautiful Garden), 285–89, 296

kidney:
    biopsy of, 175, 237
    failure of, 73, 175, 182, 232
    function of, 111, 113, 134, 238–39
    transplants of, 248–49
kidney disease, 169–77, 199, 237–49, 289
    end-stage (ESRD), 247–49, 290–95
kidney stone surgeries, 264
Kimball, Justin Ford, 61–65, 71

King (Ebonie's son), 304
Kisacky, Jeanne, 84
knee pains, 56–58, 66–68, 169–77, 237–39, 242, 245
knee surgery, of author, 75–76
Kuwait, 285

lactulose, 209
lamellar bodies, 175–76
Lancet, 276
language barriers, 11, 223
Las Vegas, Nev., 274
Lazarus procedures, 320, 323
leg prostheses, 331–32
Level 1 trauma centers, 99–100, 111
Lewy body dementia, 119
lifestyle, medical conditions and, 127–28
life support, removal from, 325
lipid (fat), 176
liquefactive necrosis, 321
listening, in doctor-patient relationship, 217
liver disease, 330
  cirrhosis in, 139–43, 205, 209
  failure in, 138, 202–7, 317–20
liver transplants, 206, 208, 295
  costs of, 140, 322, 323
  disqualification for, 207
  donors for, 320–21, 323
  historical perspective on, 320
  immediate need for, 317–19
  loopholes in, 322–23
  numbers per year of, 322
  prioritization of recipients of, 321–23
  procedures for, 321–22
low blood pressure, 324
low-carbohydrate diet, 127
Lowell, Josephine, 143
Lundeen, Suzanne, 186, 188
lupus, 175
Lyndon B. Johnson Hospital, 4, 193, 259
lysozymes, 176

malaria, 286
managed care, 50, 97
Marí (Roxana's daughter), 28, 75, 76, 91
Mariam (Roxana's friend), 311

Marseille, 287
maternal care:
  inequalities in, 298
  misperceptions about, 186
  see also childbirth; pregnancies
Maternal Early Warning System, 186
maternal-fetal medicine doctors, 183–84
maternal mortality rate (MMR), 35, 178, 181, 187, 296–98
maternity wards, 87
Mattox, Ken, 4–5, 257–61
Mayo Clinic, 170
McCain, John, death of, 159–60
MD Anderson, 3
Medicaid, 7, 34, 35, 36, 39, 52, 53, 79, 87, 88, 122, 136, 140, 144, 146, 147, 164, 180, 187, 194, 196, 201, 255, 257, 265, 272, 289, 298, 300, 305
  automated vs. case-worker based administration of, 201–2
  automatic coverage for, 206
  criteria for quality of, 188
  disqualification for, 207–10
  earning cap on, 192–93, 197, 206–7, 292, 317–19, 325
  establishment of, 47, 50, 69–70
  exclusions from, 30
  low reimbursement by, 241
  proposed cuts to, 154, 155, 158–60
  provisions of, 148
  qualifications for, 30, 140–41, 154–55
  Texas requirements for, 206–7, 283
  work requirement for, 145
Medi-Cal, 34
medical-industrial complex, 36–37
medical jargon, misperceptions in, 182–83, 285
medical judgment, financial status vs., 113
medical schools, public hospitals aligned with, 84
medical students, 117–18, 138–40
Medicare, 7, 31, 39, 88, 95, 147, 164, 165, 244, 248, 256, 290, 294
  coverage options under, 249
  cuts to, 97
  diabetes expenses of, 123
  in ESRD and dialysis, 248–49, 291–92

establishment of, 47, 50, 69–70
exclusions from, 30
paycheck deductions for, 204
per patient expenditure of, 6
qualifications for, 30
work credit for, 292
Medicare for All, 38, 39, 289, 295
medicine:
    author's three priorities of, 127–30, *130*
    unconventional approaches to, 125–33
Medicine Inc., 36–39, 50–51, 69, 113,
    148, 177, 230, 243, 256, 283, 289,
    326–27
    algorithm use in, 229
    cost as priority of, 130–33, *130, 131*,
    244
    establishment of, 70–72
    healthcare's transition to, 51
    principles of, 37–39, 132
    rationing in, 136
mental disorientation, 119
mental illness, poverty and, 143–45
meritocracy, in healthcare philosophy, 112
metastatic cancer, 221, 223, 310, 330,
    332
MetroLift, 331, 332
Mexico, 71
    healthcare in, 32, 169–70, 173–74,
    177–78, 202–4, 237, 243, 286
Mill, John Stuart, 104
minimum wage, 153, 204
minorities, 86
    unequal standards of care for, 298
miscarriages, 180
Missouri, 208
Model for End-Stage Liver Disease
    (MELD) score, 322–23, 325
moonlighting, 98
moral hazard, 64–65
morbidity and mortality (M & M)
    conferences, 259
"Morning Report" conference, 119–20
morphine, 77, 167, 238–39
mortality rates:
    of emergency room patients, 111
    in open wards, 102
mother-to-child HIV transmission, 193

MRIs, 66–67, 138, 229–30
    overuse of, 256–57
multilingualism, 133–34, 135, 150, 204
municipal hospitals, 84

Nairobi, 97
NASA, 247
National Comprehensive Cancer
    Network, 138
National Health Service (UK), 272
National Institutes of Health, 6, 247
navigators, 174–75
neck dissection, 253–54
Nelda (Christian charity representative),
    310–14
neonatal ICUs, 302, 304
nephrologists, 73, 170, 247–48
Netherlands, disaster syndrome in,
    269–71
neurologists, 181
neurosurgeons, neurosurgery, 182,
    227–28
New Delhi, 97
New England Journal of Medicine, 36, 94,
    172, 231, 249
New York Times, 232, 246, 276, 282
    author's op-ed in, 158
Nightingale, Florence, 102
Nightingale wards, 101–4, 106, 107
Nixon, Richard, 48, 50
No Evidence of Disease (NED), 267
non-alcoholic steatohepatitis, 139*n*
noncompliant, use of term, 182–84
nonemergency surgery, 154
noninterference clause, 164
nonprofit hospitals, 3, 79, 86, 88, 93, 95,
    98, 99, 104, 113, 132, 155, 175, 179,
    189, 256, 260, 295, 300, 301, 304,
    324
    tax breaks for, 86–88
    VA hospitals compared to, 164–65
Norco, 167
Norma (Christian Garza's mother),
    55–59, 66–67, 72–73, 170–77, 239,
    242, 246, 249, 286
North Carolina, 208
Northwestern University, 183

Notes on Hospitals (Nightingale), 102
Nuila, Buenaventura (author's
    grandfather), 48
Nuila, Ricardo:
    concussion of, 60–61, 68–69
    COVID response and, 275–84
    doctor-patient relationship of, 156–58,
        178–86, 208–10, 298–99
    education and career of, 8, 10–14,
        41, 75–76, 79–82, 97–98, 117–22,
        125–26, 133, 155, 178–86, 202,
        211–12, 217, 218, 226, 232–33, 275,
        278, 288
    family of, 157–58
    father of, 41–55, 76, 96, 272, 278,
        296–97
    father-son relationship of, 41–55, 69,
        96–99, 128–29, 145–47, 265–66,
        286–87
    Geronimo's eulogy delivered by, 325–28
    grandmother of, 217–25
    health insurance coverage of, 59–61
    impact of faith on, 312–17
    knee surgery of, 75–76
    personal challenges of, 226, 280
    in personal childbirth crisis, 178–80, 186
    professional style of, 151–52, 251–53
    residency of, 125, 226–27, 229, 232
    wife of, 128–29, 178–80, 186
nurse practitioners, 176
nurses, L & D responsibilities of, 185–86
nursing homes, diabetic care in, 123

Obama, Barack, 154, 260–61
Obamacare, *see* Affordable Care Act
Obermeyer, Ziad, 199–201
obstetric bleeding, 181–82
obstetrics and gynecology, 76, 100, 107,
    146, 177–89, 297
    author's father's career in, 41–45
    innovative approaches in, 185–86
Obstetrics & Gynecology, 298
occupational therapy, 331, 332
Office of Price Administration, 135–36
oncologists, 153, 166, 221–22, 267, 330
"one patient, one doctor" maxim, 46, 49
open wards, 102–4

opiates, 58
opioid crisis, 323
opium addicts, 82
opportunistic infections (OIs), 198
organ dysfunction, 10–11
organ failure, 317
    see also specific organs
orthopedics, 111
Oshinsky, David, 87
out-of-pocket costs, 170–71, 173–84, 219,
    255, 283
overtreatment, 243

pain medicines, 77, 251–52
pain specialists, 167
palliative care, 225
Palliative Performance Scale, 152
Parkland Memorial Hospital
    (Dallas, Tex.), dumping at, 93–94
parotid glands, 254, 266
patient caps, 274
patient discharge, contingency plans for,
    187–88
Paul, Mary, 195–97
payment plans, 167
PCP, 80, 81, 83
pediatricians, adult use of, 196
people, in medical priorities, 128–33, *130,
    131*
People's Clinic, 204–5, 211, 217, 231, 278
peritoneal dialysis, 245–47, 295
Permobil power wheelchair, 331
personalized medicine, 101
PET scans, 254
phantom limb pain, 309
pharmaceutical companies, 71
physical therapy, 331
physician judgment, algorithms vs., 229
placenta, blockage by, 301–5
plague, 285, 287, 288
Planned Parenthood, 36
Pocket Medicine, 118, 119, 121–22, 129,
    130, 135, 199, 212
politics, 265–66
    as divisive, 281
    in healthcare, 38–39, 90, 96–99, 113,
        159, 209–10, 243, 261, 290

poor protoplasm, 83
pop-up clinics, 90
poverty, 9, 262, 289
  mental illness in, 143–45
preeclampsia, 186
preexisting conditions, 174–75, 244
pregnancies, 33–35, 39, 177–89, 297
  emergency room treatment of, 107
  HIV in, 193–94
  uninsured in, 51–52
  see also Ebonie; maternal care
premature birth, 302, 304
premature death, impact of insurance on,
  122–23
prescription drugs, 164
preventive healthcare, 124–25, 244–45,
  275, 290
preventive medical treatment, cost
  impediment to, 121–22
price transparency, 244
pricing failures, 244
primary care clinics, 274
primary care physicians, 50, 211–12
privacy, 100–101, 263
private hospitals:
  cost of, 260
  overuse and exploitation in, 241
private rooms, 101
pro bono service, 146–47
professional patients, 251–52
profit motive, 37–39, 71–72, 88, 244,
  248, 274
prostate cancer, 262
prostheses, 310–14, 331–32
Protestants, 312
psychologists, 181
public hospitals, 88
  assumptions about, 26, 266
  neglect of, 84–88
  patient base of, 88
  procedures at, 240
  voluntary hospitals vs., 84–88
  see also specific hospitals
pulse rate, 179

qualifying life events, 59, 318
Quran, 314

race:
  as divisive issue, 281
  maternal mortality and, 298
racial bias, public health impacted by,
  298–99
radiation therapy, 166, 230, 253–54, 262,
  314, 330
radiologists, 166
RAND Corporation, billing study of,
  255–56
rationing, 135–41
Reagan, Ronald, 48, 97
Reaganomics, 50
Reddit, 249
rehabilitation centers, 329–30
reimbursement rates, government
  establishment of, 48
Relman, Arnold, 36
Renkioi, hospital at, 102
Republican Party, 257
  healthcare stance of, 154–55, 159
  Texas agenda of, 210
residency requirement, 148
restaurant businesses, 21–36, 251–52, 255,
  264
retirees, 69
retirement, of doctors, 273
Revolutionary War, 45
rheumatologists, 56–57, 66–67, 73, 173
Rise of the Modern Hospital (Kisacky), 84
Riverside Dialysis Center, 294
Roman Empire, 285–86
Roosevelt, Theodore, 65
Roxana (uninsured patient), 26–32,
  35–37, 39, 75–79, 83, 88, 91, 101,
  148–49, 155, 282, 288, 309–15
  admitted to Ben Taub Hospital, 149–54
  amputation surgery and follow-up of,
  153–54, 155–60, 309
  brain tumor of, 314
  emergency care for, 109–14
  generosity of, 313
  independence of, 331
  Muslim faith of, 312–15
  prothesis for, 310–15
  rehab of, 329–33
  resilience of, 332–33

"Roxana's Journey" (WhatsApp group), 313
rule-out diagnosis, 184
Russia:
  history of healthcare in, 15–17
  public hospitals in, 85
  tuberculosis in, 15–17
Ryan White funds, 194

safety-net hospitals, 3, 8, 91, 93, 95–96, 99, 103, 114, 154, 179, 193, 260, 289, 317
  discharge from, 187–88
  emergency rooms in, 101
  financial limitations of, 310–11
  funding for, 88–89
  limitations of, 138–41
  mission of, 88
  nonprofits compared to, 301
  patient dumping at, 93–95
  ratings of, 263–64
  rationing in, 137–38
  stress on, 178–79
  see also specific hospitals
safety-net system, 90, 98, 132, 134, 167, 183–84, 206, 212, 231, 275, 278, 293, 294, 329
  congressional threats to, 154
  faulty assumptions about, 238, 242
  financial structure of, 241
  funding for, 155
  Gold Card as entry to, 148–54
  limitations of, 323–24
  overloading of, 283
  see also Harris Health
Sakhalin Island, penal colony in, 15–17
sales tax proposal, 260
Sam (diabetic patient), 125–29, 131–32
same-day clinic, 314
San Francisco Chronicle, 172
Santana Funeral Directors, 325
Santiago (kidney failure patient), 232
satiety, 219
Save Our ERs, 111
school-based clinics, 90
science:
  applied to medicine, 287–88
  belief vs., 143–44, 313

in hospital evolution, 83–85
  in medicine priorities, 128–33, 130, 131
Science, 199
Scientific Charity Movement, 143–44, 199
Seattle, Wash., COVID pandemic in, 276
segregation, 86–87
seizure medicines, 304
seizures, 187–88, 203, 301, 304
semiprivate rooms, 101
seniors, healthcare for, 39, 69–70
shamans, 285, 287
Shandera, Dr., 293
Sharonna (Ebonie's sister), 33–34, 108, 187–88
Sheikh-Hamad, Dr., 293
shock, medical use of term, 27
shortness of breath, 134
sick benefit programs, 62
Silk Road, 285, 288
single-tier healthcare system, 295
sliding-scale payment schemes, 88–89
sobar (Mexican massage), 56
social Darwinism, 143–44
socialized healthcare, 129
social justice, 97
social risk factors, 263–64
Social Security, 46, 207
  paycheck deductions for, 204
Social Security Administration, 30, 206–7, 209, 318
Social Security Disability Insurance (SSDI), 207, 292
Social Transformation of American Medicine, The (Starr), 47
social workers, 141, 208–10
soldiers, hospital care for, 102
sophists, 286
specialists, out-of-pocket expenses for, 176
sphygmomanometers, 258
Stabilization Act (1942), 65
staph infections, 86–87
Starr, Paul, 47, 87, 104
star ratings, misleading, 263–64
statistical bias, 200–202
STDs, 83

stem cell clinics, 171–74, 176, 237
stem cells, 243, 286
step-down unit, 207
stereotypes, doctors' use of, 298–99
sterilization, forced, 143–44
steroids, 281
stigmata, use of term, 133, 285
stomach tube, 254
Sugar Land, 103
suicide, 279–80
Supplemental Security Income (SSI), 193, 197, 206, 292
Supreme Court, US:
  forced sterilization decision of, 144
  Medicaid ruling of, 154–55
surgery:
  brain, 330
  in childbirth, 186
  elective, 138, 154, 283
  lifesaving, 27
  scheduled for Roxana, 150–54
  wait time for, 154
syphilitics, 82

T3s (codeine and Tylenol), 58
Talmud, 287
Tampico, Mexico, access to healthcare in, 68, 72–74, 169–70
tax code (1954), 66
tax deductions, for hospitals, 86–88
tax incentives, 79, 88
Tea Party, 210
technology:
  advancements in, 213–14
  judgment and, 230
  overuse of, 229
  price of, 84
  as shortcut for diagnosis, 199
TEDMED talks, 274
tele-doc visits, 24
tests, overuse of, 257
Texas:
  abortion law in, 107n
  anti-dumping laws in, 94–95
  economic inequality in, 209–10
  healthcare law in, 148–49
  healthcare system in, 8–9

insurance coverage rates in, 283
maternal mortality rates in, 35, 297–98
Medicaid coverage in, 30
Medicaid expansion declined by, 155
Medicaid limitations in, 207–10
minimum wage in, 153
Seventh Congressional District of, 209–10, 317
Twenty-Ninth Congressional District of, 319
uninsured rates in, 3–4, 35
wealth in, 209–10
Texas Children's Hospital, 194
  Pediatric AIDS and Retrovirology Clinic, 196
Texas Collaborative for Healthy Mothers and Babies, 185
Texas Medicaid Provider Procedures Manual, 79
Texas Medical Center, 3, 57, 85, 101, 189, 259, 324, 329–30
Texas Medicine, 293
therapists, author's search for, 280–81
third party, AMA prohibition of, 46
tiers, 285–305
Times (London), 102
tonsil cancer, 25, 106, 253–54
tough love, 162–63, 166
tourniquets, 258
Trachelle (Aqueria's partner), 191–94
tramadol, 77
transplants, 138, 206, 291
  wait lists for, 294, 324, 325
trauma care, prioritizing of, 138
trauma centers, 99–100
triage, 100, 105, 110–11
Tropical Storm Allison, 90
Trump, Donald:
  healthcare stance of, 154
  in 2020 election, 255, 262
Trump administration, 145
  health budget cuts of, 247
tuberculosis, 15–17, 286
tumors, 36
Turkey, 102
Turntable Health, 274
two-tier healthcare system, 295–96

uncompensated care, 95
underinsured, 21–26, 59, 104
undocumented immigrants, 5, 26–32,
    79, 98, 109, 135, 148, 155, 202–3,
    311, 323
    ESRD disease among, 295
    healthcare debate over, 290–91
    healthcare for, 10, 15
    Medicare benefits unavailable to,
        292–93
    uninsured, 26–32
    see also specific individuals
unemployed, 94
unemployment benefits, 163, 265
uninsured, 26–32, 59, 69, 76, 80, 88, 94,
    98, 99–100, 103, 109, 111, 113–14,
    135, 140, 180, 186–87, 219, 288
    at Ben Taub, 41, 283–84
    in childbirth, 146–47
    by choice, 162
    Christian Garza as, 55–58
    cost of, 162
    dumping of, 93–95
    emergency room use by, 95–96
    growth of, 51
    healthcare for, 5–7, 76–79, 130–31
    lack of health maintenance care by,
        121–25
    maternal death rates in, 35
    numbers of, 30–31, 78
    preventive care unavailable to, 121, 244
    recouping costs of, 32
    stability evaluation for, 188
    three options for, 31–32
    wards for, 101
United Network for Organ Sharing
    (UNOS), 321, 322
universal healthcare, 129, 295, 327
universal health insurance, 64*n*, 129, 232
UNLV medical school, 274
unnecessary tests, 256
unprotected sex, hepatitis C and, 205

urgent-care centers, limitations of, 174
UTI, assumption of, 117–21

vasoplegic syndrome, 27
ventilators, 136, 324
Verma, Seema, 263
Veterans Affairs hospitals, 164–65
vices, as basis of need for medical care,
    84–85
voluntary hospitals, 82, 83–88
volunteerism, 52–53, 82, 89

wait lists, 294, 324, 325
wait times, 263, 264
    priorities in, 154
    rationing of, 136
    for surgery, 138
wards, 101–4
Washington, D.C., maternal mortality
    inn, 298
wasting syndrome, 191–92, 197
Wayne (hospital CEO), 76
weight loss, 191, 197
welfare, 194
West Houston, 75, 79
West Virginia, 207
WhatsApp, 313
wheelchairs, technologically advanced, 331
Wichita, Kans., private clinic in, 42–43
Wiffle ball, 59–60
Wilson's disease, 119
World War I, 16
World War II, 65
    rationing in, 135–36
worthiness, as factor for determining
    healthcare eligibility, 145, 159

YouTube, 274

Zarathustra, 287
zebras (lamellar bodies), 175–76
Zika virus, 185

About the Author

Ricardo Nuila is a writer, teacher, and practicing doctor. He is an associate professor of medicine, medical ethics, and health policy at Baylor College of Medicine, where he teaches the practice of hospital medicine and directs the Humanities Expression and Arts Lab (HEAL). Ricardo is a native Houstonian who has worked as an attending physician in the city's largest safety-net facility, Ben Taub Hospital, for more than ten years. The son of Salvadoran immigrants, he spent summers during his childhood in Central America.

Ricardo's journalistic work has been featured in *Texas Monthly* and the *Virginia Quarterly Review*, and his fiction has appeared in the *Best American Short Stories* anthology, *McSweeney's*, and *Guernica*. Ricardo covered the medical response to Hurricane Harvey, as well as the COVID-19 pandemic, for the *New Yorker*'s website. He has won awards for his teaching and advocacy, as well as for his writing, including the *New England Review*'s inaugural Award for Emerging Writers. *The People's Hospital* is his first book.

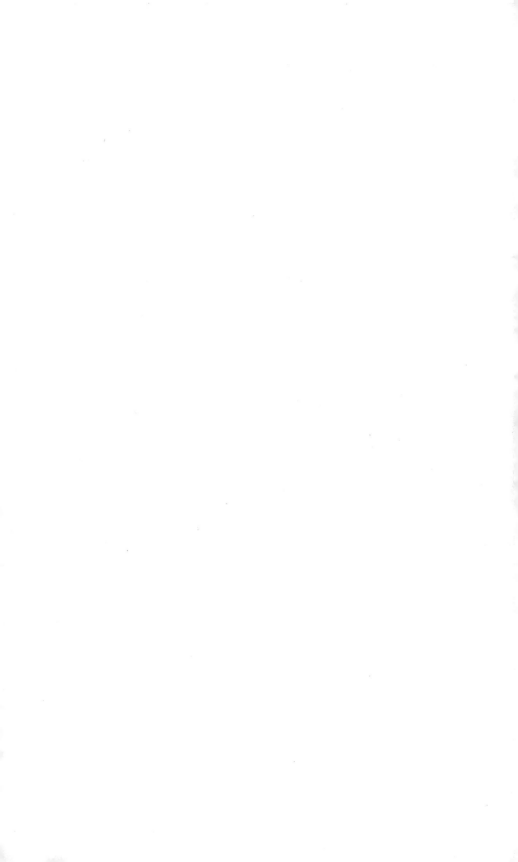